Decision Making
in Pediatric Neurologic
Physical Therapy

Decision Making in Pediatric Neurologic Physical Therapy

Suzann K. Campbell, PT, PhD, FAPTA

Professor of Physical Therapy
College of Health and Human Development Sciences
University of Illinois at Chicago
Chicago, Illinois

CHURCHILL LIVINGSTONE

A Division of Harcourt Brace & Company
New York Edinburgh London Philadelphia

CHURCHILL LIVINGSTONE
A Division of Harcourt Brace & Company

The Curtis Center
Independence Square West
Philadelphia, Pennsylvania 19106

Library of Congress Cataloging-in-Publication Data

Decision making in pediatric neurologic physical therapy / [edited by]
Suzann K. Campbell.

p.   cm.

Includes index.

ISBN 0–443–07923–4

1. Pediatric neurology—Diagnosis.   2. Pediatric neurology—Decision making.
   3. Physical therapy for children—Decision making.   I. Campbell, Suzann K.
   [DNLM: 1. Nervous System Diseases—in infancy & childhood. 2. Nervous
   System Diseases—rehabilitation.   3. Physical Therapy—in infancy &
   childhood.   WS 340D294 1999]

RJ486.D36 1999   618.92′80462—dc21

DNLM/DLC   98–38541

DECISION MAKING IN PEDIATRIC NEUROLOGIC PHYSICAL THERAPY   ISBN 0–443–07923–4

Portions of this work were previously published.

Printed in the United States of America.

Last digit is the print number: 9   8   7   6   5   4   3   2   1

To Dick,

still my mentor

and best friend—

the decision

to marry you

was the best

I've ever made.

Contributors

Jocelyn Blaskey, MS, PT
Director of Clinical Education and Clinical
  Education Research Coordinator, Rancho Los
  Amigos Medical Center, Downey,
  California
Traumatic Brain Injury

Suzann K. Campbell, PT, PhD, FAPTA
Professor of Physical Therapy, College of Health
  and Human Development Sciences, University
  of Illinois at Chicago, Chicago, Illinois
Models for Decision Making in Pediatric Neurologic Physical
  Therapy
The Infant at Risk for Developmental Disability

Martha C. Gram, MS, PT
Senior Pediatric Physical Therapist, South
  Area Special Education District, Naperville,
  Illinois; Owner, MM Therapeutics,
  Woodridge, Illinois
Myelodysplasia (Spina Bifida)

Janet M. Wilson Howle, MACT, PT
Private Practice Physical Therapist, Charleston,
  South Carolina
Cerebral Palsy

Maureen C. Jennings, MPT
Senior Clinician, Pediatric Resource Clinician,
  and Polio Clinic Coordinator, Rancho Los
  Amigos Medical Center, Downey, California
Traumatic Brain Injury

Karen Yundt Lunnen, MS, PT
Assistant Professor of Physical Therapy, College
  of Applied Sciences, Western Carolina
  University, Cullowhee, North Carolina
Children with Multiple Disabilities

Roberta B. Shepherd, EdD, MA, DipPhty, FACP
Honorary Professor, School of Physiotherapy,
  Faculty of Health Science, University of
  Sydney, Cumberland College Campus,
  Lidcombe, New South Wales, Australia
Brachial Plexus Injury

Preface

For the novice therapist, observing a master pediatric clinician is like watching a magician—it all looks so effortless, and how the effects are achieved seems a mystery. The skill with which a therapist captures a child's imagination while achieving the child's cooperation in a task requiring a great deal of endurance and strength has always held me in thrall, too, but I believe it is not beyond our capacity to understand the components. Certainly I know that the novice can achieve this same level of skill with a background of excellent training combined with perseverance, experience, and continued learning.

The skill involved in being a master clinician seems to consist, in more or less equal parts, of 1) experience, 2) physical skills, 3) creativity that arises from possessing a sense of playfulness that appeals to children, and 4) a continual accretion of knowledge based on regular review of the literature. The era of managed health care and educational inclusion of children with disabilities requires the therapist to incorporate scientific evidence into clinical practice. As a result, therapists must remain current in theory and research on best practice for achieving meaningful outcomes in the most efficient manner. Today, improving one's practice is more likely to mean implementing new models for planning and decision making for documenting outcomes, rather than gaining new technical skills in therapeutic exercise or fashioning assistive devices.

My goal in this book was to engage a group of scientific, reflective practitioners in the task of elucidating the basis of their decision making for children with a variety of the neurologic disorders commonly encountered in pediatric physical therapy. Each of the contributors has reviewed the recent literature on her topic and has presented case reports on children from her practice. In these case reports the contributors elaborate on the bases for their choices of goals, the measures used to document problems and progress, and the interventions provided. My hope is that both the novice and the experienced pediatric physical therapist will be encouraged by these reports to reflect on how their own practice might be improved, to consider new approaches to efficiently achieve meaningful outcomes for children and their families, to identify areas of need for personal continuing education, and to promise to faithfully read the literature in order to engage in evidence-based scientific clinical practice.

The opening chapter describes models for decision making that may be helpful to clinicians in reflecting on their practice. This chapter was provided to each contributor as a possible means for organizing her material. After much thought, however, no attempt was made to force the contributors to use a similar framework for presenting their material because each clearly had an effective conceptual framework already. Each contributor was, however, asked to include in her discussion information on how family members are included in decision making, what measurements she makes and how she makes them, and how to justify her choice of treatment strategies and techniques based on current theory and the research literature. I expect that it will be interesting for readers to evaluate the different ways in which clinicians frame patient problems, present clinical data, reflect on practice, and justify their plans of care. In many instances, the contributors also incorporate ideas on how they expect to revise their approach to patient problems based on new information from the theoretical, clinical, or research literature.

Each of the contributors met my expectations, and I hope they meet yours. I would especially like to acknowledge their special efforts to include photographs in the chapters to enhance your reading pleasure and to anchor the written material in a realistic context. I am grateful to the children and their families for their willingness to be photographed. Their contribution to the effectiveness of this volume is greatly appreciated. For my own chapter, I owe special thanks to Gay Girolami for photographs illustrating her Neuro-Developmental Treatment protocol for infants, and to Laura Zawacki, Gail Liberg, Kristine Johnson, Allyson Meyer, and Dena Winkleman for photography of infants participating in my research on development of the Test of Infant Motor Performance. This research was funded by grant R01 HD 32567 from the National Center for Medical Rehabilitation Research, National Institute of Child Health and Human Development, U.S. Public Health Service. During the course of editing this book, I was also partially supported by a leadership training grant MCJ# IL 179590 from the Maternal and Child Health Bureau, U.S. Public Health Service.

Suzann K. Campbell

Contents

Models for Decision Making in Pediatric Neurologic Physical Therapy

Suzann K. Campbell, PT, PhD, FAPTA

All pediatric physical therapists seek to improve treatment outcomes. The search for improved outcomes must occur within the context of changing health care and special education systems. The search must benefit, on the one hand, informed consumers, who deserve and demand an important role in decision making for their children, and on the other, families, many living in poverty, who are unable to participate optimally because they lack knowledge of child development, resources, or advocacy skills. As I engage in discussion with clinicians in continuing education programs, I am struck by the impression that what therapists think is needed in response to the dilemma of how to improve outcomes is new techniques for intervention. I tend to believe, however, that the use of more explicit decision-making paradigms with objective assessment of functional outcomes is likely to be more productive. Larin, for example, showed that clinicians employ elements of a theoretic approach to facilitating motor learning in children with neurologic dysfunction, but she believes that they may do so in a less than maximally effective way because their clinical reasoning is not explicit.[1] When a clearly articulated conceptual framework permeates all aspects of deciding how to assess and treat motor dysfunction and disability in daily life caused by neurologic impairment, techniques will be easy to develop. Within such a conceptual framework, clearly stated goals lead naturally to effective tactics for the achievement of objectives and the measurement of outcomes. With these thoughts in mind, this introductory chapter summarizes information from contemporary literature on conceptual models for decision making. The following chapters illustrate the problem-specific knowledge that is needed to implement treatment within such a conceptual model, but each chapter's authors also provide case examples in which the decision-making processes of the therapist are made explicit. The paragraph that follows outlines the essential elements that form the content of this chapter that are intended to support the condition-specific information appearing in subsequent chapters.

A variety of factors provide the keys to structuring a successful therapeutic outcome, including

1. Establishment of appropriate goals in partnership with the child's family
2. Multidimensional examination of function and the impairments that underlie neuromuscular dysfunction
3. Identification of strategies that patients are currently using to accomplish functional goals as well as strategies that might be more energy-efficient or successful
4. A strategic planning framework for designing intervention
5. Sound implementation tactics, including assessment and evaluation of outcomes

Goal development and strategic planning should actively involve and support the typical roles of family members, teachers, and other key players, whereas intervention tactics should incorporate the principles of motor development, motor control, and motor learning in an approach based on evidence in the scientific literature. Furthermore, a motivational approach is needed to fully engage children in developing skills to prevent disability in daily life roles. The need to engage children in pleasurable activity in order to motivate performance of what may be very difficult tasks suggests that a sixth important factor in producing successful outcomes is the ability of the therapist to improvise in the choice of activities during a treatment session while keeping the therapeutic goals in mind.[2]

Documentation of outcomes and the time required to achieve them in relation to preestablished goals is essential to practice in today's health care and education systems. The wise therapist will consider cost and the utilization of resources in the most efficient way. It is important to explore systematically why some goals may not have been achieved so that individual plans of care can be revised in an ongoing process of assessment, intervention, and reassessment. Such knowledge is also critical for furthering our general understanding of what works and why.

Many physical therapists have written extensively on these important aspects of a theoretical framework for intervention, so little that will be presented here is new. Those most influential in the conceptual model described in this chapter include Rothstein and Echternach,[3, 4] Embrey and colleagues,[5] Rosenbaum, Law, and coworkers,[6] Carr and Shepherd,[7-9] and Shumway-Cook and Woollacott.[10] The work of others is referred to when it illuminates certain aspects of the process particularly well. The overall framework I will use is the Hypothesis-Oriented Algorithm for Clinicians (HOAC) developed by Rothstein and Echternach and described for application to pediatric physical therapy by Palisano and associates.[11]

THE HYPOTHESIS-ORIENTED ALGORITHM FOR CLINICIANS

The HOAC is a decision model that provides physical therapists with a guide to systematic clinical planning independent of any particular theoretic approach to intervention.[3] Part 1 of the model consists of eight guides to planning intervention (Fig. 1–1); part 2 of the model addresses the outcomes of implementing the planned management program and evaluating why the preestablished goals were or were not accomplished (Fig. 1–2). Based on the judgments made in this part of the model, alterations to the plan can be devised. The section that follows describes the eight steps in part 1 of the decision-making model and elaborates on each point by bringing in perspectives from other research and clinical literature.

Steps 1 and 2: Initial Data Collection and Establishment of Goals

The first step in applying the HOAC model involves *initial data collection* from sources such as medical and educational records and the patient-family-teacher interview. Here the clinician gains knowledge of

- ▶ Functional skills and limitations of the client
- ▶ Family routines, the child's condition, and the family's concerns
- ▶ Reasons for seeking intervention

Using this information, the therapist generates a problem statement and establishes goals for the intervention that are measurable and functional and contain a temporal element defining a point by which the objectives should be accomplished. The formulation of goals *before* a formal physical therapy examination is completed is one of the unique characteristics of the HOAC. Taking the step of formulating goals before comprehensive measurement of the underlying problems of the client provides a means of ensuring that the intervention goals are functional, relevant to family concerns and interests, and aimed at reducing disability in daily life functions. As Palisano and colleagues indicate,[11] the process of goal selection in the HOAC empowers family members to act as advocates for their child through active participation in decision making and helps the therapist to

HYPOTHESIS-ORIENTED ALGORITHM FOR CLINICIANS
PART ONE

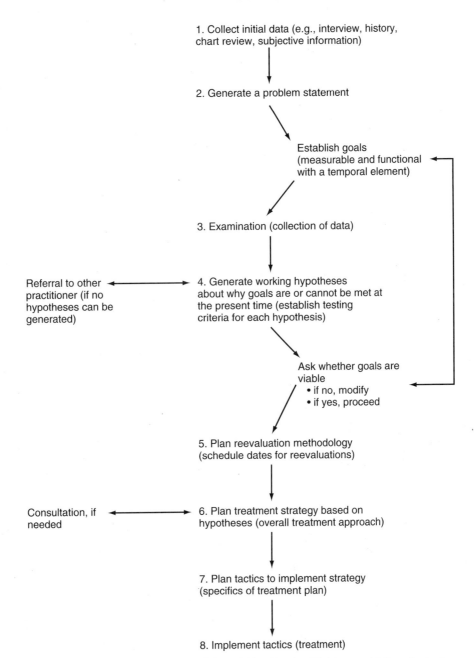

FIGURE 1–1. Part 1 of the Hypothesis-Oriented Algorithm for Clinicians: guidelines for evaluation and treatment planning. (Redrawn from Rothstein JM, Echternach JL: Hypothesis-Oriented Algorithm for Clinicians: A method for evaluation and treatment planning. Phys Ther 66:1388–1394, 1986, with permission of the American Physical Therapy Association.)

HYPOTHESIS-ORIENTED ALGORITHM FOR CLINICIANS
PART TWO

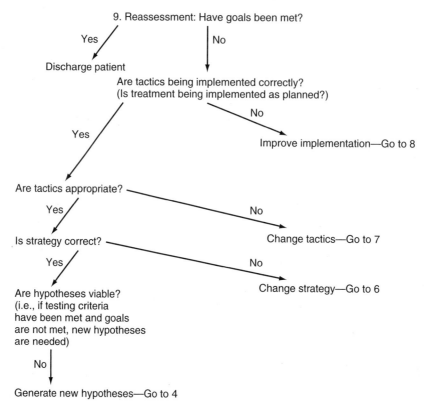

FIGURE 1–2. Part 2 of the Hypothesis-Oriented Algorithm for Clinicians: branching program. All numbers less than 9 refer to the steps listed in Figure 1–1. (Redrawn from Rothstein JM, Echternach JL: Hypothesis-Oriented Algorithm for Clinicians: A method for evaluation and treatment planning. Phys Ther 66:1388–1394, 1986, with permission of the American Physical Therapy Association.)

incorporate the family's expectations into the intervention plan. When a child has recently been diagnosed or identified as at risk for developmental disability, an initial goal is likely to be education for the family in order to provide the tools for participatory decision making in establishing therapeutic goals. In actuality, decision making is likely to involve a circular process of establishing preliminary goals, collecting data, trying out an intervention approach, reformulating goals, and so on, because both examination and treatment are part of a continual information-gathering and hypothesis-generating process.

The Canadian Occupational Performance Measure (COPM)[12–14] is a recommended tool for carrying out goal establishment within the HOAC model. This assessment guides the clients (family or teacher and child) through the process of identifying functional limitations that matter in the child's daily life, rating the limitations for importance, selecting several goals for therapeutic intervention, and rating the goals for performance and satisfaction. The assessment interview defines areas of self-care skills, work- or school-related skills, and leisure activities that are important to the client in determining productivity and the quality of life and in reducing disability in daily roles. The parents participate in goal selection using this measure, but it is important to recognize that children may have their own goals and should be allowed to participate when they demonstrate interest and the cognitive ability to do so. Barry reports that children as young as 7 years of age can identify personal goals and rate them on the 10-point scale used in the COPM (M. J. Barry, personal communication, 1996).

A further advantage of use of the COPM for the establishment of goals is that outcomes can also be used as an effective means of program evaluation. Different clients can have unique personal goals, but the same rating scales can be used to assess performance and satisfaction at the entry to intervention and again after intervention has occurred. As a result, all outcomes are quantified with the same metric. When data such as these are collected for all program clients, the results can be used for purposes such as evaluation of overall performance of individual therapists, identification of types of clients who do not appear to make satisfactory progress toward self-selected goals, or identification of types of goals that are easily or not easily reached with the types of intervention strategies and tactics used in the program.

Another well-developed approach to including the family in planning intervention is Bricker's Assessment, Evaluation, and Programming System for Infants and Children.[15] Bricker's criterion-referenced measurement system includes several types of forms developed specifically for use by families. A Family Report is used by caregivers to assess the child's skills for comparison with a similar assessment completed by professionals. A Family Interest Survey provides a response format based on research on the typical concerns of families with children with disabilities, allowing families to identify their priorities in the areas of information, garnering formal and informal support, using resources, and participating in various activities, such as learning to position their child for feeding and play. The information from these forms is used during the process of developing goals for an Individualized Family Service Plan (IFSP). An important aspect of this system is that the use of special data-gathering devices developed specifically for use by family members communicates clearly to them that their knowledge of their own child is important to service providers and that their opinions are valued in the process of goal development.

Step 3: Examination

After the development of a problem statement and goals for intervention, the next step in the HOAC model is examination of the patient, using one or more appropriate examination tools. Tests and measures should be selected to provide further insight into the problems identified by the client and family using a multidimensional approach to examination and, whenever possible, standardized tests with documented validity for the examination purpose. I recommend that clinicians use the disability model developed by the National Center for Medical Rehabilitation Research (NCMRR) as a guide to developing an individualized examination strategy.[16] The NCMRR model of the disabling process incorporates five dimensions of disability, of which three are of particular importance in the development of physical therapy plans of care. These include *disabilities* in the accomplishment of daily life roles at home, in school, and in the community; *functional limitations* in whole-body or segmental functions, such as gait, reaching, or grasping, that may contribute to disability; and *impairments,* which are specific organ system dysfunctions, such as decreased strength, endurance, range of motion, memory, or attention. Impairments are assumed to be the underlying causes of functional limitations. As an example, if the COPM has been used to identify disabilities in the daily life of a child with motor dysfunction (such as a lack of independence in community mobility), the examination process should use measures to assess the underlying problems at the level of functional limitations and impairments as well as to gain more information on roles that require mobility and the environments in which they are enacted. For children in educational settings, for example, further exploration of the effectiveness of the child's mobility in the school environment might involve working with teachers on ecologic examination of a child's mobility skills in the classroom and on the playground.[17] Play-based examination is an alternative for children being considered for enrollment in an early-intervention program.[18] At the level of functional limitations, the therapist could measure street-crossing time, test gross motor skills of standing and walking with the Gross Motor Function Measure (GMFM),[19] rate transfer skills and independence using the Pediatric Evaluation of Disability Inventory (PEDI),[20] or analyze and document the physical and cognitive strategies the child uses to manage door opening or to request assistance with doors too heavy to manage independently. Impairments that are hypothesized to be implicated in causing functional limitations, such as contractures, lower-extremity strength, and balance, would be measured with appropriate impairment-level tools, such as an electrogoniometer,[21] a dynamometer,[22] or the Pediatric Clinical Test of Sensory Interaction for Balance.[23]

Examination also includes evaluation of the client's equipment, if any; for example, whether it fits and is currently being used, and whether it meets the client's needs as defined by role functions in daily life or the prevention of contractures and deformities. Furthermore, the examination process is informed by what the therapist knows about the natural history and typical abnormalities characteristic of the patient's specific condition so that a program of prevention and anticipatory guidance for the family can be developed. Embrey and Hylton's study of clinical decision making by pediatric physical therapists revealed that clinicians regularly make use of recognizable patterns of atypical movement when selecting among treatment options for children with cerebral palsy[24] but also identified that these "movement scripts" were incomplete, containing only fragments of the salient features of movement patterns that contribute to abnormal function. As a result, the researchers' recommendations for improving practice include paying increased attention to explicit recognition of the characteristic movement patterns of these clients.[5]

Whatever tools are used, the HOAC makes it clear that measures should be appropriately selected for exploration of the individual case *based on* the previously established functional goals. Indeed, one of the reasons given by the authors for developing the HOAC was the observation that clinical decision making often lacked an obvious relationship among goals, interventions provided, and examinations used both to identify problem areas and to evaluate the outcome. Therapists need to have knowledge and skills in the use of a wide variety of tests and measurements in order to custom tailor an examination strategy for the individual client. One test does not fit all needs. Fortunately, the number of available measurement devices for use by pediatric physical therapists has grown enormously in recent years.

Shumway-Cook and Woollacott provide further elaboration on clinical assessment by suggesting strategies for using a systems-based task-oriented approach to measurement.[10] They believe that the therapist must evaluate motor behavior on three levels: objective measurement of functional skills; a description of the strategies used to accomplish these functional skills (similar to Embrey and Hylton's[24] movement scripts?); and quantification of the underlying sensory, motor, and cognitive impairments that constrain performance. Functional skills are assessed with standardized measures, such as the Alberta Infant Motor Scale,[25] GMFM,[19] PEDI,[20] or other functional tests specifically for children. Constraints are measured with impairment-level tests, such as goniometry or balance assessments. Such tests provide important quantitative documentation for professionals and third-party payers.

Unfortunately, only a small number of formal measures are available to assess the *strategies* used by patients to accomplish functional tasks. Despite a lack of a variety of formal assessments for this purpose, it is critical to measure strategies because they are largely responsible for determining the level of performance. Welford indicates that performance depends on four factors:[26]

1. The demands of the task and the person's desire for particular standards of achievement
2. Mental and physical capacities that the person brings to the task
3. The strategies that the person uses to meet the demands of the task
4. The ability to choose the most efficient strategy for a given task

Inherent in the task of the physical therapist is evaluating whether clients have chosen the most efficient strategy for accomplishing a task and whether they indeed have the capacities to accomplish the task or instead need compensatory strategies, such as the use of equipment or personal assistance. When the patient's typical strategy is so high in energy cost that other meaningful activities are compromised,[27] choosing a compensatory strategy may be preferable to the struggle to perform the task independently.

Examples of assessing strategies used by patients for mobility while maintaining balance include observation of the following: the method by which a child achieves the standing position from a chair; how the child attempts to attain maximal reach in the face of balance problems during administration of the Functional Reach Test;[28, 29] or movement patterns used during formal gait analysis. Behavioral observations during a rise to stand can be used to answer questions like the following: Does he properly position his legs and stand using only the power of his lower extremities? Or does he use his arms to push up to stand? Does he turn to face the chair when getting out or rise directly to stand? The patient's ability to adapt to changing task conditions, such as standing up from a school bus seat or from a chair on a slippery floor, must also be assessed. The Up & Go test could be used to quantify the result in terms of the time needed to accomplish the task.[30] During the use of the Functional Reach Test, some children might be observed to use a hip strategy to increase the reach distance, whereas others might use an ankle strategy or rise on tiptoes. In terms of high-tech assessments, Olney and coworkers' approach to describing power generation based on gait analysis can identify adaptations such as the use of a hip strategy to compensate for a lack of ankle plantar flexor power at push-off in the gait of children with spastic diplegia.[31]

Having defined the behavioral strategies used for accomplishing functional tasks, the therapist may need to explore the impairments that are constraining performance. For the child who rises to stand using arm pushing, constraints might include inadequate leg power to use a momentum strategy or inadequate balance. Horak summarizes the systems involved in postural control needed for tasks like standing up from a chair as including the following:[32]

- The musculoskeletal system with its dynamic interaction among linked segments and inherent passive elastic stiffness positioned over a base of support that varies according to the task
- The central neural set producing predictive control in anticipation of dynamic interactions between the body and the environment as well as between body parts during voluntary movement
- Adaptive mechanisms that change or tune posture to the task demands at hand
- Perception of vertical orientation
- Sensory interactions with flexible dependence on individual senses, again depending on the task context
- Sensorimotor strategies, that is, muscle synergies, that emerge to limit the degrees of freedom of the musculoskeletal system and optimize performance

Constraints to rising from a chair might come from impairment in any one or more of these systems, and it is important to recognize that constraints on functional performance include not only neuromuscular characteristics.[10] Because perception is essential to action, sensory and perceptual abilities must be considered. Finally, task-specific movement is performed within the context of intent and motivation; therefore, cognitive aspects of motor control must also be evaluated. These include factors such as the cognitive level, a fear of falling, attention to regulatory aspects of the task environment,[33] and motivation. A constraint to standing up, for example, might be poor motor planning because of inadequate perception of the necessary position of the feet for propulsion and acceptance of the changing center of mass during rising (a regulatory feature of the task demand). I vividly remember a high school student working under the direction of a physical therapist on practicing standing up. He tried repeatedly without success, all the while attempting to stand without his feet placed back far enough for weight acceptance. When this salient feature of the task demand was pointed out, he rose immediately, and it was obvious that what had been viewed as a problem of strength or coordination was actually a problem of perception and cognition (on the part of both therapist and client!).

Shumway-Cook and Woollacott summarize the intent of all these examinations as gaining the information needed to answer the following questions:[10] Can the impairments that constrain performance be changed through intervention? Is the patient performing optimally given the current set of impairments, or can therapy improve the strategies being used to accomplish functional tasks despite the impairments? I would add that if therapy at the impairment or functional limitations level is unlikely to lead to change, a provision of compensatory strategies, such as assistive technology, to prevent disability and to enable task accomplishment is necessary when the task is important to the child or family for daily life role performance.

Step 4: Guiding Hypotheses

Having explored aspects of the child's disability from a variety of perspectives in a multidimensional examination on community, personal, and organ system levels, the therapist is guided by the HOAC model to generate working hypotheses about why goals can or cannot be met at the present time.[3] In this step lies the true expertise of the clinician, for this is the most difficult step involving the diagnostic skill of the therapist. If impairments that constrain performance or inefficient strategies in use have been correctly identified, moving to planning of intervention to achieve the predetermined goals is not a difficult task. The therapist must, however, consider whether the client is in the process of recovery or in a stable condition before determining exactly what treatment strategy to use. When planning movement goals for children's therapy, Heriza indicates that a dynamic systems approach to intervention suggests that skills that are in flux are the most productive targets of change because instability creates the opportunity to examine the use of alternative strategies.[34] Law and colleagues, for example, use the COPM with parents in their family-centered functional approach to therapy in order to identify emerging skills, and they provide intervention *only* for skills for which parents identify readiness and motivation on the part of the child.[35] In their approach, constraints in the child, task, or environment are identified, and, whenever possible, adaptations to tasks or the environment are used in preference to attempting to change or "normalize" the child in order to enable task accomplishment.

Whatever strategy is chosen in devising a plan of care, the following overall goals should be kept in mind as potential overall outcomes of intervention:

1. Alleviation, where possible, of impairments that constrain function
2. Prevention of secondary impairments resulting from inefficient functional performance, such as reduction of the potential for overuse injury, or limiting progression of already-existing impairments caused by inactivity
3. Development or retraining of functional skills that are within the client's capacity and assistance to the child for developing effective task-specific strategies
4. Reduction of disability through compensation for necessary functions that cannot be improved or made useful through training, reduction of constraints, or selection of more efficient strategies
5. Further reduction of disability in daily life roles by attending to goals that have current priority for the patient and family (or for teachers in school-based settings), and to preparation for life with the maximal degree of self-determination attainable

Embrey and colleagues summarize these issues succinctly by suggesting that appropriate goals should be meaningful to the child and include the prevention of deforming forces and the ability to move effectively within the child's natural environment while resisting the force of gravity.[5]

Accomplishing the goal of preparing children for self-determination requires that the therapist attend, beginning as early as possible, to teaching the child and family all there is to know about the child's condition and about how to maintain health-related physical fitness while living well with a disability. Client education includes the provision of training in problem solving for dealing with typical dilemmas faced by people with disabilities, including asking for (or refusing) help or directing personal assistants. Including these general goals along with client-specific functional goals should be approached by the use of a hypothesis-oriented process for linking specific goals with the facts and hypotheses regarding the underlying causative factors and the clinical hypotheses regarding appropriate means for reducing the impact of negative factors.

According to the HOAC model, if no constraints can be hypothesized to be related to functional limitations that create disability in daily life, the problem could be multifaceted.[3] The therapist may have chosen inappropriate measures, omitted crucial tests, inadequately defined the problem, or failed to link critical observations with related performance problems. The therapist may also lack the appropriate expertise, in which case consultation or referral to another practitioner is advisable. Finally, if, because of information gained during comprehensive assessment or failure to identify a causal hypothesis, the predetermined goals do not appear viable at the present time, they should be revised in consultation with the family, teachers, or other caregivers.

Step 5: Reassessment

Once viable goals have been developed and working hypotheses formulated regarding causes and how change might be effected, the HOAC model guides the therapist to select a date and methodology for reevaluation along with criteria for assessing whether intervention has been successful. Assessments chosen should reflect the change expected as a result of intervention, be documented as reliable and valid for the intended purpose, and be cost-effective in the use of clinical time and other resources. Examination of multiple dimensions is useful to provide support for the working hypothesis of the process by which change would be expected to occur. For example, if lack of strength was identified as a restraint to standing up from a chair, documenting that strength has increased *and* that a momentum strategy for rising using the legs has replaced one relying on arm pushing provides support for the notion that the therapeutic intervention was responsible for the outcome.

Examination of short-term goal achievement need not include the use of comprehensive developmental or functional examination tools, but I recommend that such measures be used at least once a year for testing children with physical disabilities in order to identify emerging or deteriorating skills, areas of omission in therapeutic planning, and competencies that can be used to develop motivational intervention tactics to maximize the possibility of optimal cognitive and socioemotional experiences during therapy. Annual comprehensive examination is also useful as a reality check. If children with disabilities show no change over a year on a sensitive measure of motor function or disability, one should question the cost-effectiveness of continued therapy or revise the goals or strategy for intervention.

Step 6: Intervention Strategies

Next, the HOAC model suggests devising an overall treatment strategy based on the working hypotheses regarding the underlying causes of functional problems.[3] A variety of approaches are available to therapists, including Neuro-Developmental Treatment (NDT),[36] Shepherd's task-related movement science–based approach,[9] the systems-based task-oriented approach described by Shumway-Cook and Woollacott,[10] the dynamic systems approach recommended by Heriza,[34] and family-centered intervention approaches such as that of Law and colleagues.[35] Therapists must be aware that little research exists to document the efficacy or effectiveness of any of these approaches to intervention with children, but several of the most popular approaches are described here as examples of overall strategic planning. Each approach places emphasis on the importance of functional goals as the objective of therapeutic intervention, but they vary in the hypotheses guiding the selection of intervention tactics.

Neuro-Developmental Treatment and the Bobath Concept

The approach advocated by Mayston based on the Bobath concept involves techniques of handling and of guiding the client's movements with carefully graded stimulation to provide a more normal sensation of active movement that is believed to translate into function.[36] The emphasis is on the quality of movement; parent training to incorporate treatment concepts into practice during daily life experiences is considered to be essential to successful functional outcomes. The approach was originally developed for use with children with cerebral palsy who move with abnormal synergies involving extensive irradiation of muscle activity[37] and inadequate anticipatory postural reactions.[38] The techniques of handling and stimulation are used to promote those aspects of motor control that are believed to be prerequisites for automatic and voluntary activity:

- Normalized postural tone and reciprocal interaction of muscles for distal mobility
- Postural adaptation
- Graded control of antagonistic muscles during functional activity

Girolami and Campbell have demonstrated the value of the NDT approach in promoting functional motor development of premature babies at high risk for central nervous system dysfunction in a controlled clinical trial,[39] but NDT was not as effective as a more multifaceted early-intervention program for facilitating motor and cognitive development in late-treated children with spastic diplegia.[40] Therapists who use this approach should recognize that although studies exist that support its efficacy, effects have been small, and there are also a number of studies that do not provide support for its value.[41] Parents have the right to be given a balanced view of the evidence, and proponents of NDT and other approaches have the obligation to document effectiveness through well-designed research.

Sensory Integration Theory

Sensory Integration Theory is another approach used by therapists, primarily for children with mild-to-moderate learning problems associated with motor incoordination and otherwise unexplained sensory-processing dysfunction.[42] The theory postulates that learning is dependent on an intake of sensory information that is used to plan and produce organized behavior. Provision of opportunities for enhanced sensory intake within the context of active participation in meaningful activity is believed to improve the ability of the child to process and integrate sensory information leading to enhanced conceptual and motor learning. This approach is also controversial, especially among special educators.

Several therapeutic approaches are based on current information in movement science with an emphasis on the use of research evidence and the importance of task characteristics in determining methods for improving movement outcomes. These approaches are described next.

Task-Related Movement Science–Based Model

The strategic approach to intervention pioneered by Carr and Shepherd[9] and illustrated in Chapter 6 focuses on prevention or minimization of movement disorganization and learned nonuse of body segments that have impaired motor control as a result of central nervous system injury; maintenance of soft tissue flexibility; stimulation of movement; and task-related practice and exercise for increasing muscle strength, improving motor control, and learning or relearning effective action. Following Gentile,[33] goal-directed movements of two types are emphasized: (1) investigative behaviors in which the child learns to position the body parts in a way that best enables relevant information from the environment to be taken in, and (2) adaptive behaviors in which the child develops the ability to interact with the environment in a flexible manner so as to meet new challenges. Early emphasis on functional movement in erect body positions is characteristic of this approach, as is work on reducing the amount of inappropriate muscle activity used by the child during functional tasks. Treatment techniques used are derived from analysis of areas of impairment or compensation, biomechanics, the environmental context for the task at hand, and current understanding of the need for the specificity of muscle activation for functional tasks. All training is task- and context-specific. These clinicians suggest that physical therapists need to become applied movement scientists, using information from all areas of human movement science, including biomechanics, motor learning, action-perception-cognition theory, and neurophysiology, in order to effectively engage in evidence-based practice. Further information on this approach with children can be found in Chapter 6.

Tscharnuter Akademie for Movement Organization

The Tscharnuter Akademie for Movement Organization approach is another strategy for treatment with a strong emphasis on biomechanics as a tool for informing the selection of treatment tactics.[43] Instead of relating development to the maturation of the nervous system, this therapy approach emphasizes environmental forces, such as the support surface characteristics, and the child's strategies for dealing with the forces necessary to conform to the task surface, in determining how to optimize the child's self-initiated movements for efficiency and task accomplishment. The overall treatment goal is to assist the child in learning how to achieve proper orientation to the support surface and to activate the body from its support surface contacts as appropriate for the task. Through therapeutic handling, the therapist manipulates forces and torques used by the child in order to enable self-organization of adaptive movement.

Systems-Based Task-Oriented Approach

Based on their systems-based task-oriented approach to clinical assessment, Shumway-Cook and Woollacott have developed a strategic approach to intervention with individuals with disability in control of posture and movement.[10] Based on assessment results and hypotheses relating functional performance difficulties to constraints caused by impairments or the use of inefficient movement strategies, a task-oriented approach to treatment focuses on resolving or preventing impairments, developing effective task-specific movement strategies, and developing or retraining functional goal-oriented tasks. Trial-and-error learning is used to assist the client in discovering optimal solutions to many functional tasks, and the environment is carefully structured to reinforce the use of optimal strategies, including the use of augmented feedback to explicitly train skill components. Functionally relevant tasks are practiced under wide-ranging conditions to enable a transfer of skill to a variety of environments and to enable the client to develop a variety of solutions to movement problems rather than a single solution.

Task-specific requirements are key to developing treatment techniques in this approach. For example, the task requirements of gait include progression, stability, and adaptation to environmental obstacles along the intended path. A treatment plan involves attempts to decrease constraints that might impair the ability to meet task requirements as well as assisting the client to find optimal strategies to accomplish task requirements regardless of underlying impairment. An understanding of how the nervous system selects from the variety of likely-to-be-successful strategies for accomplishing task performance is essential to the use of this strategic approach to physical therapy.

Gentile[44] emphasizes the importance of task demands in her model of skill acquisition that Shumway-Cook and Woollacott,[10] like Shepherd,[9] incorporate into their strategic approach. A primary focus is on adaptive behaviors by which the individual interacts meaningfully with the environment. In goal-directed behavior, the performer attempts to mold movement to the relevant features of the environment. Those environmental features that are critical for performance are termed *regulatory conditions* because movement must conform to them to be successful. At our peril we ignore the fact that we are about to step on a patch of ice while the dog we are walking is pulling at the leash in pursuit of a squirrel! The need to recognize that the body weight must be shifted over the feet before standing up has already been mentioned as another example. My own favorite clinical example of the importance of recognizing the regulatory conditions of a task is the child with spastic diplegia who successfully walks across the room but trips on the therapy mat. If we search further, we may find that the child recognized the regulatory condition of the task (a need to lift the leg high enough to clear the foot) but is constrained by a lack of sufficient single-leg balance. On the other hand, the child may have failed to recognize the regulatory condition because of limited depth perception, cognitive ability, or visual acuity.

Because regulatory conditions change with the task, the neuromotor processes that assume critical importance in movement production also change with task conditions. Motor learning thus has an initial stage in which the performer has an action goal (a task to be accomplished) and must discover possible movement strategies commensurate with the regulatory conditions of the task in order to successfully attain the goal. Thus the overall strategy suggested by Gentile's approach is to assist the client to recognize the regulatory conditions of tasks being learned and to achieve a successful action.[44] Only with repeated practice and the feedback inherent to repetition does skill develop. Thus skill development to refine the movement characteristics and to find the optimal solution in terms of energy cost is considered to be a later stage of learning. A major contribution of this approach is a taxonomy of tasks based on the demands placed on the performer in terms of information to be analyzed and constraints on movement and neuromotor processes. The overall strategy for planning treatment tactics would thus depend on the type of functional task that is the intended goal of intervention. As illustrated in the approaches of Shepherd[9] and of Shumway-Cook and Woollacott,[10] structure of the environment and augmented feedback are used as tactics for intervention. This approach has recently been demonstrated to be effective in improving balance and functional gait, as well as reducing the risk of falling in elderly clients[45] but has not yet been demonstrated to be effective in the treatment of children.

Neurobehavioral Intervention Model

The previously discussed strategies for intervention lack specifically defined protocols for assessing progress and the achievement of intended outcomes.[46] An approach described by Horn and colleagues represents a major advance in conceptualizing outcome assessment and was developed primarily for use with children with cerebral palsy.[47] The approach also meets a criterion for effective intervention identified by Ramey and Ramey,[48] that of specific protocol guidelines for designing intervention. In the neurobehavioral approach, the development of motor milestones is viewed as the culmination of organization of underlying components of movement enabling the milestone to appear. The therapist must identify the components that are absent and present and then design tactics to assist the child in learning the needed components. A functional goal must be identified that could be achieved if the motor milestone is attained. Other skills to which the use of the movement could be applied are identified as markers that the child has *generalized* the learned skill to *new* behaviors. As intervention is provided that has been designed specifically to allow the child to attain the defined skill, the ability to achieve the functional goal and to generalize the use of the movements to other settings or stimuli is also measured. This approach, therefore, combines techniques from an NDT approach for facilitating the development of movement components needed for functional skills with a goal delineation and outcome assessment approach derived from motor learning and behavioral theory. A further strength of the neurobehavioral intervention strategy is that it has been tested experimentally and found to promote generalization of learning in all children studied.[47]

Comparing Approaches

As a summary of approaches to reviewing various strategies for intervention with children with disabilities, the therapist should consider the following major points of potentially different emphasis in each approach:

1. Who selects goals and what kind are they?
2. Are valid and reliable examinations recommended for problem identification?

3. Does intervention stress changing the child, the task, or the environment?
4. Is generalization of a skill to a variety of environments explicitly planned?
5. What outcomes have been validated by sound research and how are they documented in clinical practice?

Not only therapists but also families and referring or collaborating professionals should have this knowledge as a basis for their own decision making.

Step 7: Selection of Intervention Tactics

After the selection of an overall strategy for approaching intervention, a specific plan of treatment is developed and implemented. Tactics selected are obviously based on the goals of the plan of care, and a myriad of approaches might be selected within the context of an overall strategic framework. Here the creativity of the therapist can shine forth, but often parents are able to devise the most creative tactics for use with their children when the goals of treatment and working hypotheses are clearly communicated. This is the best of all possible worlds and allows the therapist to teach and coach, rather than provide more costly direct treatment. Strategic approaches such as those described previously suggest, however, that elements of any treatment plan should be based on the principles of motor learning, task analysis, constraints, and typical movement strategies of the client, as well as the age and mental level of the child. Many resources exist on these topics that are not covered in any detail here, but they are described in the condition-specific chapters to follow. Two points, however, should be emphasized. First, Embrey and colleagues have shown that therapists tend to use repeatedly a rather small set of techniques that they have found to be successful.[5] As a result, Embrey and colleagues recommend that therapists build and refine their repertoire of treatment ideas. Second, I emphasize the psychosocial aspect of providing not only an environment that is structured to facilitate task performance, but also one that draws children in because of its motivational appeal. It is a maxim of pediatric physical therapy that "play is the work of children" and that therapy should be playful in order to be inherently motivating. This is probably the major difference between treatment plans for children and those for adults and between the clinical skills of novice and experienced therapists,[24] and it is deserving of more scientific research than has been hitherto applied to the problem.

One aspect of selecting tactics for intervention that appears to be important, particularly for work with infants and toddlers, is choosing activities that will create an optimal psychologic experience, or what Csikszentmihalyi calls "flow."[49] Psychologic flow is what we experience when we are so deeply immersed in an activity that an objective sense of time is lost, concentration on the present is intense and complete, and we engage in the activity with an enjoyment so deep that we will expend a lot of energy just to experience it. An example from childhood is the repetition of activity children engage in as a new skill emerges, which was elegantly illuminated by Thelen's research.[50] Darl Vander Linden shared an example of his daughter Abby's repeatedly going up and down a 4-inch step from the house to a screened porch, insistently demanding that her parents open the screen door to provide her access to the step while resisting all attempts to interest her in another activity.[51] This almost obsessive interest in performing an activity for its own sake disappears once the activity has been mastered and becomes an automatic part of the child's repertoire. Even animals engage in this type of intense concentration on a single act. I remember my Labrador retriever barking to go outside, and then immediately barking to come back in, about a dozen times within the space of an hour, when she first learned the association between her woof and the door being opened. Although one might expect that adults would experience flow primarily during pleasurable leisure activities, actually people report that flow experiences are more typical of activity engaged in at work. Furthermore, the experience of flow does not even require that the activity be pleasurable.[49] People who have successfully endured long incarceration frequently report that the ability to induce flow experiences through concentration on activities that allowed the sense of exercising control in a situation of almost total loss of self-determination was crucial to their survival.

In addition to the characteristics of flow activities already described, other elements of importance to producing such experiences have been identified. These include engagement in a task one is capable of completing that also has clear goals and immediate feedback. A reward is not necessary because the sense of flow can be its own reward, and the goal does not necessarily have to be a *functional* goal because children practice skills for the sake of practice, as demonstrated by Vander Linden's child. We must be able to concentrate on the task, and engaging in the task provides the experience of exercising a sense of control over one's own actions. Concern for self disappears during the activity but paradoxically emerges stronger after completion of the act. Flow activities need not be physical, but when they are, the physical activity is accompanied by intense cognitive attention and processing that make one feel at one with the environment. Appropriate activities require an investment of psychic energy but cannot be done without the requisite physical and cognitive skills.

For application to the planning of therapeutic activities, the requirements for generating a flow experience suggest that activities with just the right amount of challenge relative to the individual's skills are those that need to be chosen. As previously mentioned, Law and colleagues specifically incorporate the idea of readiness for skill development in selecting goals in their family-centered approach to intervention.[35] The therapist needs to understand the child's cognitive abilities as well as physical abilities, and keep in mind the overall goals of intervention during the intense interaction that occurs during a therapy session, but also be able to recognize when the child is engaged in a flow experience that should be allowed to continue even when a previously intended short-term goal of the session might need to be discarded for the day.[5]

Able-bodied children are natural seekers of flow experiences and they "know" what activities to engage in that present the appropriate amount of challenge. When repetition of an activity starts to get boring, they "up the ante" to increase the degree of difficulty. Whether children with physical and cognitive disabilities are as capable of seeking out and engaging in flow activities is unknown, but clearly therapists can set up a therapeutic environment to stimulate such activity if they have a deep knowledge of a child's well-developed skills and emerging skills, often acquired from parents' observations. Embrey and Nirider have also shown that more experienced therapists demonstrate greater psychosocial sensitivity to children than novice therapists, so skill in this area also appears to develop with practice.[52] During the therapy session, they can recognize when the child "needs" to repeat an activity over and over again without interruption, or when the child is getting bored or overwhelmed with an activity and needs to have the challenge level appropriately adjusted, as well as when it is time to move to a new activity.

Modern motor control theory suggests that the therapist should adjust the challenge by structuring the environment to elicit the movement skills desired rather than use handling of the child to guide the child through the process, but one can also envision the possibility of aiding a child's ability to achieve a flow experience by structuring the *movement,* as in the NDT approach, for optimal energy cost and successful task attainment. The therapist who has command of both the science of movement (and its abnormalities in the condition under treatment) and an intuitive sense of the child's engagement with the process and creative ways to engender the sense of flow is a pleasure to watch in action because one develops a sense that the players are mutually engaged in a flow experience. This intuitive ability to synthesize a variety of factors, that is, the art of therapy, really cannot be planned in advance because it happens during the therapist-client interaction. The improvisational nature of treatment leads Embrey and Adams to suggest that decision algorithms are not likely to be helpful in this situation.[2] This point is well taken, but I believe that it is equally likely that the thought and planning entailed in using the HOAC to envision tactics to achieve goals based on an underlying working hypothesis about causality, when firmly in mind just below consciousness during a therapeutic interaction, frees the therapist to be fully engaged with the patient and most likely to be able to take advantage of fortuitous observations that can be turned to therapeutic advantage in the production of an optimal experience. Such an experience would involve child-generated activity that the therapist assists through a variety of tactics to maintain an appropriate level of challenge to guarantee success but also to facilitate motor learning to attain a new level of skill.

Carter has described the ability of the master clinician, when compared with the novice practitioner of NDT, to anticipate the child's needs by providing an inhibitory stimulus when movement seems likely to go wrong or a facilitatory stimulus (whether handling, verbal guidance, or physical placement of equipment or toys) to change the level of challenge.[53] Novices tended to provide stimulation at less appropriate times and were perhaps concentrating on their own activity too much because it had not yet become automatic. The master clinician holds an intuitive level of knowledge and skill that we need to articulate better in order to speed the process along for novice therapists, and Embrey and colleagues' work on clinical decision making is an excellent beginning.[5]

Another area of theory and research that needs to be consciously applied to the planning of therapeutic tactics is motor learning. Larin has described its elements that fit well with the concept of creating optimal psychologic experiences.[1] These include

- Attention to the context in which learning will occur (physical environment, promoting initiations by the learner, reciprocity and shared control, and provision of responsive feedback)
- Motivation through prior knowledge of the activity and its goal and through establishing an appropriate level of challenge
- Stimulation of creative behavior through flexibility in therapy and using cognitive challenges to attempt new movement behaviors
- Learner engagement in goal setting
- Careful use of instruction and modeling
- Sequencing of tasks using repetition and feedback for skill development as well as use of mental practice in ways demonstrated to be most effective in stimulating long-term retention rather than immediate performance

Gentile also suggests that a taxonomy of tasks be used to select those that combine the elements of the environment (stationary versus motion, and variable versus stable), degree of body stability (with or without manipulation), and degree of body transport (with or without manipulation) required by the task to select activities for meeting therapeutic functional goals.[44] The therapeutic process would emphasize accomplishing the task for the new learner while repetition for skill improvement is the appropriate objective of the learner who has "gotten the idea" but needs to become more efficient or more consistently effective.

In my invited lecture at the World Confederation for Physical Therapy, I suggested that therapy programs for children should also be structured to create effects to last a lifetime.[54] These ideas were developed as a result of a conference that increased my awareness of the problems of young adults with cerebral palsy or spina bifida that could perhaps be prevented with a more future-oriented approach to planning intervention experiences for children.[55] Based on the stated needs of adults with these conditions, therapy programs need to

1. Encourage a sense of self-esteem through an ability to engage with and control the environment in age-appropriate ways
2. Teach families and children themselves all there is to know about their condition so they become owners of their problems as well as capabilities
3. Emphasize the needs that adults with disabilities find most salient, such as community mobility[56] and communication
4. Prevent overuse syndromes and musculoskeletal conditions that can lead to pain and increased disability in adulthood
5. Provide access to counseling on proper nutrition and other aspects of a healthy lifestyle
6. Include in therapy programs activities that can be used to promote lifelong physical fitness, stress reduction, and social engagement through activity

These should be overarching goals for the reduction of disability in daily life apart from, but no less important than, the specific functional goals needed for self-care and mobility at the moment. Because of the intense interaction between children, parents, and therapists in the typical therapeutic relationship, significant education on these issues can be easily incorporated into treatment sessions as well as included specifically in plans of care, especially at important points of transition, such as graduation from grade school or high school.

Step 8: Implementation

Implementing treatment also requires decisions about frequency and who will provide the intervention. We have little research to draw on here, but the increasing restrictions of health care payment systems require new ways of thinking about implementation of therapeutic goals, including the use of physical therapist assistants and family members more extensively than has previously been the case. To begin with, we should think more systematically about what needs to be done by a therapist and what should be turned over to the family or to an assistant or aide. A basic guideline that seems practical is that when a child is able to accomplish a functional activity but needs to become more skilled or automatic in its performance, this activity should be turned over to the home environment for daily and frequent repetition that can happen in only that setting. Emerging skills need to be identified by persons familiar with the child and guided toward further development by professionals, but a structured environment for practice can frequently be provided in group therapy or under the supervision of an assistant who has been well trained.

The frequency-of-treatment decision is more complex. If a child is receiving services in a public school, frequency is dictated by the Individualized Educational Program (IEP), and failure to provide that level of service can be a cause for legal action.[57] As a result, careful thought must be given to the frequency specified. But what is the basis for making that decision? Giangreco maintains that the best practice in a school-based setting should be based on a value system oriented to providing supports that are "only as special as necessary" rather than a "more-is-better" approach or a "return-on-investment" approach based on providing more services to those with the most favorable prognosis.[58]

Therapists also need to think about whether intensive therapy for short periods can be more useful in certain situations than regular but less frequent therapy over prolonged periods of time.[59] Once again, families that are empowered with full knowledge of their child's condition and with anticipatory guidance about expected future development or possible impairments, such as worsening contractures during growth spurts, can become personally responsible for identification of the need for timely professional consultation but can otherwise implement much of a typical treatment plan, thereby reducing the frequency of direct therapy. In any case, current limitations placed on service provision, capitation service delivery models, and the need to match therapeutic goals to educational needs in school settings are examples of service dilemmas that require a serious look at issues such as when and how often to treat, when to consult or monitor, and when to discharge. The final part of the HOAC model suggests explicit reflection on such issues.[3]

Analyzing and Reflecting on Outcomes

The second part of the HOAC model involves reassessment and reflection on the plan of care after therapy has been implemented and reevaluation of goal attainment has occurred (see Fig. 1–2).[3] Embrey and Yates[60] and Larin[1] have shown that therapists reflect on practice seriously and frequently, but often not explicitly, and that there are differences between experienced therapists and novices both in frequency of reflection and in whether reflection is on positive or negative aspects of performance. According to the HOAC, the patient should be discharged if the goals have been attained and no new goals are identified, an infrequent occurrence in the practice of pediatric physical therapy. If the previously established goals have not been met, the therapist sequentially examines whether the tactics were implemented correctly, whether the tactics were appropriate, whether the strategy was correct, and whether the hypotheses on which treatment was originally predicated were actually viable. If any question is answered in the negative, revisions are made and reassessment planned for a later date.

HOW DOES THE HYPOTHESIS-ORIENTED ALGORITHM FOR CLINICIANS MODEL FIT WITH "BEST PRACTICE" OPTIONS FOR PEDIATRIC SERVICE DELIVERY?

The families of today's children with disabilities have a multitude of service delivery options to choose from, although the choice may obviously be curtailed by limitations imposed by poverty, insurance plans, and government-determined rights to access. Today's models of service delivery may define appropriate goals in different ways, but one can often find an especially good fit with the HOAC model's recommendation that goals should be established in consultation with the consumer *before* formal assessment.[3] Giangreco goes further in emphasizing that in decision making for related services in school settings, it is essential that a consensus on goals be reached *among* professionals,[58] rather than each discipline having distinct and perhaps different, or even conflicting, goals. Because services must be educationally relevant and necessary, however, all service providers must be aware of the content of the educational program, a significant difference from service provision in a typical medical model and one not acknowledged in the HOAC approach. In the Choosing Options and Accommodations for Children approach to planning related services in public school settings,[61] goals encompass three categories of educationally relevant services:

1. Priority learning outcomes that are family-selected, individualized, discipline-free, and reflected in the IEP in annual goals and short-term objectives
2. Additional learning outcomes determined jointly by team members to ensure that the student has access to a broad range of learning outcomes from across elements of the curriculum, such as creative activities or inclusion in regular physical education
3. General supports that need to be provided to allow access to education or facilitate participation, including personal needs, physical needs (e.g., positioning), sensory needs, teaching others about the student, and providing access and opportunities (e.g., inclusion in regular class activities)

Classification of services into these three components makes it clear, for example, that positioning is a support, not a learning activity, and would be considered necessary and educationally relevant only if connected with facilitation of learning outcomes specified in the IEP.

Bundy emphasizes that the choice of service delivery model is intimately related to the expected outcomes, once again making the point that careful goal delineation is essential as the starting point in the decision-making process even though she places goal setting in the second stage of her model of service delivery options (Fig. 1–3).[62] The choice of service delivery model can be considered a part of the process of determining *strategy* in the HOAC model,[3] but the relevant issues are not directly addressed by the model. A consultation model is chosen when the expected outcome is that the school environment will change in ways that enable successful learning despite functional limitations. Indirect service involves teaching an aide, parent, or teacher to implement a necessary technique and then monitoring the performance and outcomes. Expected outcomes include refinement of a student's skill, a maintenance function, or the provision of a needed support for learning or other school activities such as personal care. When direct service is selected, an expected outcome is that the student will change to meet the expectations of the environment or will gain skill. If the service is not provided in the classroom, the skill should be seen as critical enough to justify disruption of school participation and, of course, must be educationally relevant. If the service is provided in the classroom, it must contribute to the child's ability to engage in the learning activities and emphatically *not* consist of "therapy" that is unrelated to the

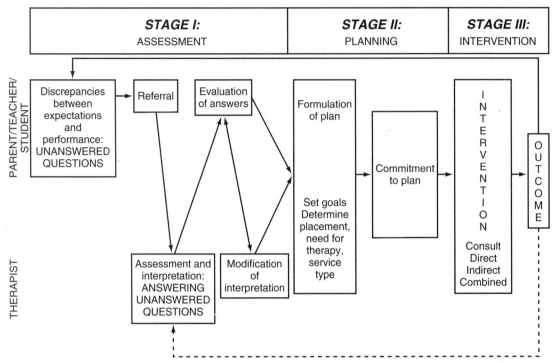

FIGURE 1–3. Bundy's conceptualization of a service delivery model for educational settings. (Redrawn from Bundy AC: Assessment and intervention in school-based practice: Answering questions and minimizing discrepancies. Phys Occup Ther Pediatr 15(2):72, 1995, copyright 1995, The Haworth Press, Binghamton, NY.)

classroom agenda. Because in surveys classroom teachers often express a preference for pullout services, Bundy believes that they typically find intervention by therapists in the classroom to be disruptive rather than enhancing of learning performance of students.[62]

Students have reported a problem with the disruption involved in pullout services.[63] Only half of the subjects in a survey of children with disabilities who received school therapy services reported positively anticipating therapy sessions, even though most of the subjects expressed their appreciation for the value of therapy and liked their therapists. The primary reason for the lack of positive anticipation was the disappointment in being interrupted while involved in other activities. Being involved in therapy was also a source of embarrassment for some children when dealing with peers. These issues make it clear that the HOAC model does not address the broader context of settings in which many children receive therapy and does not take into account the roles of other professionals whose activities are ultimately affected by the decisions made by pediatric therapists.

Service delivery within a managed care system presents entirely different dilemmas to therapists serving children with disabilities and their families. The National Coalition for Family Leadership has developed criteria for parents to use when evaluating managed care plans for children with disabilities or chronic illnesses.[64] The coalition stresses that families must be considered to be the core of any health system and that managed care systems must recognize that outcomes for children with special health care needs will improve when families and professionals make decisions jointly. Children with special health care needs should be provided with a coordinated system of comprehensive community-based services and have unconditional and equitable access to primary care; preventive, habilitative, and specialty health care services; and equipment at reasonable cost. Decision making should be flexibly based on the unique circumstances of the child and family. Access should include, when needed, in-home care and equipment and referrals to interventions outside the network for specialized care.

Although the HOAC model does not specifically address issues of access in decision making, its stress on having the therapist identify hypotheses for what is problematic and how change can be effected should be useful to primary care providers in a managed care system for identifying when specialized consultation and services outside the network are needed. Therapists contracting with such systems can play a helpful role by clarifying the types of services they provide, outcomes expected as a result of specific amounts of intervention, and why a specialist is needed to provide care for children with disabilities.

The NCMRR framework can also be used profitably by therapists working with managed care systems when they need to provide education to case managers regarding the differences between goals that can be accomplished in early-intervention programs, which usually operate primarily on an educational model, and in physical therapy programs, either integrated in an educational model or serving primarily health-related, rather than educationally relevant, needs. Much confusion continues to exist regarding where responsibility (including financial responsibility) lies for various types of interventions to meet the complex needs of children with disabilities, and the use of an explicit decision-making model can be helpful in communicating across disciplinary and role boundaries.

Although in a managed health care system the therapist may play a role in helping to clarify the need for therapy to meet health-related needs, the opposite may be true for the therapist working in a technologically oriented neonatal intensive care unit. Here the attention of highly skilled health professionals may be unswervingly devoted to the growth and survival of fragile infants, whereas the therapist may play an important role in supporting families emotionally while also helping them to attend to and advocate for their baby's developmental needs. Once again, the explicit structure of both the HOAC and the NCMRR model provides a framework to enhance communication across disciplinary and role boundaries for the benefit of children with special needs, despite failing to address these issues directly.

Not yet common for physical therapists in pediatric practice is the use of critical pathways (also called clinical pathways or care paths).[65] Critical pathways display time-ordered goals for patients, delineating the ideal sequence and timing of professional actions in order to efficiently achieve desired outcomes. The term *critical* is used because this type of care plan evolved from industrial efforts to identify rate-limiting processes in the production process that, if tackled effectively, could significantly reduce costs and time. In medical care, critical pathways are developed to select best practices when practice styles vary unnecessarily, to define standards of care, to allow all disciplines to use the same time-saving forms for the documentation of care, and to improve patient satisfaction by incorporating plans of care into educational programs for patients and their caregivers. When done well, critical pathways incorporate the evaluation of current methods of care, use evidence to decide on actions and their timing, and allow study of why variations in outcomes or the achievement of short-term goals occurs so that the critical pathway can be revised and improved. In some cases, critical pathways have been transformed into pictorial care plans that are especially useful for educating patients with low cognitive functioning or language barriers in the stages to be expected in their plan of care.[66] Furthermore, effective critical pathways have been developed for use in multiple stages of care, including transitions from hospital care to home health care. Because I have found frequent complaints from practitioners in *both* community-based settings and in tertiary care hospitals related to a failure of others to communicate care goals and plans to their counterparts in other settings, such multisetting pathways would be highly advantageous to introduce into the care of children with chronic disabilities who frequently need surgery or other inpatient care.

In summary, it is my firm belief that therapeutic outcomes can be improved by explicit engagement in thoughtful decision making using a decision algorithm and a conceptual framework for understanding disability, coupled with a commitment to collaboration with families in understanding and meeting their needs. Models describing service delivery options specific to pediatric practice fill in the basic outline for planning and reflection by elaborating on setting-specific issues. Subsequent chapters in this volume aim to make such use of reflection on practice explicit, thereby offering the reader a unique opportunity to review how experienced pediatric physical therapists describe and analyze their past and current actions on behalf of children and families with a view toward improving outcomes and efficiency for the best practice in the new millennium. In the following chapters, master clinicians discuss how they develop goals, select strategies and tactics for successful plans of care, and document outcomes that matter in the lives of children with special needs and their families.

REFERENCES

1. Larin HM: Motor learning: Theories and strategies for the practitioner. *In* Campbell SK, Vander Linden DW, Palisano RJ (eds): Physical Therapy for Children. WB Saunders, Philadelphia, 1994, p 157.
2. Embrey DG, Adams LS: Clinical applications of procedural changes by experienced and novice pediatric physical therapists. Pediatr Phys Ther 8:122, 1996.
3. Rothstein JM, Echternach JL: Hypothesis-oriented algorithm for clinicians: A method for evaluation and treatment planning. Phys Ther 66:1388, 1986.
4. Echternach JL, Rothstein JM: Hypothesis-oriented algorithms. Phys Ther 69:559, 1989.
5. Embrey DG, Yates L, Nirider B, et al: Recommendations for pediatric physical therapists: Making clinical decisions for children with cerebral palsy. Pediatr Phys Ther 8:165, 1996.
6. Rosenbaum P, King S, Law M, et al: Family-centred service: A conceptual framework and research review. Phys Occup Ther Pediatr 18(1):1, 1998.
7. Carr JH, Shepherd RB (eds): Movement Science: Foundations for Physical Therapy in Rehabilitation. Aspen, Rockville, Md, 1987.
8. Carr JH, Shepherd RB: A Motor Relearning Programme for Stroke, 2nd ed. Heinemann, London, 1987.
9. Shepherd RB: Training motor control and optimizing motor learning. *In* Shepherd RB (ed): Physiotherapy in Paediatrics, 3rd ed. Butterworth-Heinemann, Oxford, 1995, p 42.
10. Shumway-Cook A, Woollacott M: Motor Control: Theory and Practical Applications. Williams & Wilkins, Baltimore, 1995.
11. Palisano RJ, Campbell SK, Harris SR: Clinical decision-making in pediatric physical therapy. *In* Campbell SK, Vander Linden DW, Palisano RJ (eds): Physical Therapy for Children. WB Saunders, Philadelphia, 1994, p 183.
12. Law M, Baptiste S, McColl MA, et al: The Canadian Occupational Performance Measure: An outcome measure for occupational therapy. Can J Occup Ther 57:82, 1990.
13. Law M, Baptiste S, Carswell-Opzoomer A, et al: Canadian Occupational Performance Measure Manual. CAOT, Toronto, 1991.
14. Toomey M, Nicholson D, Carswell A: The clinical utility of the Canadian Occupational Performance Measure. Can J Occup Ther 62:242, 1995.
15. Bricker D (ed): Assessment, Evaluation, and Programming System for Infants and Children, vol. 1. AEPS Measurement for Birth to Three Years. Paul H Brookes, Baltimore, 1993.
16. National Institutes of Health: Research Plan for the National Center for Medical Rehabilitation Research. NIH Publication No 93-3509. US Department of Health & Human Services, Washington, DC, March 1993.
17. Linehan SA: Ecological versus developmental assessment: Influences on instructional expectations. J Assoc Persons Severe Handicaps 16(3):146, 1991.
18. Linder TW: Transdisciplinary Play-Based Assessment. A Functional Approach to Working with Young Children. Paul H Brookes, Baltimore, 1993.
19. Russell D, Rosenbaum P, Cadman D, et al: The Gross Motor Function Measure: A means to evaluate the effects of physical therapy. Dev Med Child Neurol 31:341, 1989.
20. Haley SM, Coster WJ, Ludlow LH, et al: The Pediatric Evaluation of Disability Inventory: Development Standardization and Administration Manual. New England Medical Center Publications, Boston, 1992.
21. Hazlewood ME, Brown JK, Rowe PJ, et al: The therapeutic use of electrical stimulation. Dev Med Child Neurol 36:661, 1994.
22. Damiano DL, Vaughan CL, Abel MF: Muscle response to heavy resistance exercise in children with spastic cerebral palsy. Dev Med Child Neurol 37:731, 1995.
23. Deitz JC, Richardson P, Crowe TK, et al: Performance of children with learning disabilities and motor delays on the Pediatric Clinical Test of Sensory Interaction for Balance (P-CTSIB). Phys Occup Ther Pediatr 16(3):1, 1996.
24. Embrey DG, Hylton N: Clinical applications of movement scripts by experienced and novice pediatric physical therapists. Pediatr Phys Ther 8:3, 1996.
25. Piper MC, Darrah J: Motor Assessment of the Developing Infant. WB Saunders, Philadelphia, 1994.

26. Welford AT: Motor skills and aging. *In* Mortimer J, Pirozzolo FJ, Maletta G (eds): Scientific Bases for Neurophysiologic Approaches to Therapeutic Exercise. FA Davis, Philadelphia, 1977, p 13.

27. Franks CA, Palisano RJ, Darbee JC: The effect of walking with an assistive device and using a wheelchair on school performance in students with myelomeningocele. Phys Ther 71:570, 1991.

28. Donahoe B, Turner D, Worrell T: The use of functional reach as a measurement of balance in boys and girls without disabilities ages 5 to 15 years. Pediatr Phys Ther 6:189, 1994.

29. Niznik TM, Turner D, Worrell TW: Functional reach as a measurement of balance for children with lower extremity spasticity. Phys Occup Ther Pediatr 15(3):1, 1995.

30. Podsciadlo D, Richardson S: The timed "Up & Go": A test of basic functional mobility for frail elderly persons. J Am Geriatr Soc 39:142, 1991.

31. Olney SJ, Costigan PA, Hedden DM: Mechanical energy patterns in gait of cerebral palsied children. Phys Ther 67:1348, 1987.

32. Horak FB: Motor control models underlying neurologic rehabilitation of posture in children. *In* Forssberg H, Hirschfeld H (eds): Movement Disorders in Children. Med Sport Sci vol 36. Karger, Basel, 1992, p 21.

33. Gentile AM: Skill acquisition: Action, movement, and neuromotor processes. In Carr JA, Shepherd RB (eds): Movement Science: Foundations for Physical Therapy in Rehabilitation. Aspen, Rockville, Md, 1987, p 115.

34. Heriza C: Traditional and contemporary theories. *In* Lister MJ (ed): Contemporary Management of Motor Control Problems: Proceedings of the II STEP Conference. Foundation for Physical Therapy, Alexandria, Va, 1991, p 99.

35. Law M, Darrah J, Pollock N, et al: Family-centred functional therapy for children with cerebral palsy: An emerging practice model. Phys Occup Ther Pediatr. 18(1):83, 1998.

36. Mayston MJ: The Bobath concept—Evolution and application. *In* Forssberg H, Hirschfeld H (eds): Movement Disorders in Children. Med Sport Sci vol 36. Karger, Basel, 1992, p 1.

37. Leonard CT, Hirschfeld H: Myotatic reflex responses of non-disabled children and children with spastic cerebral palsy. Dev Med Child Neurol 37:783, 1995.

38. Nashner LM, Shumway-Cook A, Marin O: Stance posture control in select groups of children with cerebral palsy: Deficits in sensory organization and muscular coordination. Exp Brain Res 49:393, 1983.

39. Girolami GL, Campbell SK: Efficacy of a Neuro-Developmental Treatment Program to improve motor control in infants born prematurely. Pediatr Phys Ther 6:175, 1994.

40. Palmer FB, Shapiro BK, Wachtel RC, et al: The effects of physical therapy on cerebral palsy. N Engl J Med 318:803, 1988.

41. Ottenbacher KJ, Biocca Z, DeCremer G, et al: Quantitative analysis of the effectiveness of pediatric therapy: Emphasis on the neurodevelopmental treatment approach. Phys Ther 66:1095, 1986.

42. Fisher AG, Bundy AC: Sensory integration theory. *In* Forssberg H, Hirschfeld H (eds): Movement Disorders in Children. Med Sport Sci vol 36. Karger, Basel, 1992, p 16.

43. Tscharnuter I: A new therapy approach to movement organization. Phys Occup Ther Pediatr 13(2):19, 1993.

44. Gentile AM: The nature of skill acquisition: Therapeutic implications for children with movement disorders. *In* Forssberg H, Hirschfeld H (eds): Movement Disorders in Children. Med Sport Sci vol 36. Karger, Basel, 1992, p 31.

45. Shumway-Cook A, Gruber W, Baldwin M, et al: The effect of multidimensional exercises on balance, mobility, and fall risk in community-dwelling older adults. Phys Ther 77:46, 1997.

46. Horn EM: Basic motor skills instruction for children with neuromotor delays: A critical review. J Spec Educ 25:168, 1991.

47. Horn EM, Warren SF, Jones HA: An experimental analysis of neurobehavioral motor intervention. Dev Med Child Neurol 37:697, 1995.

48. Ramey CT, Ramey SL: Effective early intervention. Ment Retard 30(6):337, 1992.

49. Csikszentmihalyi M: Flow—The Psychology of Optimal Experience. Harper & Row, New York, 1990.

50. Thelen E: Kicking, rocking, and waving: Contextual analysis of rhythmical stereotypies in normal human infants. Anim Behav 29:3, 1981.

51. Campbell SK: The child's development of functional movement. *In* Campbell SK, Vander Linden DW, Palisano RJ (eds): Physical Therapy for Children. WB Saunders, Philadelphia, 1994, p 3.

52. Embrey DG, Nirider B: Clinical applications of psychosocial sensitivity by experienced and novice pediatric physical therapists. Pediatr Phys Ther 8:70, 1996.

53. Carter RE: A behavioral analysis of interactions between physical therapists and children with

cerebral palsy during treatment. Unpublished doctoral dissertation. Northern Illinois University, DeKalb, Ill, 1989.

54. Campbell SK: Therapy programs for children that last a lifetime. Phys Occup Ther Pediatr 17(1):1, 1997.
55. Lollar DJ (ed): Preventing Secondary Conditions Associated with Spina Bifida or Cerebral Palsy. Spina Bifida Association of American, Washington, DC, 1994.
56. Butler C: Augmentative mobility: Why do it? Phys Med Rehab Clin North Am 2:801, 1991.
57. Rapport MJK: Laws that shape therapy services in educational environments. Phys Occup Ther Pediatr. 15(2):5, 1995.
58. Giangreco MF: Related services decision-making: A foundational component of effective education for students with disabilities. Phys Occup Ther Pediatr. 15(2):47, 1995.
59. Bower E, McLellan DL: Effect of increased exposure to physiotherapy on skill acquisition of children with cerebral palsy. Dev Med Child Neurol 34:25, 1992.
60. Embrey DG, Yates L: Clinical applications of self-monitoring by experienced and novice pediatric physical therapists. Pediatr Phys Ther 8:156, 1996.
61. Giangreco MF, Cloninger CJ, Iverson V: Choosing Options and Accommodations for Children: A Guide to Planning Inclusive Education. Paul H Brookes, Baltimore, 1993.
62. Bundy AC: Assessment and intervention in school-based practice: Answering questions and minimizing discrepancies. Phys Occup Ther Pediatr. 15(2):69, 1995.
63. Jewell MW, Roush SE: Students' perceptions of their school-based physical therapy. Pediatr Phys Ther 7:161, 1995.
64. Managed care standards and criteria for children with special health care needs. Except Parent August:74, 1996.
65. Pearson SD, Goulart-Fisher D, Lee TH: Critical pathways as a strategy for improving care: Problems and potential. Ann Intern Med 123:941, 1995.
66. Ignatavicius DD, Hausman KA: Use of clinical pathways in a variety of health care settings. *In* Clinical Pathways for Collaborative Practice. WB Saunders, Philadelphia, 1995, p 34.

Cerebral Palsy

J a n e t M. W i l s o n H o w l e, MACT, PT

Physical therapists who are responsible for planning programs and treating children with cerebral palsy (CP) are faced with overwhelming decisions regarding the quality of care and the quality of life for these children and their families. Changes in managed health care and health care funding have added to the complexity of these decisions. In order to make the most appropriate decisions based on research, experience, and clinical knowledge, therapists must develop their knowledge of the following key concepts that contribute to a problem-specific, comprehensive, cohesive clinical practice:

1. *Define the problem.* What is CP? How early can this diagnosis be made? Can CP be described in a way that immediately brings to mind a clinical picture of the child? Does the description have predictive value? How does CP change over a lifetime?
2. *Develop a theoretic framework for understanding motor control.* How does normal movement occur? How is it controlled? How does it develop? How does movement in a child with CP differ from movement in normally developing children? What are the constraints on movement in a child with CP? What aspects of movement can be changed with intervention?
3. *Develop a disability model that can be used to direct and prioritize the examination process, treatment goals, and strategies.* Is it possible to define a model that precisely describes the fundamental movement problems of a child with CP and is flexible enough to account for the changes over a lifetime?
4. *Organize an examination and treatment approach that is logical and consistent with both the theoretic elements and the research evidence but also meets the practical needs of the family and the child.* Do the problems that are assessed derive directly from the problems and concerns identified by the family and the needs of the child? Do the problems outlined in the process of examination lead directly to the treatment goals? Do treatment goals specify treatment strategies? Is it possible to measure successful outcomes of the treatment? Can treatment address lifelong problems?

This chapter leads the reader through these essential components and provides guidelines on both theoretic and practical processes for successful decision making in managing the child with CP.

DEFINING THE PROBLEM

What Is Cerebral Palsy?

Cerebral palsy is the term most commonly used to describe children with disorders of posture and movement that are usually evident in early infancy. CP itself is not a diagnosis, but rather the description of the clinical sequelae resulting from a nonprogressive encephalopathy in an immature brain whose cause may be pre-, peri-, or postnatal.[1] CP is characterized by impairments of the neuromuscular, musculoskeletal, and sensory systems that are either the immediate result of the existing pathophysiology or are indirect consequences developed to compensate for the underlying abnormality. The signs often appear to be progressive because the abnormality affects a changing organism in which a developing, albeit abnormal, central nervous system (CNS) attempts to interact with and influence other maturing systems. The expression of the impairments and the resultant disabilities and handicaps change throughout the life cycle as the child grows, develops, and compensates for underlying abnormalities.[2] At the same time, the environment and the people in it place changing demands on the child, requiring increasingly complex movement strategies in order to participate in tasks that are specific to the demands of the environment.

Although the hallmark of CP is impaired posture and movement, CP is often complicated by mental retardation or learning disabilities (50 to 75 percent), speech and language disorders (65 percent), auditory impairments (25 percent), seizure disorders (25 to 35 percent), and visual disorders (25 percent).[3, 4] Sociopsychologic and family problems often occur secondary to the presence of the primary problems.[3]

CP is the second most common neuroimpairment in childhood, after mental retardation. The causes of CP have been changing over time, although the overall incidence has remained much the same.[5-7] A figure of 2 per 1000 births represents the average of data in industrialized countries.[8, 9] Understandably, CP is more common in underdeveloped countries with low levels of pre- and postnatal care and high levels of nutritional deficiency.[10, 11] The prevalence of CP has not declined despite improvements in obstetric and perinatal care. This may be due to an increasing incidence of CP in preterm infants as a result of the increased survival rate of very preterm babies.[12-16]

Accurate diagnosis of CP at a young age is important for economic, social, emotional, and medical reasons. Although very low birth weight and preterm infants have an increased risk of CP, even the most sensitive neonatal screening does not identify all infants who develop neuromotor dysfunction. The problem is development itself. Similar insults to the developing brain of the fetus or newborn can produce strikingly different problems depending on the structure and physiology of the brain at the time of insult. In addition, developmental changes of the brain can lead to recovery from dysfunction, whereas ongoing maturation can disclose sensorimotor dysfunction that is not recognized until the infant develops movement against the force of gravity.[17-20] Many neonatal assessments have been developed to provide earlier predictors to accurately identify infants who are at the greatest risk for developing CP.[20-22] Most recently, Prechtl and coworkers have developed a promising assessment technique based on the examination of the quality of spontaneous movement.[19, 23, 24] Many investigators have related delayed motor milestones at 4 months combined with a history of premature birth or other medical complications as predictors of CP.[25-30] Except for very mild cases, most cases of CP can be identified by 6 months of age through the use of repeated developmental examinations, a combination of tests, careful medical and developmental history, and listening attentively to the ongoing concerns of the parents. The earlier the diagnosis is made, the sooner the family can begin the process of coping, adapting, and accessing support systems and resources for intervention.[31]

Classification

Classification of CP by clinical types and the topographic distribution of movement impairment was adopted by the American Academy for Cerebral Palsy (now the American Academy for Cerebral Palsy and Developmental Medicine) and remains the most widely used descriptive system of classification.[32] This system relies heavily on clinical judgment and clinical experience but is useful to physicians, parents, and physical therapists because it provides a "diagnostic label" based on the topographic distribution and type of movement impairment.

Types of Impairment

Children are divided by the type of impairment into the categories spasticity, dyskinesia, ataxia, and hypotonia.

Spasticity is characterized by muscles that are perceived as stiff in which velocity-dependent resistance to passive movement produces increased muscle tone; selective control is limited, producing abnormal and limited movement synergies; the active range of motion (ROM) is limited by coactivation of muscular activity; and the timing of muscle activation and postural responses is abnormal.[33, 34] Spastic CP is the most common type of CP. Spastic diplegia is the most common type of spastic CP.[8, 35–38] Combined with spastic hemiplegia and quadriplegia this group makes up 75 percent of all children with CP. Spastic CP results from insult to the motor cortex or white matter projections to and from cortical sensorimotor areas of the brain; however, in all cases of CP a correlation between clinical findings and neuroanatomy is possible only to a limited degree.

Dyskinesia is a group of disorders in which movements are perceived to be uncontrolled and purposeless. This group includes athetosis, rigidity, and tremor. Athetosis is the most common of the dyskinesias and accounts for 20 percent of all cases of CP. Athetosis always involves involuntary movement; movements that are poorly executed in timing, direction, and spatial characteristics; impairment of postural stability and abnormal coactivation of muscles that produces abnormal timing and coordination in reversal of motion, as well as increased latency of onset of movement; and oral-motor dysfunction involving feeding and speech production. These problems may or may not be accompanied by abnormal muscle tone, primarily hypotonia in infancy, and asymmetric postural alignment.[39–43] Rigidity is much less common than athetosis, and, as with spasticity, movement is impeded. There is, however, continued resistance to movement throughout the ROM in both the agonists and antagonists, and this phenomenon is not velocity dependent. This type of hypertonicity is often called "lead pipe" rigidity because the tone is increased throughout the range during repeated flexion and extension of an extremity.[7] Tremor is rarely seen as an isolated type of CP. Dyskinesia is associated with impairment of the basal ganglia, their connections to the prefrontal and premotor cortex, and their role in the selective activation or suppression of complex movement sequences.[44–47]

Ataxia is primarily a disorder of balance and control in the timing of coordinated movement. Ataxia represents less than 10 percent of cases of CP. Ataxia results from deficits in the cerebellum. The specific symptoms relate to the area of the cerebellum that is affected. The primary characteristic of ataxic CP is impaired postural control. This includes impairments in postural alignment, impaired anticipatory postural adjustments during movement, and abnormal postural stability. In addition, there is usually hypotonia, impaired force and power production during voluntary movement, and impaired motor planning affecting sequencing for speech (dysarthria) and the rhythm and orderly progression for reciprocal gross (dysmetria and ataxia) and fine movements (dysdiadochokinesia). Because the cerebellum's inputs and outputs connect with the motor cortex and the brainstem, ataxia is often seen in combination with spasticity and athetosis.[45–47]

Hypotonia is characterized by diminished resting muscle tension, a decreased ability to generate voluntary muscle force, excessive joint flexibility, and postural instability. It is often seen as a transient stage in the evolution of athetosis or spasticity. Hypotonia has not been related to a particular neural lesion.[48]

Topographic Distribution

A second part of the descriptive classification of CP includes the topographic distribution of abnormal tone, posture, or movement and includes *diplegia,* involving the lower body and legs to a greater degree than the arms; *hemiplegia,* involving the arm and leg and one side of the body; and *quadriplegia,* involving the entire body, with equal or greater involvement of the arms and upper body. The term *double hemiplegia* is sometimes used to indicate a type of quadriplegia in which the arm and leg on one side are significantly more impaired than those on the other side. The designations *mild, moderate,* and *severe* are often applied within types to further define the motor disability. These terms are often poorly defined and based on the individual examiner's experience. Although other investigators have related severity ratings to functional abilities in attempts to better define the motor problems of children with CP,[36, 49, 50] the disability model developed by the U.S. National Center for Medical Rehabilitation Research, described in Chapter 1, can serve as a functional framework to describe the child's current abilities and limitations in gross motor function in a four-level classification of severity:

1. *Mild.* This term is used for children who have sensorimotor impairments that lead to poorly coordinated and inefficient movement when compared with normal peers, but whose functional limitations are found only in those most advanced gross motor skills used in daily life at the child's present age level. These children do not require special assistance or equipment but may require extra time to carry out age-appropriate skills such as crossing the street, dressing, grooming, eating, or writing.

2. *Moderate.* This term is used for children who have sensorimotor impairments that produce functional limitations in whole-body functions, such as walking, sitting, changing postures, hand use, and speech. They are unable to attain motor milestones within normal age limits. With modifications in the time needed to perform a task; their environment; or equipment, or when given physical assistance, they can participate in most age-appropriate activities.

3. *Severe.* This term is used for children whose disability restricts them from performing activities necessary to fulfill normal life roles, such as managing doors for school and other public buildings, using school and public restrooms, climbing onto school buses or using public transportation, or carrying a cafeteria tray, bookbag, or briefcase because of dependence on assistive devices for mobility. These children are unable to be independent in daily living skills because of a lack of balance or an inability to use their arms and hands for skilled movement, or both. They are unable to participate in play or family activities independent from an adult because of deficiencies in the ability to communicate. The quality of life of both the children and their families may be seriously affected.

4. *Profound.* This term is used for children who have no useful or purposeful motor ability and therefore are prevented from having access to their community and society. These children cannot perform even the most basic motor functions, such as changing their position, sitting independent from special equipment, using their arms and hands for feeding or self-care, or using speech for communication. They are unable to function independent of a caregiver. They are dependent on technology, mobility aids, and special equipment for all daily activities. Health issues are serious complications.

Adding these definitions to the terms *mild, moderate, severe,* and *profound* should enhance communication among professionals and families as they clarify the child's functional abilities and limitations and assist the family in setting realistic expectations for themselves and their child.

Evaluating Classification Systems

The system of classification adopted by the Academy for Cerebral Palsy is well recognized, but it is limited in two aspects. First, it does not take into account changes that occur during the development of the child with CP. For this reason, it is possible for an infant to be described as having mild, hypotonic CP, and at 1 year of age, as the child begins to crawl and sit, to be described as having moderate spastic diplegia, whereas at 4 years of age, as the child pulls to stand, attempts to walk, manipulates toys, and struggles with self-care, the child may be described as having severe spastic quadriplegia. None of these descriptions are wrong. This child actually presented quite differently at various developmental stages and chronologic ages, and within the demands of various environments. The changing "diagnosis," however, may lead to confusion and mistrust between the parents and the professional expert and a lack of credibility in the perception of some professionals on the part of other professionals.

The second problem in classifying CP according to clinical types is the inability to provide clues for a reliable prognosis. Because the value of early intervention has not been clearly established, the accurate identification of the prognosis is essential to evaluate the independent effects of treatment and maturation and to provide realistic expectations for the family. Palisano and colleagues have attempted to address this issue with a new system of classification based on the concepts of disability and functional limitation.[51] The Gross Motor Function Classification System describes self-initiated movement with particular emphasis on sitting and walking. The authors use a five-level classification system with clinically meaningful distinctions in motor function among levels. Level 1, the highest level, represents one end of this continuum of children with mild neuromotor impairments—those whose functional limitations are less than those typically associated with CP—whereas level 5, at the other end of the continuum, represents children who lack the most basic antigravity postural control. This classification system based on abilities and limitations in gross motor function was designed to assist in determining a child's needs, making management decisions, and describing the development of children with CP. If the system is found to have predictive validity, it would prove helpful in providing information for the reliable prognosis of functional gross motor outcomes.

DEVELOPING A THEORETIC FRAMEWORK

The next step in making appropriate clinical decisions is describing a theoretic framework for motor control. Physical therapists who can define the problems and needs of the patient based on a theoretic framework for motor control are better able to develop consistent strategies for assessing and planning treatment sequences, both within a single treatment session and over time. All clinicians base their examination and treatment on assumptions about motor development and motor control, whether they articulate it well or not. Theory guides most of our decision making and biases our examination, treatment, and evaluation of outcomes. It shows in what the therapists select to assess and how they examine it. Theory guides the therapist during treatment. Keshner describes how various theories have influenced physical therapy.[52] The theoretic models therapists use to design their treatment approaches are based on clinical experience, developmental and clinical studies, and scientific understanding. Horak describes the various motor control models currently used in neurologic rehabilitation.[53] This chapter describes examination and treatment based on nine assumptions about normal and abnormal motor development and control. These assumptions borrow heavily from dynamic systems theory described for the clinician by Horak, Shumway-Cook and Woollacott, Heriza, and Thelen and colleagues.[47, 53–55] My clinical experience and understanding of movement, however, influenced the formulation of these assumptions.

The Nine Assumptions About Normal and Abnormal Motor Development and Control

Assumption 1. Movement is organized around behavioral goals.

The same movement may occur for a variety of reasons. For example, a 10-month-old baby rolls to her side in the process of sitting up. A 7-year-old child rolls to his side when getting out of bed to get ready for school. A 35-year-old man rolls to his side to make love to his wife. An 80-year-old woman rolls to her side to relieve a painful shoulder. Goals must be meaningful both in real time and in developmental time. In fact, movement patterns drop out of the individual's repertoire if there is no longer a reason for the pattern to exist. Other patterns are reinforced if the purpose of the movement becomes more and more generalized in usage over time. For example, I have not had any reason to do a cartwheel since I was 14 years old and briefly had the desire to become a professional clown, yet I have become more efficient and skilled at rapid finger movements as I have learned to play the piano, type on my computer word processor, and communicate in sign language.

The same goal can produce quite different movements. For example, the goal to walk independently produces different movements in an 11-month-old baby who is taking his first steps, in a 2½-year-old who slips his mother's grip and runs through the aisle of the grocery store, and in a 72-year-old woman who cautiously discards her walker after hip surgery.

Movement may be self-directed or goal-directed, or both. Infants often engage in movement that appears to be purposeless when viewed by an adult. This is particularly true of newly learned movement in which the child engages in the movement over and over "for no apparent reason." Adults usually refer to this as play or practice; however, these activities are functional behaviors representing important components of motor learning and motor development.[56, 57] These self-directed movements of infants and young children should be viewed as meaningful to the child within the child's stage of development even when the movement cannot be identified by an adult as purposeful or goal-directed. This concept is particularly important when observing movement in infants and children with neuromotor disabilities because they often need more practice time to incorporate self-directed movements into goal-directed activities. On the other hand, a child who is allowed to perseverate in using one particular movement pattern may exclude the use of other patterns of movement, thereby limiting functional variability. For example, many children practice trunk extension in the supine position, arching backward while retracting the shoulder girdle and extending the hips and knees. Some children with CP begin to scoot on the floor using this pattern. If this is practiced *to the exclusion* of creeping and crawling, patterns that incorporate weight shifting, precise timing of reciprocal movement, and interlimb coordination, the child will not practice these components, which are correlated with the achievement of walking.

The purpose of a movement may not be obvious to an observer and may not represent a conscious decision on the individual's part. For example, as a child is lifted out of the bathtub by a caring father's arms, he struggles, wiggling, and finally cries. The movement appears to indicate personal displeasure or even being uncooperative. In actuality, the father's watchband scratched the child's side, causing unexpected, sudden pain. The purpose of the movement was simply to get away from a painful stimulus. In another scenario, a child with athetoid CP who does not reach out and pick up her spoon when presented with a favorite food may have the goal of maintaining a sitting posture as a higher priority than reaching, even when she would like to get the spoon.

Assumption 2. Movement emerges as an interaction among different systems or subsystems, each contributing different aspects of control.

In motor planning, multiple systems are organized according to the inherent requirements of the task being performed and the current status (postural, motivational, emotional, cognitive, and so forth) of the actor. The CNS is seen as a necessary but not sufficient component to explain movement changes.

The control of movement includes neurologic systems for comparing, commanding, and recording motor control as well as respiratory-cardiac, autonomic, biomechanical, musculoskeletal, sensoriperceptive, cognitive, and psychologic systems within the individual and all the subsystems within these systems. The importance of each subsystem changes continuously both before and during a movement as determined by the goal of the movement, the strategy that the individual uses to accomplish the goal, and the social environment in which the movement takes place.

Assumption 3. The organization of the various elements of control of movement is determined by the specific elements of the movement, prioritizing and resolving conflicts within the control systems and the environment in which the movement takes place.

The nervous system must adapt to and predict constraints placed on movement by the physical laws associated with the musculoskeletal system and its environment, such as the reactive forces created by the contracting muscles or unpredictable events in the environment.

For example, if a child reaches out for a toy that has been placed within the child's sitting base of support, such as between the thighs, there is less demand for balance and postural control than if the same toy is placed outside the base of sitting stability, when balance must be maintained as the center of mass is shifted outside the base of support during reaching. In both situations the child reaches for the toy. The limit of reaching is governed by the length of the child's arm; the extensibility of joint ligaments; muscle strength in the trunk muscles; postural adaptations to disequilibrium; motivation to get the toy; and the placement of the toy in the environment. In the second situation, the demands on postural control and balance are much greater than in the first situation—so much so that a 7-month-old child can get the toy if it is placed between the legs but is unable to get the toy if it is placed just a short distance away to one side (or the child who tries may fall).

Assumption 4. The environment presents a powerful incentive or disincentive for movement.

A great deal of change in movement can occur simply by manipulating the environment. I continue to be amazed at how much movement, and what quality of movement, occurs when children are comfortable and secure in their environment. If, on the other hand, the children feel a threat to their balance or posture from the environment, such as being required to sit on a chair in which the seat depth is greater than their thigh length so that their feet do not touch the floor, functional movements of the arms and manipulation skills of the hands decrease.[58, 59] Physical therapists often do not take full advantage of the environment. The use of assistive technology is one approach to using the environment to facilitate function. Adapted seating and mobility aids have long been considered an important *adjunct* to therapy, a method to increase carryover of therapy goals into the home and classroom setting. More recently, assistive devices have been considered "enabling technology," which can actually generate new opportunities for movement and function.[60] Children who are moderately involved show immediate changes in posture and gait characteristics when using posterior walkers.[61–63] Children with severe or profound CP often spend most of their waking hours in special chairs or in other equipment that may have a stronger influence on their posture and movement than the few hours of direct therapy they receive weekly. The environment can be used to promote changes in motor control rather than producing changes by physically manipulating the child. For example, in the section Organizing Treatment and Management, which illustrates treatment, Stephanie is shown to have little disassociated movement of the lower extremities and has incomplete hip extension in standing. However, when she is motivated to "climb on the fire truck to be the fire chief," she shows excellent hip extension on the right side with hip and knee flexion of the left leg (along with weight bearing through the right arm and trunk rotation) to climb over the straddle seat and seat herself (see Fig. 2–2F–H). The environment must be structured, prepared, and controlled to promote changes in motor control when a child is engaged in self-directed activities. It requires a great deal of awareness and skill on the therapist's part to ensure that the child remains motivated, succeeds in the activity, and is meeting specific movement goals.

Assumption 5. Strategies for moving emerge from interactions between the individual and the environment to accomplish the functional task.

Individuals solve motor problems with different strategies depending on both their inherent physical makeup and the environment. Left-handed people orient to their environment differently than right-handed people. Tall people fit into and perceive their environment differently than short people. A small child might have to stand on tiptoe and stretch an arm up overhead to reach a tabletop to get a glass of juice, whereas a 6-foot 4-inch teenager would have to bend over and reach down. If the juice is in a paper sip-box rather than a glass, the grasping strategy must be different. The strategies individuals use must take into account their unique personal characteristics and the regulatory features of the task. A strategy used at one time in life may not work at another time. New strategies must be constantly explored as the individual changes in ways that may seem only remotely connected to motor control.

Assumption 6. Movement is linked to sensory input in two distinct ways.

First, sensory feedback or closed-loop control is required for learning movement. Tactile, proprioceptive, and visual input are necessary for learning complex, discrete movements that require accuracy. This is probably why a child moves more slowly when trying out new movements. Second, sensory feedforward or open-loop control is used for rapid well-learned automatic movements.[64] This concept has been a guiding principle in physical therapy for children for many years.[65, 66] Physical therapists facilitate or inhibit movement through carefully directed manual tactile and proprioceptive input, but once the movement becomes part of the child's functional repertoire, the therapist allows the child to produce and practice the movement with only verbal cues or with no dependency on sensory inputs from the therapist.

Assumption 7. Under conditions of optimal neuromotor control and environmental conditions, the emergent motor behavior is efficient, energy saving, and effective.

Massery describes how interactions between the mutual musculoskeletal components for breathing and transitional movement of the trunk normally work in harmony to produce efficient movements.[67] On the other hand, breath holding requires the trunk muscles to work in isometric patterns, inhibits the dynamic patterns needed for the transition from one position to another, and sets up conflicting responses in the muscles of the trunk that lead to inefficient, energy-expending, stiff movements. It is generally accepted that children with disabilities use more energy while walking than able-bodied children.[68, 69] Programs that involve muscle strengthening and fitness have been introduced for children with spastic CP to determine if conditions can be changed to increase the efficiency of movement as measured by the performance of daily activities.[70]

Assumption 8. Practice or repeated opportunities for movement to occur in a task-specific context increase the efficiency, stability, and flexibility of performance.

Efficiency of movement occurs when multiple neurons, muscles, joints, and bones of the body are constrained to act together in a self-organizing manner to accomplish a task.[64] The more often a coordinated pattern occurs in a given situation, the greater the stability of that pattern in performance while at the same time strengthening the flexibility of the coordinative pattern to adjust to a variety of environmental demands.

As I sit at my keyboard, I can't help but be aware of my typing speed and accuracy. I am driven by deadlines (task specific) and the need for revisions (practice). My speed and efficiency have increased dramatically in the past few months. Although the coordination of my pattern for striking the correct keys has improved, so has my flexibility to type under different circumstances, with background noise, in various sitting postures, and with interruptions. I no longer have to wait until everything is "just right" to get at this project. Vulpe discusses the problems of transference of skills from one environment to another in children with disabilities.[71] The inability of children with CP to adapt to various environments and work under different circumstances is one of the frustrations all therapists experience when facilitating the generalization of treatment-specific functions to use as daily living skills.

Assumption 9. Normal motor milestones, common to all children, emerge from the ability of various sensory, neural, and musculoskeletal subsystems to organize themselves according to each system's individual maturation, development, and continuous interactions yet are limited by the basic intrinsic characteristics of each system in the developing human.

The neural structures, including neural pathways, are well described for some motor behaviors, but in other situations there does not seem to be a correlation between the motor behavior and any particular neural structure. Many of the same behaviors exist in both prematurely born and full-term infants, modified by the effects of gravity and shaped by a variety of subsystems, including the specific body size and configuration of the infant.[72, 73] This suggests that certain movement patterns are preferred (but not obligatory) by most infants because they are adaptable within environmental demands. This assumption accounts for the general "sameness" of motor milestones, general timing, and progression of skills among children but also accounts for the individual differences that define the personal signature of the individual child.

Considering the Advantages

The advantage of these assumptions in a contemporary model of motor control is that they account for the flexibility and adaptability of motor behavior in a variety of environmental conditions. Such a theoretic framework allows the clinician enormous flexibility in choosing treatment methods because movement can be influenced by manipulating the child, the task, or the environment. This model does require therapists to be clear about the functional goals and to make certain that demands on the various systems of control are compatible and appropriate for accomplishing the task in both real time and developmental time. One word of caution: Although systems models are appealing, the information in support of this theoretic approach has *not* been gained by research with children with neuromotor disabilities. It would be inappropriate to expect that children with sensorimotor impairments can gain normal motor skills simply by setting the goal, manipulating the environment, and waiting for optimal movement to occur. Many unanswered questions remain, both about movement in normally developing children and about movement in children with CP. We can use this current thinking to add to our understanding of how movement occurs, how it is controlled, and how it develops, and to add new concepts to existing clinical practice. In this way, we can broaden our approach to the examination and treatment of patients and merge theories of clinical practice with theories of motor control.

MODELING THE EXAMINATION PROCESS

In the United States, interdisciplinary, multidisciplinary, or transdisciplinary team approaches are the current standard of practice for the assessment of CP. The individual personnel and the professions they represent may vary depending on the child's age, developmental level, and degree of involvement, the physical setting, and the system of service delivery. The physical therapy examination must fit within this context and provide a systematic method for decision making that addresses the evaluation of examination results and treatment planning. In this chapter, the theoretic framework used to describe the process is the Hypothesis-Oriented Algorithm for Clinicians (HOAC) model that is described in Chapter 1.[74]

Data Collection

The first part of the examination consists of the initial data collection. This should include a review of medical records, any previous assessments and treatment plans, and educational records, as well as interviews with the family regarding their questions and reasons for seeking physical therapy services. The information obtained in this stage includes the following:

- *Medical history.* This includes a prenatal history and problems in pregnancy, such as premature birth; a perinatal history, including medical complications at birth, multiple births, anoxia, and birth trauma; the postnatal course, including the length of the hospital stay, seizures, feeding problems, irritability, and a lack of or inappropriate responsiveness.
- *Developmental history.* This includes milestones for locomotion, sitting and standing, language and speech, self-help skills, and hand use, as well as the current developmental status.
- *Basic senses and functions.* This includes information on vision and hearing; behavioral and physiologic characteristics including orientation and attention to tasks, learning style and preferences, adaptability to personal and environmental demands, motivation and cooperation, temperament and emotional stability, and energy levels and endurance.
- *Family and environmental characteristics.* This includes the size of the family and household; the stability of the family environment; cultural standards; the family's understanding of the disability and expectations for change or improvement; and internal and external resources including financial, emotional, and intellectual supports.

The initial data collection provides the physical therapist with information about the child's current developmental level and rate of development, and the impact of any limitations on other areas of performance, as well as the context and relationships that will shape the child's development.

Statement of the Problem

The second part of the assessment involves generating a problem statement to guide the selection of goals. This should reflect the family's reasons for seeking help. When a child with CP is referred to a physical therapist at 3 or 4 years of age, this is generally not a difficult problem. The family is familiar with the diagnosis of CP and is usually able to be clear in describing their reasons for seeking help. When a child is referred at 3 or 4 months of age, however, with no clearly described problem or prognostic indicator but only a history of prematurity and a periventricular hemorrhage, and the family does not even know what to expect of any infant at that age, the problem becomes much more difficult. There are situations in which a family does not have enough information to fully participate as an advocate for the child; however, the initial collaboration between the family and the therapist in developing a problem statement begins a pattern of establishing the importance of the family's opinions and concerns as part of ongoing interactions between the family and professionals. The collaboration between professionals and the family is mandated in the United States by the Education of the Handicapped Act of 1968 (Public Law 99-457) and the Individuals with Disabilities Education Act of 1991 (Public Law 102-119), but, more importantly, the trust and credibility between the family and the therapist sets into motion patterns of thought and behavior that will last for years.

Selection of Goals

The third part of the assessment is the selection of goals that are measurable and functional and that include a time frame for achievement. Although this aspect of the HOAC model may seem the most foreign to pediatric physical therapists who are more comfortable with examination of the patient as the next step, it is really the next mental step most therapists currently take. Even before a new patient is even seen, the therapist should review in his or her mind the problems that have been either described in the medical and educational reports or included in the family's comments and decide what the goal or goals of therapy will be if it is initiated. For example, a child who walks on his toes on the left foot and holds his left arm with the elbow flexed and the hand fisted is referred with a diagnosis of spastic hemiplegia. Before examining the child, the therapist plans to change his ambulation so that the child no longer walks on his toes when walking at a normal speed and uses an arm swing when he walks. The HOAC model requires two new ways of thinking: First, this model requires the therapist to set goals (which are certainly modifiable and tentative), stated in behavioral terms, indicating what the child and, in many cases with very young children, the parents and the therapist hope to achieve. The goal is stated in terms of the patient's outcome so that the expected purpose of physical therapy is clear to everyone—the family, the child, the physician, and third party payers. Second, a time frame is defined so that everyone knows when it is reasonable to expect the accomplishment of the goal and either discharge the child or move to other goals now that this goal is completed. If the goal has not been met, the decision-making process proceeds to evaluation—Why? This leads to a change of treatment strategy or tactics if the goal still seems reasonable. This process keeps the physical therapist focused on understanding the child's and the family's expectations and on helping them to be realistic yet optimistic in expecting changes in the child.

Examining the Child

Functional Skills

The next step is examination of the child, which begins with assessment of the child's functional skills and any limitations in those skills. The physical therapist may select either norm- or criterion-referenced tests to assess the motor functions in an infant or child with CP. A norm-referenced test is one in which a child's performance is compared with the performance of other children the same age, using a standard format. The following are examples of standardized tests commonly used with infants and children with motor problems:

- Alberta Infant Motor Scale (AIMS)
- Gross Motor Function Measure (GMFM)
- Pediatric Evaluation of Disability Inventory (PEDI)

The AIMS assesses the motor development and postural control of infants from birth to 18 months.[21] It is a performance-based, norm-referenced, observational tool for the motor assessment of the developing infant and can be used to diagnose developmental delay in order to document the need for therapy. The 58 items incorporate the components of motor development that are deemed essential for the identification and treatment of at-risk infants. A graph is provided to plot the infant's total AIMS score. From this graph, the examiner can determine the percentile ranking of the infant's motor performance compared with the normative sample of same-age infants. Because items on the AIMS cannot be passed if performed with an abnormal quality of movement, the AIMS cannot be used to record developmental progress of infants with CP but is useful to identify them as having delayed gross motor development.

The GMFM is a standardized criterion-referenced instrument designed and validated to measure changes in gross motor function over time in children with CP.[75, 76] It cannot be used for the diagnosis of motor delay because it has not been normed. The GMFM measures motor skills in five dimensions regardless of the quality of motor performance: lying and rolling; sitting; crawling and kneeling; standing and walking; and running and jumping. Skills cover the age range from birth to about 5 years in normally developing children. Within each dimension, activities sensitive to the special problems of children with CP, such as difficulty with trunk rotation, have been included. Because this test was designed to measure change, a total score, which can be expressed as a percentage score across all dimensions as well as a percentage score for each dimension, can be calculated. Those dimensions targeted as "goal areas" for an individual child, that is, areas in which change is expected as a result of intervention, can be reassessed for the percentage achieved as a way to rate progress based on the goals for the individual child.[77] It is possible to test with aids or orthoses in use when this is appropriate.

The PEDI is a functional assessment for the evaluation of disabled or chronically ill children ranging in age from 6 months to 7 years (or whose development falls into this range if older).[78] It can be administered through a parent interview. A series of reliability and validity studies have been completed by various investigators.[78–81] The PEDI measures functional status and functional change in three areas: a self-care domain, which contains items related to feeding, grooming, dressing, and toileting; a mobility domain, which contains items related to car, chair, tub, and toilet transfers and to indoor and outdoor locomotion and stairs; and a social function domain, which contains items related to comprehension and speech, peer interactions, and home and community functions. Separate scales assess the assistance needed from persons or equipment. This test can be scored in two ways. Normative standard scores allow the child to be compared with an age-matched peer group, whereas scaled scores provide data comparing the child's performance with a total possible score of 100. The latter is a criterion-referenced score representing the degree to which the child has accomplished all skills appropriate for a 7-year-old child. This scoring allows retesting to show improvement in the various areas of development over time and is particularly valuable for children with severe handicaps and slow development who simply fall further behind when compared with their age-mates across time. In summary, the PEDI can be used both for the diagnosis of functional limitations in self-care, mobility, and social functions (normed-referenced scores) and for assessing progress in therapy (scaled scores).

Several other criterion-referenced tests can also be used when assessing motor function in children with CP. These tests compare a child's performance to a predetermined behavioral criterion and report the child's performance in terms of what the child can do. Although criterion-referenced tests are not normed, they do provide a way to track a child's progress over time. The primary usefulness of these tests is in the planning of developmental intervention programs and evaluating functional skills the child does or does not have at any point in time.[82]

Two commonly used tests of this type are the Vulpe Assessment Battery (VAB)[71] and the Carolina Curriculum for Handicapped Infants at Risk[83] and its companion for older children, the Carolina Curriculum for Preschoolers with Special Needs.[84] The VAB comprises items that attempt to cover comprehensively essential areas of child development from birth through 6 years of age.[71] The VAB assesses basic senses and functions, gross motor behaviors, fine motor behaviors, activities of daily living, and speech and language comprehension. This examination is comprehensive and is not a screening tool. It is not necessary for the entire battery to be administered at any one time, and it is possible for several different therapists (physical, occupational, and speech) to give the appropriate parts of the test. The test is achievement-oriented so that the child can succeed. Scoring of the child's performance considers the teaching technique used and the child's learning style; therefore, it is possible to use the VAB for examination and for programming. One of the unique characteristics of this assessment is the scale that rates the children's performance based on their independence from assistance, either physical, verbal, or environmental. This rating scale makes it possible to show progress within a developmental level, that is, how independent of assistance a child becomes, even when the child is not gaining new skills or changing developmental levels.

The Carolina Curriculum for Handicapped Infants[83] and for Preschoolers with Special Needs[84] was developed to provide appropriate intervention strategies for children with developmental delays. An assessment log accompanies the curriculum and includes items in the areas of gross and fine motor skills; activities of daily living; speech and language; social interactions; and personal development. The items are based on normal sequences of development that appear on most norm-referenced tests. The items in each domain are subdivided into logical teaching sequences based on how one skill builds on another. Modifications of items are suggested in order to accommodate the child's particular sensorimotor limitations. The examination leads directly to curriculum planning and the development of intervention.

Both these tests as well as many others provide therapists with a way to collect and record information about a child's functional skills and limitations in a systematic and objective manner. This information serves as a baseline measure of function at a given time and as an aid to evaluating the functional change resulting from applying a specific intervention over a specific period of time. When functional limitations have been identified, the therapist must then identify impairments that act as constraints on function and contribute to the development of functional limitations or disabilities.

Examination of Neuromuscular Impairments

The neuromuscular impairments that contribute to functional limitations in CP are described earlier in this chapter. The examination of these areas is discussed here as it relates to understanding functional limitations and treatment planning. The neuromuscular impairments encompass a diverse group of problems that represent a major constraint on the control of movement and posture. This information, no matter how it is organized, describes how a child moves. This section of the examination makes it possible to anticipate how a child's existing control of posture and movement will influence, either positively or negatively, the child's continued development. Generally this information is gathered as a child moves spontaneously during an examination. The child should be encouraged, through play, to assume as many postures and transitions requiring resistance to the force of gravity and control of the center of mass during dynamic movement as possible. Given a comfortable situation and adequate time, children will do what they can do. It is possible to gain a representative sample of a child's motor behavior only if the child is cooperative and unthreatened. The examiner should question the parent as to whether observations represent typical behavior.

Alignment and Patterns of Weight Bearing

Abnormalities in alignment are the first clues to abnormalities in motor control. *Alignment of the body* refers to the arrangement of body segments with respect to one another, as well as the position of the body with reference to the force of gravity and the base of support. *Weight bearing* refers to the distribution of the body weight at rest and in anticipation of movement. Normal alignment is so fundamental to human behavior that any deviation from it is easily recognized. Before feeling a child's stiffness or observing any movement, it is possible to anticipate problems in movement strategies by observing abnormalities in alignment.[47] The focus in this section of the examination is on the repetition across activities and postures of abnormal or normal components of postural alignment, rather than positions, because concern for specific consistently observed patterns is descriptive of current typical movement strategies and predictive of future development and the potential for orthopedic problems.

Abnormalities in alignment should be observed both when the child is comfortably at rest and while alert and attentive to the environment. The process of alerting changes the alignment because the entire body "alerts" as the child anticipates movement. An absence of this characteristic is often noted in children with CP. They do not show changes in body alignment (or muscle tone) with alertness, which can be misinterpreted as a lack of interest in a new stimulus in the environment.

This section of the examination also includes description of the patterns of weight bearing, noting how the child shifts and bears weight in anticipation of movement in each position. Anticipatory postural adjustments in typically developing children take place in advance of potentially destabilizing voluntary movements and are small weight shifts in the direction opposite the anticipated voluntary movement that ensure that stability of the center of mass is maintained throughout the entire movement sequence, and the appropriate body segments are unweighted and free to move. The inability to activate postural muscles in anticipation of voluntary movements has been described in children with CP.[47, 85] Symmetry or asymmetry in weight bearing is noted because persistent asymmetric weight bearing to one side limits the movement of that side and can contribute to the development of structural deformities. In addition, the therapist must note the child's ability to adapt to the weight-bearing surface. Efficient contact with the support surface is necessary as a foundation for movement from that surface. The child often cannot conform to the surface so that the body part that does take weight is in fact only a very small surface of the body part that is in contact with the surface. This limitation in weight bearing is a further limitation on movement.[86] Abnormal stiffness or spasticity can also limit stability for weight bearing. Often the side that appears most stable for weight bearing is, in fact, the stiffer side; once tone is reduced in treatment or through surgery, it may turn out to be the less stable side. Stiffness has perhaps developed as a compensation for inadequate stabilizing forces.

Muscle Tone

Abnormalities in tone, including spasticity, stiffness, and hypotonia, have been found to be consistent and predictive findings in young children who are at risk for CP, as well as hallmarks of children described as having CP.[87] Investigators have attempted to define and measure spasticity and other aspects of muscle tone in many ways. The difficulty of assessing muscle tone in developing children is compounded by the fact that muscle tone normally changes drastically in the premature infant as development progresses through the first year of life. Saint-Anne Dargassies has described the changes in muscle tone in the normally maturing premature infant and uses these changes as a guide to evaluating normal or abnormal distribution of tone in premature infants.[88] Amiel-Tison has used a similar method of assessing tone in small-for-date babies.[89]

Abnormal muscle tone ranging from hypotonicity to hypertonicity may limit a child's ability to control posture against the force of gravity, leading to limitations in upright posture, that is, sitting, standing, or hands-and-knees positions. Abnormal tone may lead to problems in the control of movement so that hand functions, crawling, or walking is abnormal in coordination, sequencing, or timing. The extent to which abnormal muscle tone is a limitation in controlling movement is currently under considerable debate in the literature as methods to normalize tone, such as surgery or drugs, do not change movement coordination problems. Most examiners assess spasticity by the amount of resistance a muscle gives when rapid movement through the range is manually applied by the examiner because spasticity is velocity dependent.[22, 90–93] The Ashworth Scale for grading hypertonicity is often used to rate spasticity.[94] However, this scale, which evaluates changes in tone when passive motion is imposed on the muscle, is not specific to spasticity.[95] Others recommend that measures of muscle tone should capture the effect of tone on the adaptability of muscles during active movement.[4, 96, 97] The ways in which spasticity interferes with the execution of movement may be associated with positioning and the child's effort to move. The detailed assessment shown in Box 2–1 allows the therapist to describe both resistance to passive movement and constraints on active movement by the child.

In addition to describing the severity of tone, it is important to describe the distribution of tone over the body and limbs. Muscle tone is described in one part of the body relative to other body parts. Generally, the tone in the head, neck, and trunk is compared with that in the extremities; the right side is compared with the left; the upper extremities are compared with the lower extremities; and the distal parts of the extremities are compared with the proximal parts. Any asymmetries, including facial asymmetries, are described.

Changes in tone with speaking, laughing, crying, excitement, a change in the environment, and play are noted. This information is particularly important to a therapist when planning treatment. For example, a child who gets very stiff when asked to talk should not be engaged in complicated language games during difficult movement activities and vice versa.

The therapist needs to note the effect that various sensory stimuli have on the child's tone. Spasticity is caused by abnormalities in processing segmental stretch reflex inputs. This may be an increase in alpha motoneuron excitability that results in an increased response to stretch, or contraction-evoked input from muscle spindles and Golgi tendon organs, or a disorder within the stretch reflex mechanism itself that could alter the threshold or the gain of the stretch reflex.[47] Some children have a low threshold to tactile input and are unable to inhibit motor responses to exteroceptive and muscle proprioceptive inputs. Touch or pressure over muscles actually increases tone in these children. Children who have not been treated are often fearful of movement and become stiff when handled. In addition, the therapist will note the influence of the speed, direction, and force of vestibular input on the changing patterns of the child's tone. In an initial examination, it is important to attempt to find the amount and type of sensory input and movement a child can tolerate while maintaining relatively normal muscle tone.

An interdependent relationship between muscle tone and movement patterns has been accepted by most therapists and used as a basis for treatment.[87, 98] It has been suggested that spasticity limits a child's ability to initiate motion and move quickly and interferes with movement control because activation of the stretch reflex mechanism is velocity dependent.[99] More recently, however, a number of research studies reporting on neuromotor disorders provide evidence that inadequate recruitment of agonist muscle motoneurons may be the primary basis for disorders of motor control.[100–102] Although these studies examined adult patients, there is growing evidence that even in the presence of normal muscle tone, children with CP still have problems with the initiation and speed of movement.[100, 103] This section of the examination gives the therapist the opportunity to comment on the influence of tone on movement in various positions in which the force of gravity must be resisted. Some children get much stiffer when they attempt to move, and the degree of tone at rest does not correlate well with the interference experienced during movement. Other children become less stiff with movement. Although movement is not the only factor affecting the child's tone, treatment

Assessment of Muscle Tone

−3: Severe Hypotonia

Active: Inability to resist gravity; lack of cocontraction at proximal joints for stability; apparent weakness

Passive: No resistance to movement imposed by examiner; full or excessive passive range of motion (ROM); hyperextensibility

−2: Moderate Hypotonia

Active: Decreased tone primarily in axial muscles and proximal muscles of the extremities; interferes with length of time posture can be sustained

Passive: Very little resistance to movement when imposed by examiner; less resistance encountered in movement around proximal joints; joint hyperextensibility at knees and ankles on weight bearing

−1: Mild Hypotonia

Active: Interferes with axial muscle cocontractions; delays initiation of movement against gravity; reduces speed of adjustment to postural change

Passive: Some resistance to joint changes; full passive ROM; hyperextensibility limited to joints of hand, ankles, and feet

0: Normal Tone

Active: Quick and immediate postural adjustment during movement; ability to use muscles in synergic and reciprocal patterns for stability and mobility depending on task of moment

Passive: Body parts resist displacement; momentarily maintain new posture when placed in space; can rapidly follow changing movement imposed by examiner

NOTE: The examiner should be cautious in using the term spasticity *unless it is possible to determine that resistance to movement passively imposed is velocity dependent. The term* hypertonicity *may be more appropriate as a general description of muscles that resist passive movement.*

+1: Mild Hypertonia

Active: Increased tone causes delay in postural adjustment; movements are slow; coordination may be affected

Passive: Resistance to change of posture in part of or throughout range; poor ability to accommodate to passive movements

+2: Moderate Hypertonia

Active: Increased tone limits speed, coordination, variety of movement patterns, and active ROM at some joints

Passive: Resistance to change of posture throughout range; limited passive ROM at some joints

+3: Severe Hypertonia

Active: Severe stiffness of muscles in stereotypic patterns; limited active ROM; little or no ability to move against gravity; great effort needed to overcome stiffness when moving

Passive: Passive ROM limited; unable to overcome resistance of muscle to complete full range without modifying position or stabilizing other body parts

IT: Intermittent Abnormal Tone

Active: Occasional and unpredictable resistance to postural changes alternating with normal adjustment or lack of resistance; may have difficulty initiating active movement or sustaining posture; sudden collapsing

Passive: Unpredictable resistance to imposed passive movement alternating with complete absence of resistance planning requires that the therapist know what to expect when the child begins moving. If a child is stiff (or floppy) before treatment is begun and gets stiffer (or floppier) with movement, the therapist needs to find positions and movements that do not increase (or decrease) tone as well as alter the demand for speed and the application of stimulation to accommodate tone changes. In addition, some children are much more able to manage movement without abnormal tone changes in some positions against gravity than in others. By observing the interaction of tone and movement in various positions, the therapist will be able to identify whether muscle tone is a major impairment of posture and movement coordination in any individual child with CP.

Selective Motor Control

Children with CP move in patterns that are more or less predictable based on the clinical description, age, extent of involvement, and their own prior movement experiences. The selection, sequence, and timing of muscle groups influence how the movement looks. It is important to note how the child moves, emphasizing both normal and abnormal movement patterns. Some children may move quite normally in lower-level developmental positions and show abnormal movement patterns only when standing and walking. Knowing the positions in which the child has the best motor control allows the therapist to build on these normal movement experiences when planning treatment sequences.

The inability to initiate movement with the body part appropriate for the task causes distortion in the control of movement patterns. Hemiplegic children often initiate movement with the sound side. The diplegic child often initiates movement with the head, neck, upper trunk, or arm while the legs follow through passively but stiffly. Some children attempt to initiate movement with the same side (or extremity) they are using for weight bearing or support. In addition, the speed of initiation and effort of movement are noted. Many children show a long latency of response that can be confused with a lack of understanding or motivation rather than motor control problems. Excessive effort to initiate movement may contribute to poor general exercise endurance. This section of the examination also evaluates the child's ability to inhibit a movement on command once the movement is started. Many children are unable to stop, slow, or reverse a movement once it has begun. This is the result of poor timing of agonist and antagonist muscle activity and alteration of their normal reciprocal relationships.[103]

Irradiation of activity in multiple muscles, both in the same segment and in muscles far removed from the prime movers, is an additional problem of selective control. Irradiation may inhibit the normal reciprocal relationships between agonist and antagonist muscles during voluntary movements[104, 105] and make it impossible for the child to move the muscles of one joint without movement of the entire extremity. This contributes to the abnormal quality of dynamic movements that often appears worse as the child makes more effort and works harder.

The persistence of primitive reflexes as an influence on selective movement control in CP has been described by many researchers. The examination of these reflexes and their appearance, disappearance, and impact on normal and abnormal development have been much debated.[106–108] These stereotypic movements are initiated by exteroceptive and proprioceptive stimuli. Assessment of developmental reflexes provides information on how a child responds to specific sensory input applied in a systematic way. If these early reflex patterns dominate the child's movement, the child will have little variety of movement, a decreased ability to isolate movement in a body part, and an inability to inhibit the effect of sensory input on motor responses. Fetters suggests that primitive reflexes serve specific needs for the infant at a particular time in development and are utilized when no other movement patterns are available.[109] This concept is not inconsistent with evaluating these motor responses in children with CP because the important issue is whether these movements in response to specific sensory stimuli are adaptive for the child or whether they inhibit the expression of more complex motor responses. For example, one may see that the only way a child can extend one arm is by initiating it with a head turn toward that arm. The influence of the asymmetric tonic neck reflex prevents other variations of arm extension and dissociation of movements of the head from those at the shoulder and arm.

Recognizing the influence of primitive reflex patterns during spontaneous movement requires close observation and a great deal of experience. If the tester records the way a child moves as part of this assessment, examination of the recurring patterns may reveal a consistent and overpowering influence of the primitive reflexes, preventing the development of more adaptive movements. The importance of recognizing whether arm extension with head turning is in fact the persistence of the asymmetric tonic reflex, a visual problem, or habit pattern, is important in treatment and educational planning. Habit patterns can often be modified through a behavioral modification approach. A visual problem can be corrected with lenses or surgery. A persistent tonic neck reflex can be modified only with maturation and perhaps through specific handling techniques that carefully combine selectivity in the degree, force, and speed of sensory input and body position with movement. Although it is unclear how developmental reflexes contribute to or interfere with motor development and motor control, recognizing their presence in children with CP and the strong relationship of these movement patterns to specific sensory input may aid in clarifying reasons underlying the presence of typical and predictable patterns of movements in these children. The presence of predictable movements whenever a specific tactile or proprioceptive sensation is applied provides information about the child's inability to modify responses to sensory input and develop selective motor strategies to meet changing tasks and environmental conditions. For the severely involved child who has little voluntary or spontaneous movement, a reflex test will determine if movement can be elicited through proprioceptive and exteroceptive stimulation. For less involved children, a specific reflex test may not be necessary but will aid the examiner in recognizing the more subtle ways that reflexes interfere with motor control.

Balance and Postural Control

Postural control involves controlling the body's position in space for 1) *equilibrium,* maintaining the center of mass within the base of support; 2) *orientation,* the ability to maintain an appropriate relationship between the body segments and between the body and the environment for a task; and 3) *protective reactions,* the ability to break the fall if stability limits are exceeded when the center of mass of the body is displaced outside the base of support.[47] Although the neural mechanisms underlying posture and balance are not well understood, it is not surprising that children with CP always have some difficulties with balance. Balance depends on inputs from visual, somatosensory (proprioceptive, cutaneous, and joint receptors), and vestibular systems and on the ability of the CNS to interpret the relative importance of each input. The neural mechanisms must activate, time, and execute synergistic muscles at mechanically related joints to ensure stability while allowing mobility at other joints to allow compensatory movements, all while comparing the executed movement with the intended movement. All this is done moment to moment while the child attends to functional goals without giving any thought to posture and balance.

Although normal postural control is seen as a well-integrated motor response, it is possible to separate some of the components of the postural reactions and evaluate these separately. The orienting reactions that bring the head and body into "normal alignment" when assuming an upright posture or when changing positions are called *righting reactions.* For testing purposes, they are divided into reactions that orient the head in space or in relation to the body, or those that orient one body part to another in relation to the support surface.[107, 108] Together, these reactions allow the body to follow the head or the head to follow the body automatically when, for example, the child rolls over, assumes a sitting position, and moves to a standing position. These reactions can be initiated either by proprioceptive or tactile inputs as a result of changes in the body in relation to the support surface or through activation of the vestibular system as the head is moved in space. Normal movements always involve rotation around the longitudinal axis of the body. These postural reactions are the hallmark of the normal rotational and counterrotational movements of the shoulder and pelvic girdle during walking and during transitions involving resistance to the force of gravity.

The reactions that provide stability when the location of the center of mass relative to the base of support is challenged are called *equilibrium reactions*. They require input from the visual, somatosensory, and vestibular systems as well as the ability to organize muscle activity in response to normal background postural sway and to perturbations of balance caused by reactive forces during movement.[110, 111] These reactions lag the development of the ability to maintain a posture in various positions against gravity. For example, the child must have experience in sitting (and falling) before equilibrium reactions are developed in the trunk and must practice standing before equilibrium reactions to maintain balance in standing develop in the hips, legs, feet, and ankles. Several studies have indicated that young children rely more heavily on visual inputs when developing postural control than on proprioceptive inputs, whereas the opposite is true of older children and adults.[112–114] Children with CP and associated visual problems are often delayed in developing reliable equilibrium reactions. Although most children with CP have some ability to maintain an upright posture, often these movements are poorly developed and depend on the speed, directions, force, frequency, and duration of sensory input. Equilibrium may be ineffective in providing a stable posture to resist the force of gravity in response to transient perturbations, even those caused by one's own movement. A child who has poor equilibrium reactions in a sitting position frequently places one hand on the floor in a supportive response, thereby limiting two-handed use for dressing or play. A child who is posturally insecure often develops one way to perform a task, and the child's movements are thus stereotyped and limited in variety. It is important to describe under what conditions a child can or cannot maintain balance and posture because this information leads directly to understanding functional limitations caused by lack of effective balance and postural reactions.

The automatic responses of the extremities that occur when the center of mass is displaced outside the base of support and equilibrium reactions are inadequate to maintain or restore stability are called *protective reactions*. They are provoked by stimuli to the vestibular and somatosensory systems and involve extension-abduction movements of the upper and lower extremities on the side opposite to but in the direction of displacement. Fully developed, these are two-phase reactions, the movement phase of the extremity and a support phase to protect against falling. They are often considered backup responses to equilibrium reactions. If the perturbation is so strong or rapid that the center of mass cannot be maintained within the base of support, protective reactions are available to prevent falling and injury and to recover postural alignment. Children with CP may have limited functional use of these protective responses because of faulty interactions of the timing and sequencing of the intralimb joints and muscles during the movement phase, lack of power and force during the support phase, or an inability to instantaneously recruit and change the activation patterns of the appropriate motor units for patterns of mobility followed by stability.

Strength

Strength is probably the single most difficult area to examine in children with CP because of many perceptual, cognitive, neuromuscular, musculoskeletal, and biomechanical factors that influence the child's ability to understand and demonstrate the power to initiate, complete, or repeat a movement. Strength depends on properties of the muscle itself as well as the appropriate recruitment of motor units and the timing of their activation. Traditional methods of isolating a single muscle's ability to resist the force of gravity or perform against a resisting force are not effective in children with CP. Whether strength is considered part of the neuromuscular impairment assessment or an aspect of the musculoskeletal assessment depends on the therapist's judgment of whether the primary reason for weakness is impaired motor control from a centrally mediated imbalance of muscle strength or secondary to the peripheral effect of muscle imbalance due to musculoskeletal growth. Strength can be assessed in children with CP in functional developmental positions using movements that the children have demonstrated that they can perform. The therapist must keep in mind the muscle group or specific muscle that is to be assessed. It is important to know the child's available ROM, selective muscle control, and passive and active muscle tone as any or all of these factors may limit the force of the movement being tested. These factors complicate strength testing and require the therapist's creativity in factoring out confounding variables.

There are three ways in which problems in muscle strength can limit a child's posture and movement, and testing strength needs to address each of these components:

1. *Isometric strength.* This is the ability to hold a position against the force of gravity or a known resistance. Most often the muscle is tested by applying force in its shortened range. In children with CP, it is often important to test the ability to hold a midrange position as well.
2. *Isotonic strength.* This is the ability of the muscle to move through its range with resistance applied throughout.
   a. *Eccentric strength.* This is the ability to resist a force as a muscle is lengthening.
   b. *Concentric strength.* This is the ability to resist a force as the muscle is shortening.
3. *Endurance.* This is the ability to continue to produce adequate power for a given number of repetitions.

For example, hamstrings can be tested for isometric strength if the child is placed supine, legs in the hooklying position with arms across the chest, and asked to make and hold a bridge by raising the hips off the floor. Eccentric and concentric strength can be tested if the child is placed on the hands and feet with the weight distributed across the metatarsal and metacarpal heads and asked to slowly bend the knees to gain a hands-and-knees position and then return to a hands-and-feet position. Endurance can be tested with the child in the same position by asking for 10 repetitions. The positions and movements selected can be used in test-retest situations or before and after surgery to monitor progress.

Hand-held dynamometers have been used to assess strength in children with CP. They have been shown to be reliable in the measurement of isometric strength in children and can be used to provide more objective measures of changes in strength.[115–117]

Examination of Musculoskeletal Impairments

Assessment of musculoskeletal impairments includes examination of the ROM and the use of orthoses, adaptive equipment, and assistive devices. Postural alignment and strength are often considered an aspect of the musculoskeletal system. In infants and young children with CP these problems appear to be related to problems in control by the neuromuscular system. In older children and teenagers, disuse atrophy may complicate problems of motor control, and in that situation, or in situations following muscle-lengthening procedures that produce weakness, strength assessment should appear in this portion of the examination.

One of the primary effects of treatment for children with CP might well be the prevention of contractures and deformities. In a study of correlates of physicians' decisions to refer children with CP to physical therapy, Campbell and colleagues found that 70 percent of the physicians believed that the value of physical therapy for children with CP was in the prevention of contractures and deformities.[118] If untreated, these impairments would lead to functional limitations and possibly to disability if they persisted for long periods of time and could not be compensated for by therapeutic or surgical means. The ROM is assessed using slow passive motion to avoid stretch reflex activity. The test position should be recorded because abnormalities of tone and the presence of primitive reflexes, which vary by position, may influence the ROM. To compare the results over time, the same test position must be used each time. Joint range can be measured with a goniometer while keeping in mind that the joint range may vary with age. Assessment of the ROM includes information on the potential influence of the current posture and movements on the future development of deformities and contracture. For example, a child who habitually sits between the heels is at risk for hip adductor contracture and medial femoral torsion.

Individual joints and the neural and nonneural influences on them, as well as on the spine and long bones, are examined. Bleck, Samilson, and others have written extensively and clearly regarding the musculoskeletal and biomechanical problems in children with CP.[49, 119] Knowledge of potential orthopedic problems common in CP will help the therapist to understand the value of evaluating the ROM. If joint deformities or muscle contractures exist, they are described in this section of the examination.

If the child has splints, braces, or other orthotic appliances or has had surgery, these are noted in this part of the musculoskeletal assessment. First, there is a description of surgical procedures and their influence on the child's neuromuscular and musculoskeletal impairments. The timing, dates, and goals of surgery are included as well as the effect on function. Second, information on orthoses is noted, including how long they are worn and for what purposes they are worn. Movement with and without the appliance is described.

Many children with CP use adaptive equipment and assistive devices or mobility aids to increase their function and decrease their disability in daily life roles. Appropriate mobility aids can alter a child's gait pattern, reduce energy expenditure, and promote independence in walking.[63, 120, 121] Seating systems and wheelchairs can add to comfort, freedom, and functional abilities.[122, 123] Any equipment currently being used should be described with the purposes clearly defined. The PEDI[78] is useful for objective documentation of assistance and equipment modifications.

Summary of Examination

The examination summary includes a list of the child's strengths. This may include information regarding both internal and external resources. Internal resources include intelligence, interest, attention, motivation, cooperativeness, self-concept, and functional skills. The family's size, interest, level of understanding of the child's abilities and functional limitations, goals, energy available for interaction and therapy, and financial resources may be noted as examples of external resources.

After a list of strengths, the therapist formulates a list of problems and hypothesizes reasons for the problems. This includes the neuromuscular and musculoskeletal impairments underlying the functional limitations but also may include behavioral, cognitive, perceptual, social, and environmental causes as well. The procedure of enumerating strengths and problems allows the therapist to focus on how the strengths can be used to facilitate changes in the problem areas.

Listing the problems and family aspirations leads directly to a list of goals for therapy and of treatment methods designed specifically to meet the goals listed. The following section illustrates how the evaluation of examination results and the lists of strengths and problems are integrated with a treatment plan.

ORGANIZING TREATMENT AND MANAGEMENT
Life-Cycle Approach

Whether physical therapy, medical or surgical treatment, or educational or employment options are described, the management of a person with CP must reflect a life-cycle approach. Treatment must take into account the child's age, capabilities, needs, and values and accept that just as every person changes during the progression from infancy through adulthood, so does the person with CP. Programs designed to serve children throughout their lifetime must not only include goals and methods that are appropriate for the present but also educate clients to take responsibility for directing the quality of their own lives, including health, physical fitness, and motor learning.[3, 124]

Treatment and management in infancy focus on clarification of the problems and integrating this information into a family structure and value system. The family is the primary developmental setting, and the focus must be on assisting the family to facilitate growth and development of their infant in response to being loved and nurtured by the parents. The preschool years provide an opportunity to review the child's abilities and limitations in a wider environment as the child begins to interact with places and persons outside the family. There will be new expectations from the child and new demands from the environment. What has worked previously may not be adequate anymore. The school years provide new areas of concern and opportunity. The child is more strongly influenced by the peer group and by educational expectations.

Physical growth as well as emotional and intellectual development affect the problems of CP. Adolescence is a time for establishing identity and independence, goals that can be very difficult to attain for the teenager with a disability and his or her family. Adulthood is a time for establishing employment and independence in a new home and work environment. Full participation in contemporary society for adults with disabilities is especially difficult because provisions for support are scarce compared with those available to children.[125, 126] Issues of retirement and aging have hardly been addressed as they relate to the person with CP. The transitions along the life cycle are reciprocal. Children with disabilities change those around them and at the same time are changed by the continuously changing environments and persons in it. Accepting this dynamic situation, it is possible to outline guidelines that are important to follow if treatment is to remain effective throughout the life cycle.

Guidelines for Treatment

1. *Treatment goals are designed to meet specific problems within a specific time frame.* These vary with age, family concerns, and the extent of signs at the onset of treatment. Establishing a reevaluation schedule is a critical part of the decision-making process.
2. *Treatment goals change with changes in the presenting problems.* For example, an infant with hemiplegia may initially present with hypotonicity in the upper extremity leading to limitations in reaching. By 6 or 8 months, once the child begins to move against gravity, the child may present with hypertonicity. To gain reaching, the therapeutic goal therefore changes from increasing tone in the involved upper extremity to decreasing tone in the upper extremity.
3. *Treatment goals are set by the family, the child, and the therapist.* Goals are stated in terms of function. Older children participate in deciding on goals for therapy. This approach helps the child and the family to focus on what is and is not a reasonable expectation within a given time. In my experience, young school-aged children are able to describe reasonable goals. For example, I began treating a 7-year-old boy with a diagnosis of mild spastic diplegia. He was attending regular second grade and had no special assistance. The first time I saw him, I asked what he wanted to accomplish with me before the school year was over. (His mother referred him to me in February when his school therapist moved out of town.) He told me he wanted to be able to play soccer and to jump rope. He told me these two things were important to him because he was always the last to be picked for soccer. None of the children wanted him on their team because he often missed the ball when he tried to kick it, and he couldn't dodge and move quickly on the field. He wanted to jump rope because this is what the other children did at recess. Both of these were reasonable goals, and he had the basic movement skills to accomplish these goals within the time frame.
4. *Treatment methods and techniques change with the child's age, need for independence, and function as well as motor impairments.* A young baby enjoys being held for play, therapy, dressing, and feeding. A natural environment is the mother's lap, and a great deal of baby treatment can effectively take place there. Because a 2-year-old child needs to develop

independence, dressing can be done on a bench or chair (with appropriate support), and treatment requires much more mobility, exploration, and self-initiation. A 10-year-old child needs to function independently in areas of self-care and mobility. Teenagers are assisted in finding methods, through sports and physical activity, to integrate fitness into their lifestyle. An 18-year-old headed to college needs methods to maintain flexibility and strength independent of special equipment or other people. The treatment changes to provide this young adult with methods to monitor his own movements and to maintain his ROM, strength, and endurance while specifically addressing his capabilities and disability.

5. *Families are given information regarding the child's problems and management as they are able to understand and assimilate the information.* The role of the family in treatment and care is described in detail in the section Family-Centered Intervention. Families may understand and accept the child, the child's problems, and their responsibility toward the child in different ways at different times throughout their child's life. Just because the family has adjusted well to having a preschool child with CP does not necessarily mean that they will adjust easily as their child becomes school age and is visible in the community environment, attending public school. The adjustment process is ongoing and reflects the individual capabilities of the parents and their particular pattern of response to life stresses. What one family handles easily may represent a major disruption to another.

6. *Suggestions to the family are as practical as possible.* The therapist must remember that parents have responsibilities toward their other children, to each other, to themselves, to jobs, and to their community as well as to their child with a disability. Parents repeatedly tell me that they are more inclined to do regularly activities that can be easily incorporated into the daily care routines that they do normally with their child, such as doing a ROM of the upper extremity as the child stretches out an arm to put on a coat or pull off a T-shirt.

7. *Treatment is geared to the functions the child needs as the child grows and develops.* Functions used in activities of daily living, including dressing, feeding, and personal grooming, are important to address with therapeutic techniques. These are real-life activities and are meaningful to the family and the child. Treatment described in terms of function focuses on preventing disability and handicap even if underlying impairments are lifelong problems.

8. *Therapy is designed to use the child's strengths, recognizing that every child has competencies.* If a child has good imaginary play and language skills, story telling can focus the child's attention and imaginary play can provide a framework for moving. Focus on the child's strengths builds self-esteem and centers everyone on the capabilities of the child at any age.

9. *Sensory stimulation is integrated with motor output.* Loud or vigorous auditory and visual stimuli can be used to evoke attention and produce forceful movement. Multisensory stimuli, however, should not be used with highly distractible or emotionally volatile children. Tactile or vestibular hypersensitivity or hyposensitivity can have a profound effect on the movement outcome. Changing the type and level of sensory input can have a direct effect on improving the quality of motor response. Sensory stimulation should never be given as an isolated therapy but should be paired with the motor response directed to functional activities that require the child to adapt to the environment.

10. *Therapy is designed to evoke active responses from the child.* Passive movement is less effective than active movement in producing changes in tone, movement patterns, or motor learning. Active movement, however, does not necessarily mean voluntary movement. For example, postural

reactions performed automatically during balance activities require a great amount of strength and endurance.

11. *Play is integrated into therapy to provide motivation and purpose to reinforce and direct movement responses.* Play must be carefully monitored during treatment so that it does not overstimulate the child and interfere with the desired movement response or produce abnormal increases in tone. Simulated sports or dance is appropriate play for school-aged children and teens. Music develops rhythm, timing, and endurance. These are highly motivating activities and are functionally oriented.

12. *Whenever possible, movement is initiated by the child.* The control of movement is maintained by the therapist, but the child leads the treatment and initiates the activity. For example, if the goal is to improve reaching in a sitting position, the therapist sets up the environment, placing the child in a seated position and providing stimulating toys at various positions in space that require changing, adjusting, and correcting muscle length and alignment of the joints, stabilizing the trunk, shoulder, arm, and hand as it moves through space, and providing opportunities to develop accuracy in orienting the hand to objects. The child initiates reaching for and engaging in play with various items, often unaware that the therapist has provided the structure.

13. *Treatment includes planning and solving motor problems.* Motor planning begins with one-step goal-directed problems and progresses to multistep open-ended functions, as demonstrated by the progression revealed in first asking "How are you going to get your arm in your sleeve?" then later, "How are you going to organize your clothes and get dressed in time for school?" Self-initiated problem solving transfers the responsibility and ownership of movement sequences from the therapist to the child. Each child eventually must work out ways to perform various tasks based on the child's own musculoskeletal, biomechanical, and neuromuscular limitations as well as motivation and the priority and necessity for the task. No two people plan and carry out a motor task in exactly the same way, and a single person alters the plan and solution for a motor problem according to the specific task and the environmental constraints at the moment.

14. *Repetition is an important component in motor learning.* Motor activities that are task specific, repeated throughout a session and in functional ways at home, have a better chance of becoming part of the child's habitual repertoire than infrequently practiced skills. Therapists need to wait while a child "practices" an activity during therapy. Older children can be encouraged to find "another way" or "more ways" to do a task, as repetition does not necessarily mean doing the same thing, the same way over and over, but rather finding a variety of strategies to accomplish functional goals.

15. *A single treatment session progresses from positions in which the child is most capable to ones that are more challenging.* Within each treatment session a child should have the opportunity to work in various developmental positions appropriate to the child's age, but the progression from one position to another must be carefully controlled so that as the child is challenged by the force of gravity, speed, or effort, the child continues to produce movement directed toward broadening the movement options. Treatment should end with positions and activities that are functional for the child and provide a cooldown period after a vigorous exercise session. One of the most difficult aspects of therapy for the therapist is knowing when to push for difficult components of movement and knowing when to back off. The guidelines for this change not only as the child develops, but also from day to day, depending on many other life factors of which the therapist may lack knowledge. For example, I began a treatment session with a 10-year-old girl whose abilities were well known to me. On this particular day, she was

not able to do activities during our warmup that were moderately difficult but possible with concentration. When I finally said, "Becky, this just isn't going well," she burst forth with an emotional response describing how a few children in her class were acting up and the teacher had made all the members of the class stay in during recess. Becky felt she had been treated unfairly because the disruption didn't involve her. Her emotional state had a profound impact on her physical ability in the therapy session.

16. *Movement in one position prepares for movements in another.* Through experience with an individual child, the therapist will find positions and activities that have a positive effect on the child's movements. These activities are used early in a treatment session to give the child the feeling of control in positions in which movement is easier before attempting movement in positions that are difficult or new for the child. Children will persist in attempting difficult movements if they experience success with less difficult movements.

17. *As a child is able to perform movements independently, the therapist provides time in a treatment session for the child to move freely.* It is important for the child to feel movement produced through the child's efforts without the control of the therapist. Only in this way will the child incorporate these movements into daily living. It is equally important not to interrupt the child's spontaneous play activity in order to adhere to a planned sequence of therapeutic activities. It is important for children to work out their own strategies for play and for therapists to accept their ability to find "the best way" for them at the time. Self-initiated and self-controlled movement gives the message that the children are in control of their world and can learn from their own activity.

18. *The environment is conducive to cooperative participation and support of the child's efforts.* Because therapy will be an ongoing part of the life of a child with CP, it should be pleasurable. If children enjoy movement, they will be more inclined to make movement, through exercise and recreation, part of their lifestyle. The environment can be used to stimulate the child to move in ways that achieve the therapeutic goals and encourage the child to engage in self-initiated play. When interviewing a young woman with spastic diplegia who was headed to college, I asked her in what ways physical therapy had had a positive impact on her life. First, she apologized for not being able to respond by listing specific exercises or physical activities that had a positive impact; then she told me that physical therapy had given her the discipline to place exercise as a high priority in her life—for all her life!

19. *Individual treatment sessions are designed to evaluate the effectiveness of treatment within the session.* This can be done informally by motivating the child to demonstrate an activity, movement, or posture at the beginning of treatment and again at the end in order to determine subjectively whether changes have occurred, or through the use of more formalized methods (see the section Evaluation of Outcomes). Knowing that change has occurred is motivating to the child and reinforcing for the therapist and the family.

20. *Physical therapy is coordinated with the goals and activities of all other medical and educational disciplines involved with the child.* Treatment is integrated with the goals and methods of occupational therapy and speech therapy, orthopedic and neurosurgical management, and educational and home management. At different times in the child's life, the focus and importance of the various disciplines will change so that one discipline will have a higher priority than another. Collaboration between professionals and the family has been mandated by law in the United States (Public Law 102-119); this law empowers the family to act as advocates for their child through active participation in decision making regarding the prioritization of treatment goals.[127]

CASE STUDY

To illustrate how these principles of examination and treatment are integrated into a specific program, a case study is presented, following the child from examination through a treatment progression and outcome assessment.

EXAMINATION FINDINGS AND SUMMARY

Pathophysiology and Description of the Problem

Stephanie D. is a 4-year-1-month-old girl, born 10 weeks prematurely after her mother was seriously injured in an automobile accident. She has a history of a grade III periventricular hemorrhage, respiratory distress syndrome, neonatal seizures, and hydrocephalus. She has a shunt and is currently on carbamazepine (Tegretol) for seizures, which recurred when she was 2 years old. Her motor disability is classified as level III spastic diplegic CP according to the Gross Motor Function Classification System.[51]

Developmental and Family Characteristics

Stephanie was referred to the Parent and Child Training Program when she was 5 months old. This program included physical therapy. At 2 years of age, she began attending the Learning Center, a community program for preschool children with special needs. She receives twice-a-week therapy in this setting. Both of her parents work. She is the third child in a family that includes four children. The older two children are her half-siblings, as this is a second marriage for her mother. Both parents are proud of the progress she has made but hope that someday she will walk independently of aids and have better use of her right hand.

Statement of Concerns

The parents' chief concern is whether Stephanie will be able to attend her community school kindergarten when she turns 5 because her physical limitations affect her age-appropriate mobility, manipulative skills, and daily living skills, as well as her personal-social interactions.

Strengths

1. A cooperative, social, inquisitive child
2. Speaks in short simple sentences to express wants and desires
3. Motivated to move if the goal is clear and immediate
4. Not fearful of movements
5. Has apparently normal vision and hearing
6. Has an emotionally supportive family, interested in her well-being and progress but limited in time and financial support

Functional Skills and Limitations

Delayed functional capabilities as determined by the PEDI and GMFM (Tables 2–1 and 2–2).

Stephanie's standard scores (compared with a normative mean of 50 with a standard deviation of 10) indicate that she is performing significantly below expectations for

Pediatric Evaluation of Disability Inventory Composite Scores

TABLE 2–1

Domain	Raw Score	Normative Standard Score	Standard Error of Measurement	Scaled Score	Standard Error of Measurement
Self-care	43	19.2	2.8	57.4	1.6
Mobility	29	<10	—	50.5	2.1
Social function	45	26.6	2.7	58.6	1.6

Gross Motor Function Measure Summary Scores

TABLE 2–2

Dimension	Score (%)
A. Lying and rolling	100
B. Sitting	95
C. Crawling and kneeling	90
D. Standing	17
E. Walking, running, and jumping	15
Total score (A + B + C + D + E ÷ 5)	64
Goal Total Score (D + E)	32

her age in self-care and mobility. The self-care score is more than 3 standard deviations below the mean score for her age and specifically indicates limitations in

1. Using utensils
2. Pouring liquids
3. Brushing teeth
4. Grooming hair
5. Washing and drying hands, face, and body
6. Putting on shirts, pants, shoes, and socks
7. Manipulating buttons and fasteners
8. Self-toileting

The mobility score is more than 4 standard deviations below the mean score for her age and specifically shows limitations in

1. Independent walking indoors and out
2. Toilet, tub, chair, and car transfers
3. Carrying objects
4. Walking on uneven surfaces
5. Managing stairs

The social function score is slightly more than 2 standard deviations below the mean score for her age but could place her in the low-normal range when considering the standard error of measurement (2.7) for her obtained score. This area demonstrated specific limitations in

1. Sentence complexity and syntax
2. Functional use of sentences and expressions of thoughts and feelings
3. Connecting sentences to tell a story
4. Problem solving
5. Complex play involving rules
6. Providing directions
7. Orienting to time
8. Completing household tasks
9. Understanding self-protection
10. Exploring the community
11. Meeting expectations of the school and community setting

Her scaled scores show a distribution typical of a child with spastic diplegic CP who has significant motor impairment and resulting functional limitations. Mobility scores are significantly worse than either self-care or social function scores. These scores may be more appropriate than the standard scores to chart progress during therapy because her standard mobility scores are so low that they are not likely to be sensitive to changes that can be expected in a reasonable time frame.

The GMFM adds information regarding the underlying sources of Stephanie's functional limitations by exploring her movement capabilities in a variety of positions (see Table 2–2).

The individual dimension scores are more significant than the total scores because scores on the first three dimensions are so much better than the last two. As a result, the total score distorts the perception of her capabilities. Specifically, in the standing domain she is unable to stand independently, lift a foot in standing, attain standing from a bench without use of her arms, attain kneeling from high kneel, or reach to the floor or squat from standing. In the walking/running domain she is unable to do any of the activities that involve walking independently. Those areas that need to be targeted as goal areas (dimensions D and E) are clear from her score distribution, and retesting in 6 months or a year should show an increase in the percentage score for the Goal Total Score. This will be helpful in measuring outcomes and changes in outcomes over time.

Neuromuscular Impairments

1. *Abnormal alignment and distribution in weight bearing.* Stephanie sits with more of her body weight on the left side and aligns herself within a broad base of support. Any anticipation of movement increases this asymmetry and the stiffness of her lower extremities and right upper extremity relative to her head and trunk. She cannot conform to the support surface, further limiting her movement options.

2. *Abnormal muscle stiffness.* Tone is increased, more on the right than on the left, more in lower extremities and the right upper extremity (+ 3) than in the trunk and left upper extremity (+ 2); distal parts of the extremities are stiffer than proximal parts. There is sustained clonus in both ankles. Excessive cocontraction in the trunk muscles prevents movement of the rib cage for respiration and trunk rotation.

3. *Impaired selective motor control.* Movement is initiated by the head and the upper extremities. There are very limited and predictable patterns of movement in the lower extremities. She is unable to move joints of the lower extremities independent of each other. There is limited speed and prolonged latency of initiation of movement. She often cannot initiate movement with her body part appropriate for the task. There is limited active joint excursion during movement. She has active opening and grasping of the right hand but is limited in range, force, and complexity. Irradiation inhibits normal reciprocal relationships during voluntary movement. Movement decreases with speed, excitement, or the difficulty of the task.

4. *Impaired balance and postural reactions.* She has limited righting reactions with no trunk rotation when changing position. Equilibrium responses are limited in the sitting position, absent in the standing position. She has overuse of protective responses in the sitting position to compensate for a lack of equilibrium. Inadequate postural reactions inhibit an anticipatory weight shift when initiating movement. Balance is inadequate for functional movements in standing.

5. *Impaired strength.* Weakness (combined with stiffness) in her right hand limits all bilateral skills. She cannot alter the power of grasp or release needed for the task. Full hip extension is limited by an inability to move fully through the ROM against the force of gravity. She cannot sustain power to maintain hip and knee extension while performing skills in the standing position. She has poor endurance and cannot repeat movements without deterioration in the quality of the movement.

Musculoskeletal Impairment

1. *Limited passive ROM.* Her passive ROM is limited to 65 degrees in hamstrings, 60 degrees in hip adductors, and neutral in gastrocnemius-soleus muscle groups bilaterally. The right shoulder flexion ROM is limited to 120 degrees. Inactivity in the rib cage and chest wall appears to be, in part, limited passive ROM.

2. *Limited active ROM.* She has limited active extension ROM in the thoracic spine. Thoracic rounding is a musculoskeletal compensation for problems in sitting alignment and postural control. Immobility of the ribs for respiration and trunk rotation appears to be both a result of a limited passive ROM and a postural alignment compensation. A limited active ROM in shoulder flexion results from both limited passive ROM (on the right) and poor disassociated scapular-humeral movements.

Figure 2–1 illustrates Stephanie's motor problems.

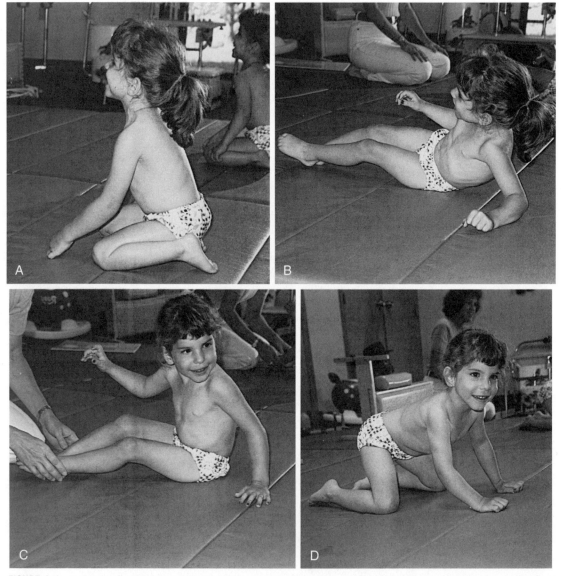

FIGURE 2–1. *A,* This is Stephanie's preferred sitting posture. She can sit independently on a bench, but on the floor she prefers to sit between her legs, which gives her a wide base of support and allows movement within a safe base of support. In this sitting posture, she can use her hands for play without fear of falling. *B,* When asked to assume sitting from the supine position, movement is initiated by her head and upper trunk over her left side. The stiffness in her lower extremities increases with the stress of the activity, limiting the movements of her legs. *C,* In long sitting on the floor, weight is on her left side. Notice that only her hand, hip, and heels contact the floor. This is not a stable or secure position for play. *D,* Stephanie can assume the hands and knees position and crawl using a reciprocal motion. Notice that weight is on the heels of her hands and on her knees. The distribution of her weight is shifted to the left and backward. Excursions of movement are small when crawling in order to keep her movements safely within a comfortable base of support.

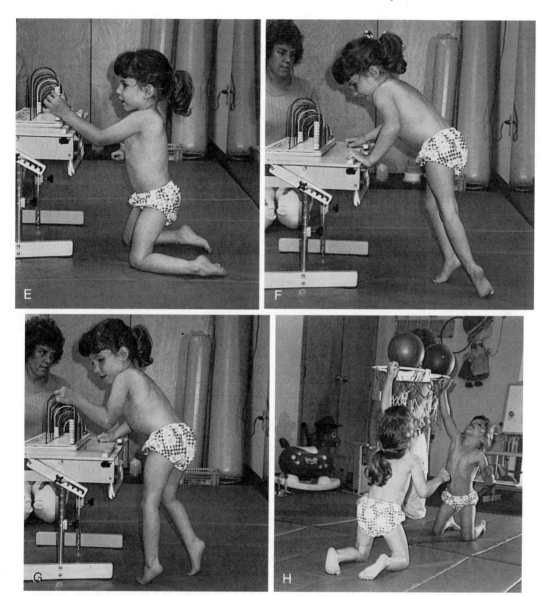

FIGURE 2–1 *Continued. E,* Stephanie can kneel upright and balance. The base of support is shifted toward her left side, and contact with the floor is minimal. In all illustrations the high rib cage is apparent with little activity in the abdominal oblique muscles. The shoulders and scapulae move as one unit. A lack of scapular stability is apparent. Play is limited to her left hand, which also serves as her weight-bearing arm. Notice no involvement of her right arm or hand in the play activity. *F,* A pull-to-stand shows poor disassociated movements of her legs. Work is initiated by her arms and shoulders. Stiffness has increased with effort as evidenced by plantar flexion in her feet. *G,* Standing to play is very difficult because of an abnormal alignment, a lack of balance, an inadequate base of support, and an inability to adjust her posture through her legs. Incomplete hip extension is apparent here and in *E* and *F. H,* Effort, speed of movement, and excitement increase Stephanie's problems with tone, alignment, and balance. High tone in the right upper extremity has eliminated the possibility of using this extremity in play. Excessive neck extension is used to compensate for a lack of thoracic and hip extension. The quality of movement has deteriorated with effort against the force of gravity.

TREATMENT GOALS, STRATEGIES, AND TACTICS

In the HOAC format for clinical decision making, each therapist asks herself or himself the following questions to link goals, strategies, rationale, and outcome.

1. What do I want to accomplish (change, improve) today? What are my single-session goals?
2. How do I plan to accomplish this? What treatment strategies and tactics am I going to use?
3. Why do I want to make these changes? What is my rationale? What longer term goals do I have in mind?
4. How long will it take to accomplish change?
5. What will I do if I do not accomplish my goals? (reevaluation of goals, strategies, and tactics)
6. What new goals or strategies will I select when I do accomplish these goals?

Bower and colleagues showed that the factor most strongly associated with increased motor skill acquisition was the use of specific measurable goals.[128] Movement can be facilitated through verbal cuing; manual cuing, which includes graded tactile and proprioceptive input; manipulation of the task; or environment and behavioral reinforcements. During any treatment session the therapist has the opportunity to use any or all of these methods to help the child maintain posture and produce movements that the child cannot do independent of assistance. The specific method or combination of methods depends on both the therapist's experience and training and the responsiveness of the child to various types and degrees of sensory stimulation.

In this case study, the strategies used to accomplish the goals include movement facilitation and therapeutic handling consistent with a Neuro-Developmental Treatment (NDT) approach accompanied by manipulation of the tasks and structuring of the environment, drawn from the assumptions about motor control and motor learning described earlier in this chapter. Stephanie's goals, the rationale for their selection, a time frame for their accomplishment, and examples of a treatment sequence follow. The longer time frames represent the time when it is reasonable to expect the goal to become a part of the child's functional repertoire.

Goal 1: Improve Alignment and Postural Control in Sitting

Rationale. Stephanie is 4 years old, attending preschool, and preparing for integration into her community kindergarten. She needs to sit securely when using her hands for school readiness skills and to have a position in which to interact well with children and adults. Better sitting will assist her voicing and increase her independence in hand use appropriate for her age. Moving within a sitting position also prepares her for moving in standing.

Time Frame and Short-Term Goals. Within a treatment session, Stephanie will have the opportunity to sit on various surfaces and play. Within a month, she will be able to sit on a bench with no additional support and maintain good alignment while doing simple activities with two hands, such as catching a ball, using rhythm instruments in time to music, imitating various "Simon Says" hand and arm movements, assisting with clothing and shoes, or eating a snack.

Goal 2: Increase Movement in the Lower Extremities

Rationale. Stephanie moves her legs very little to adjust her posture within a position or to initiate a change of position. She needs to use her legs in weight bearing when rising to stand and when shifting her weight as she moves in standing and walking. In addition, she is at risk for developing contractures and deformities in her hips, knees, and feet if she does not move them actively through wide ranges of motion.

Time Frame and Short-Term Goals. In each treatment session, Stephanie will experience a variety of positions and activities that will require her to use disassociated movements of her legs when changing positions. Presently she is uncomfortable if one hip is passively flexed and the other extended. She will be able to maintain positions that require this and assist when asked, "Stephanie, can you help me bend just your right leg?" (when moving into a half-kneeling position and preparing to stand). She will begin to be responsible for moving her own legs to adjust her posture in floor and bench sitting and for pushing down with her legs to stand up with only verbal cuing (such as "fix your feet" or "are your legs ready to stand up?") within a month.

Goal 3: Develop Rotation Around the Longitudinal Body Axis with Weight Shift During Transitions

Rationale. Using the trunk for the initiation of movement and rotation during a weight shift will free her upper extremities for skilled movements and her lower extremities for weight bearing. Rotation about the body axis contributes to smoother, easier transitions from one position to another and will make her movements more fluid. She needs these transitions to move onto and out of her classroom chair and onto and off the toilet and to transfer independently into and out of her walker.

Time Frame and Short-Term Goals. In one treatment session, Stephanie will be given the opportunity to reach for and play with toys placed on either side of her. The therapeutic environment will be structured to provide this opportunity. Within a month, Stephanie will be able to rotate her trunk in a sitting position to reach toys placed to either side without placing her hands on the seat to assist. Within 3 months, she will be able to move from her walker to a bench or child's chair and back to her walker by rotating her trunk and appropriately adjusting her posture around her legs and feet.

Goal 4: Initiate Movement with Appropriate Body Part for the Task

Rationale. Stephanie has already developed the habit of initiating all movement with her head and upper extremities. Being able to stabilize one body part and initiate movement with another will increase the speed and variety of her movements. An increasing variety of movement will provide more options for solving movement problems she faces during daily life.

Time Frame and Short-Term Goals. In one treatment session, selective initiation must be done with physical and verbal cues because Stephanie has developed habit patterns that have decreased her options for moving and she doesn't seem to know how to move differently. It will take several months to see any changes in her spontaneous movements, and then only when she is comfortable and concentrating on her movements.

Goal 5: Increase the Variety of Movement Patterns in the Right Upper Extremity and Hand

Rationale. Stephanie has little active movement in the right upper extremity. Her hand is often fisted with the elbow flexed and forearm pronated. This posture interferes with the most basic grasp patterns, weight bearing through this extremity, and manipulation skills that involve the use of two hands. She has been unable to develop basic preschool skills or self-help skills including dressing, grooming, and toileting because she cannot use her right hand. She is at risk for developing contracture at the elbow and hand.

Time Frame and Short-Term Goals. In one treatment session, Stephanie will take weight on an open hand when sitting or supported in standing. This will first be done with physical manipulation and visual cues and later in the session with verbal cues. "Stephanie, do you see all your fingers?" She will engage in bilateral arm and hand movements in which she assists movements of her right arm and hand with her left. This is to establish a lifelong habit of self-ROM and a sense of responsibility for maintaining her own flexibility. In 3 months, she will do these simple ROM activities with a verbal prompt such as, "Stephanie, time out for a good stretch." (See illustrations of a single-session evaluation, Figure 2–3.)

Goal 6: Increase Strength and Endurance, Particularly in the Lower Extremities

Rationale. Stephanie tires easily and still requires long afternoon naps. She frequently has upper respiratory infections. She has little mobility of her rib cage, and this may compromise the depth of respirations or limit changes in patterns of respiration needed for rapid or difficult movements. Stephanie's parents want to enroll her in the neighborhood kindergarten next school year but are concerned that the daily routine there will be too exhausting for her. They know that it takes her considerable effort to move and believe that all her life she will need to be aware of general fitness and wellness.

Time Frame and Short-Term Goals. In each session, Stephanie will be required to initiate movements against the force of gravity, constantly changing positions and increasing the number of repetitions. Activities that require her to move from a sitting to a standing position and move in a standing position will strengthen her legs. Riding a therapeutic tricycle will be part of her school day to increase muscle and cardiopulmonary endurance. Within 3 months, Stephanie will be able to keep up with other preschool children when riding her bike outside during the school day. She will nap only as appropriate for her age.

Goal 7: Provide Opportunities for Age-Appropriate Skills Needed for Self-Care and Play

Rationale. Stephanie is interested in age-appropriate activities, including identifying pictures in books; matching, sorting, and naming colors and shapes; and imaginary play. These activities, however, need adult supervision because of her limited movements and lack of balance in standing. Her parents are concerned that she is too passive and believe that this is related to the fact that she cannot select toys or choose where or with whom she wants to play. It is important that she become more assertive and confident in her ability to select her own play and learning activities when she is attending preschool. Her teenaged siblings need to interact with her in age-appropriate ways. Because she is dependent in daily activities at home and is small for her age, they tend to treat her like their 2-year-old brother.

Time Frame and Short-Term Goals. In each therapy session, Stephanie will be given a choice of activities. Once she selects what she wants to do, this decision will be respected. Each session will end with the remark, "Think about what you want to do next time you come." The following session will begin with asking her what she wants to start with. During each session, the therapist will say, "O.K., now it is your turn to pick an activity," or "Show me a different way to do this (game, activity, movement)." The therapist will structure how it is done to make certain the therapeutic goals are met. The therapist will model age-appropriate language and social interactions to make her a more active participant in her home as well, requiring her to make choices regarding clothing, food, daily activities, and play. Over the next 6 months, her two teenaged siblings will also attend therapy sessions to increase their understanding of Stephanie's limitations and capabilities and to observe and participate in interactions that will develop Stephanie's self-reliance and independence. A time frame for specific behavioral changes will not be enforced since this requires changes in all family members and their interactions with Stephanie in their home environment. The therapist will ask her parents specific questions regarding Stephanie's home behavior such as, "How many evenings this week did Stephanie feed herself dinner? Did she fasten and unfasten her seat belt on the way to school this morning? Did she pick out the clothes she is wearing? Did she walk with her walker from the car into therapy?" These questions will serve as reminders to the family without being too intrusive or judgmental regarding family values and priorities.

In summary, Stephanie's list of goals addresses impairments in postural control, alignment and weight bearing, selective movement patterns, strength, and endurance underlying her functional limitations in sitting, standing, and hand use. All these goals can be addressed in each treatment session by combining facilitation of components of movement through specific handling and positioning consistent with NDT with the application of the principles of motor learning and motor control utilizing prompting, reinforcing, and the practice of specific tasks in a controlled environment.

ILLUSTRATION OF TREATMENT

It is somewhat artificial to pair each goal with specific treatment tactics because each goal represents one component of the overall approach to the posture and movement problems seen in a child, and treatment methods necessarily overlap among goals. If we accept the premises outlined in Developing a Theoretic Framework, a change in one area of motor control will have a significant effect on other areas. Yet without approaching the problems systematically and attempting to link problems and possible causes with treatment strategies and tactics, therapists will not advance in sorting out effective treatment approaches and "best practice procedures" from those that are less successful.[129, 130] Figure 2–2 illustrates a progression of treatment activities designed to meet the goals described here. Photographs were taken in a single treatment session to show treatment tactics and progression. Notice throughout the series of illustrations how the environment, task, imaginary and real toys, and the therapist actively facilitate achievement of the goals for posture and movement.

Single-Session Evaluation

Each treatment session is structured to include informal, subjective methods to evaluate how effective the treatment was in producing change in the child's posture, movement, and function. The therapist observes a posture, movement component, or function before treatment and again at the end of treatment (Fig. 2–3). By observing changes at the end of a session, it is possible to assess whether the goals for treatment are appropriate, whether the tactics selected are meeting these goals, and what problems continue to exist. The HOAC model suggests that the parents and the child, if appropriate, be involved in deciding whether the goals have been met and whether they see targeted changes in their child's movements and functions. If change has not occurred or the goals have not been met within this treatment session, the therapist and the family must decide if the goal is appropriate, if the treatment strategies and tactics selected are appropriate, and if the means of evaluating outcomes are realistic. Horn showed that when the intervention was focused on movement components used to perform specific actions (defined by NDT), children were able to develop and execute a variety of movement patterns and generalize use of these movement components to functional skills.[131] When this approach is used to evaluate a single treatment session, it helps the therapist to decide which goals and activities to continue and which ones to discard for the next treatment session. Methods to assess longer-term outcomes are described in Evaluation of Outcomes.

Additional Therapeutic Components

Family-Centered Intervention

The involvement of the child's family as active participants is critical to the success of the overall intervention program. To be effective in involving the family in an intervention program, physical therapists must recognize that a family consists of a system of relationships that has undergone an unexpected change with the addition of a child with CP. The needs of the family and their resources to cope with these needs change over time, reflecting both continuity of family development and changes in the structure and function of the family unit.

When planning family-centered physical therapy, the therapist must recognize and accept that children grow up in different subcultures that have their own values, expectations, patterns of interpersonal relationships, manners, and styles of intellectual operations and communications. Programs for groups of culturally distinct or economi-

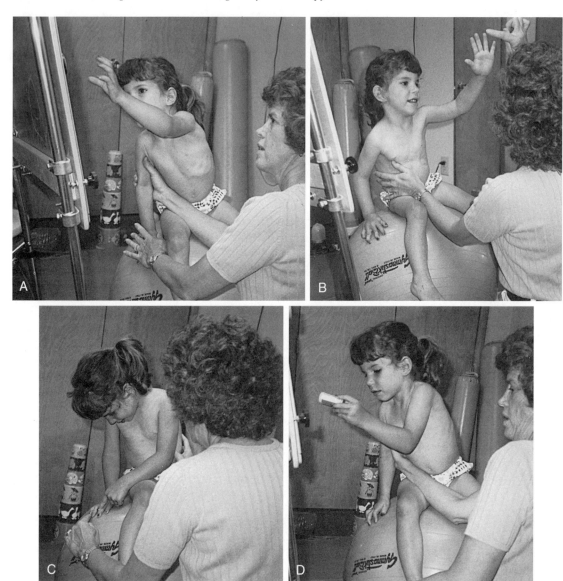

FIGURE 2–2. Treatment. *A,* This day therapy begins on a ball to provide a mobile surface for sitting that makes it possible to adjust weight bearing in sitting and prevent Stephanie from using her habitual pattern of weight bearing to the left. The therapist assists weight bearing on Stephanie's right arm with Stephanie's hand open as Stephanie reaches across her body to remove magnetic pieces from the board. The placement of the easel and magnets is important if Stephanie is to initiate and incorporate trunk rotation into her movement in sitting. The therapist controls the speed, direction, and amount of movement and gauges the level of movement in play that permits these patterns of reaching with trunk rotation to occur naturally. *B,* Once Stephanie has given the therapist the magnetic block, her weight is maintained primarily on her right side and time is taken to "count her fingers," requiring her to hold her left arm elevated in space and pay attention to her hand. The therapist continues to control alignment over the right hip and right arm. Notice Stephanie's open right hand. Head and trunk are properly aligned for visual attention to her hand. *C,* To focus Stephanie's attention on her right hand, the therapist now asks her to count the fingers on her right hand using her left. Movement of her head and trunk as she attends incorporates rotation with extension then flexion. Notice that she is able to maintain her open hand and extended elbow when she is focused and motivated. Her own cognitive and verbal reinforcement are added to maintain the posture that was initially facilitated by the therapist. *D,* Now she is asked to shift her focus once again to place the magnetic piece. Weight bearing on the open hand and alignment are relegated to the background of automatic postural alignment, and her attention is on precise grasp and placement of the toy. (She must place the piece correctly in a circle, square, or triangle that was drawn on the board.)

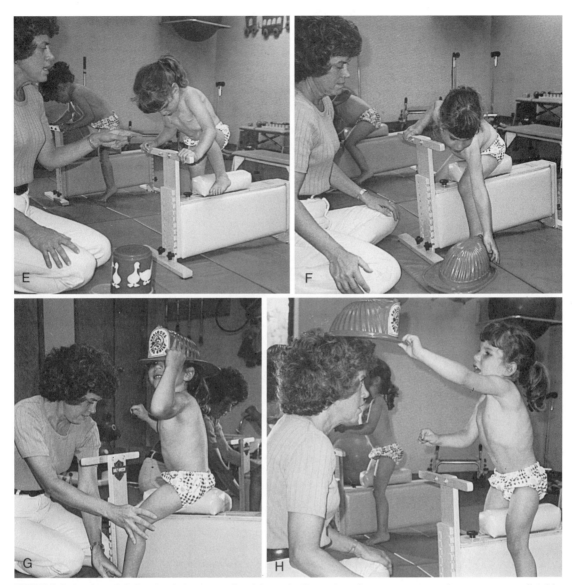

FIGURE 2–2 *Continued. E,* Stephanie is too comfortable on the floor, where her movements and posture are predictable. She needs to develop a greater variety in her movement in the upright position and practice balance against the force of gravity. She asks to wear a firechief's hat. The activity is structured to work on the following neuromuscular impairments: balance in sitting, trunk rotation, weight bearing over her right side (building on the goals in the first activity, *A–D*), independent leg movements, and prevention of breath holding by combining talking and moving. Here the therapist asks her to "climb onto the fire truck." She gets on from the right side, showing extension of her right leg and hip and left knee flexion while taking weight on her right hand and moving her trunk around these support points. *F,* As she reaches down to the left, Stephanie must balance her weight between her right hip and left leg or her body will simply follow her reach and she will fall off the fire truck. Her goal is to get the hat, but she must work equally hard to maintain her seated position as her upper body moves around her base of support. She works for both postural control and active reaching. *G,* After she has achieved her goal, the therapist assists her in placing her feet so she can rise to stand by shifting her weight forward over her feet and stand up without the use of her arms. Independently, Stephanie can get into a standing position only by pulling up with her arms and allowing her legs to follow passively, as shown in Figure 2–1*F* and *G. H,* Rather than manually facilitating a forward weight shift of her trunk over her legs, the therapist moves slightly backward while asking Stephanie to place the firechief's hat on the therapist's head. She follows the therapist's body movement and experiences this movement independent of any physical assistance. The straddle seat controls her tendency to adduct her legs and gives her the security to rise to stand. Notice, however, that the stress of the activity has once again increased the stiffness in her right arm. This sequence has combined active trunk movements of flexion, rotation, and extension with active leg movements, patterns she does not use independently.

Illustration continued on following page

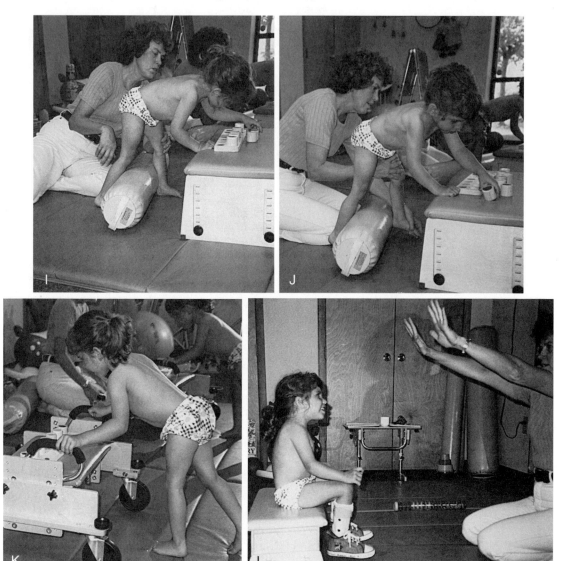

FIGURE 2–2 *Continued. I,* Now that Stephanie has become more active with her legs, the following activities will require her to develop better disassociated movements at the hips in preparation for a longer stride and a weight shift from one leg to the other needed to adjust her posture in standing and while walking. Stephanie is asked to place colored cylinders in matching holes. The placement of the toy requires her to shift her weight from right to left. The therapist places her in step position over a bolster. Throughout the session, the toys, along with imaginary play, are appropriate for her age and development. While she is encouraged to make her own choices and indicate preferences, the possible choices have been preselected to develop a variety of preschool skills. *J,* The therapist rolls the bolster forward and back as she completes the matching, requiring her to shift not only from side to side, but also forward and back from her right foot to her left. She prefers to always have her hips slightly flexed and similarly aligned (see Fig. 2–1*E–G*). This is a difficult position for her to tolerate, and the amount and speed of movement must be carefully graded so she can maintain knee extension and experience weight bearing appropriately from her heels across the metatarsal heads as her weight shifts forward. Notice her feet in Figure 2–1*G* as she stands to play. *K,* Now that she has experienced disassociated movement in the step position, Stephanie has the opportunity to feel this on her own. Walking with her trunk upright is still too difficult if she is expected to take long steps and transfer weight across the foot from heel to toe. She pushes this rolling seat on a mat to give added resistance and slow down her movements. Her weight forward onto her arms aids in trunk symmetry and extension so she needs only to shift her weight from one leg to the other. She "delivers" the completed matching toy, walking slowly so it does not tip over. This demand to avoid tipping the toy gives her time to change her walking pattern to use extension on the weight-bearing side and a longer stride on the swing side than is typical. *L,* Ultimately, Stephanie needs to use her legs for weight bearing and walking and free her arms and hands for skills. Even though she has no balance in standing and cannot walk without a walker, therapy is a time to practice emerging skills. She is asked to touch the therapist's hands, requiring her to lean forward, bringing her pelvis over her femurs and shifting her weight onto her feet.

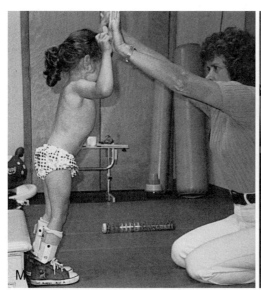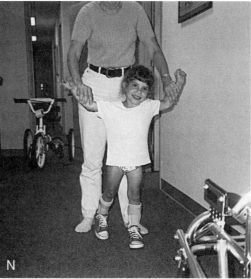

FIGURE 2-2 *Continued. M,* Stephanie rises to stand, pushing down with her legs yet ending with her hands in contact with the therapist's as a support surface for balance. As the therapist pushes against Stephanie's hands, Stephanie must resist collapsing and use her legs to maintain standing. *N,* To give her the feeling of walking without using her arms for support, the therapist uses Stephanie's abducted arms to facilitate her weight shift onto the stance leg while controlling speed to encourage a long step. Shoulder rotation that gives her the appropriate trunk rotation is facilitated. She leaves the therapy room in this way.

cally disadvantaged families have been notable failures when planned by white middle-class professionals, partly because of the lack of attention to individual needs and the failure to understand attitudes of the group to be served.[132–135] Parents of children with disabilities do have specific needs and priorities as well as expectations of the professionals with whom they are involved. Parents want an active role in the rehabilitation process involving their child, a say in decisions concerning the child's program, and information regarding test results and changes in the child's progress and program.[133] Parents generally are becoming more knowledgeable consumers of services they and their children require. Moreover, parental compliance with home programs has been shown to be more strongly related to their relationship with professionals than knowledge of the therapeutic regimen.[134] This focus is consistent with the current emphasis on family-centered services, in which the care offered to families should be concordant with their needs, wishes, and values.

Recognizing and responding to the parents' needs may require the therapist to reorder priorities to initiate realistic plans for meeting the family's goals. The most effective way to influence the development of children is to provide professional support for the parental care of children.[135] If the family's goals are actually detrimental to the child, the therapist may need to seek advice or intervention from a social worker or psychologist to help the family recognize the differences in their need and goals and those that will promote autonomy in their child. The family spends the greatest amount of time with the child; therefore, keeping the total child in mind, it makes sense to teach the parents to understand normal and abnormal development and to make use of the available knowledge about care and management that is pertinent to their child. When beginning family-centered intervention, it is important, when appropriate, to imitate the interactive style of the parents rather than require that the parents give up their accustomed methods of handling their child to follow a prescribed approach that may be incompatible with their own natural style. This way the parents can learn child care routines that will reinforce and maximize the child's skills while continuing to feel adequate as parents.[136] Parents who are taught basic concepts of development and who understand general principles of intervention are equipped to generalize handling and

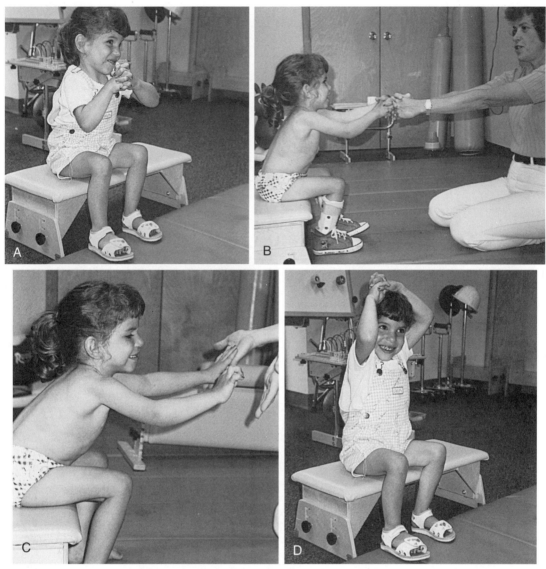

FIGURE 2–3. Treatment evaluation. *A,* Before treatment, Stephanie was asked to clasp her hands, interwining her fingers, and to stretch her hands out in front of her, then raise them over her head (see *D*). The difficulty of this task is evident both in the lack of movement in her arms and hands and in the stress shown on her face. *B,* After therapy she is asked to do the same task. She is much more capable of equal movements of her arms and can extend her right elbow through a greater range, and the motion is performed with less effort. Notice also the improved position of her right scapula and better trunk extension. *C,* She is now asked to do the same activity without the assistance of her left arm. She can now extend the right arm in space, with wrist extension and partial finger extension. Again notice the improved position of her scapula for this task. *D,* Before therapy Stephanie attempts to raise her arms overhead. She is able to get them on top of her head only by bringing her head forward.

teaching techniques to accommodate various situations that arise as the child grows and develops, as well as to assimilate these methods of management into their own parenting style.

Evidence is accumulating that the child's own parents are the best choice as caregivers to facilitate long-term gains.[137] If, however, the internal and external resources of the family are inadequate to provide an optimal learning environment, a parent surrogate can be substituted if the person can provide a stable, stimulating situation.[138] Extended family members and child care personnel are common sources of help. Sparling and colleagues stress that today's contemporary families, which include single-

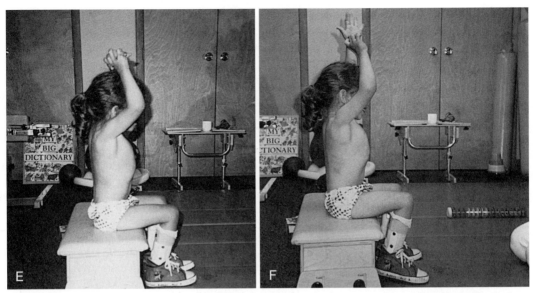

FIGURE 2-3 *Continued. E,* After therapy she attempts the same task. She is now able to extend her arms so that she clears her head. The movement is confined to her shoulders and arms, her back remains extended (notice even some lumbar lordosis), and her head is in line with her body. *F,* Finally, Stephanie is asked to raise both arms above her head without using her left to assist her right. Although she is not able to fully extend the right, her range of motion is more complete, and she is able to open her hand.

parent families and families with dual-career parents, may require identification of support persons with interest in assisting with the responsibilities of child care.[31]

Some of the success of the home management aspect of a family-centered intervention program depends on how effectively the parent is instructed. The initial interaction of parents with the therapist and the therapist's attitude and concern are as important to the overall performance of the parents as are the actual methods of written or oral instructions. Redman-Bentley found that the professional's personal traits are important.[133] Parents preferred a professional who was honest and knowledgeable and who listened to information provided by the parents. King and colleagues found that both mothers and fathers valued the enabling aspects of caregiving and the partnership aspect between the parent and the professional.[139] The physical therapist must realize, in deciding which daily care routines or therapeutic techniques should be included as part of the home program, that parents represent the entire range of social, emotional, and intellectual behaviors. Some parents have high intellect, have good motor skills, and learn easily, but children sometimes have parents who are retarded, emotionally disturbed, alcoholic, or preoccupied with basic physiologic or financial needs. The confluence of stress and support in contemporary families defines the uniqueness of each family and demands an individual approach to addressing a family's needs, concerns, and priorities. Bricker has outlined these various factors for guiding intervention with families experiencing change themselves and change in relation to their children with special needs.[140]

Many therapists have a preconceived notion that managing a child with CP places additional stress on the family, but the validity of this statement is unclear from the literature. Lonsdale interviewed the parents of children with developmental delay about their reactions and the effect of the child on family relationships.[141] More than half the parents interviewed reported marriage difficulties resulting from the birth of the child with a handicap. Floyd and Zmich also reported added stress and negative feelings in families with children with disabilities.[142] High rates of physical and mental ill health among parents of children with disabilities have been reported as well.[143–145] On the other hand, the majority of the studies reviewed by Dunlap and Hollingsworth did not support the perception that having a family member with a disability has a substantial effect on family life.[146] Other investigators have shown that the presence of a child who was developmentally delayed did not appear to change the family routine to any large extent. These studies showed that family unity increased as the family worked together to meet the challenges presented by including a child with a disability as a family member.[147, 148] Taanila and colleagues found that only 7 percent of parents reported a negative effect on their marital relationship.[149] They also reported that adequate information, a realistic notion of the disability, and practical advice for everyday life were protective factors for the marital relationship.

Simeonsson and McHale[150] and, in a separate publication, Stoneman and Berman[151] reviewed the effects of a child with a disability on sibling relationships. These reports demonstrated that there is a great diversity of effects on the sibling relationship. Some studies showed that the presence of a child with a disability in a family results in problems of adjustment and development for siblings,[152] whereas other studies indicate that siblings of children with disabilities may benefit from their experience and are often well adjusted.[153, 154]

What are the implications for the therapist? First, the therapist should not assume that the presence of a child with a disability necessarily disturbs the structure, function, or development of a strong family unit. However the child is perceived by the family, parents are able to accommodate the problems of raising a child with a handicapping condition to a considerable extent and most often assume a successful parenting role with their child.

Second, the therapist must be able to achieve effective parent involvement as appropriate for the individual family. Therapists should not have preconceived ideas about what parents should do for their children but must accept what a parent can do for a child and capitalize on these abilities. The therapist must help the parents put the intervention program into the proper perspective so as not to disturb the parent-child relationship or the family unit and its functions. Focusing attention exclusively on the child's disability may hamper rather than foster overall development and place undue focus on the parent's inability to parent the child with a handicap. All efforts must be made, rather, to stress the competencies of the child and the parents.

Third, therapeutic tactics must be adapted to the skills of the parents and may consequently differ from the techniques and standards the therapist applies to the same activity. Some parents have the time, energy, and skills to carry out complicated therapeutic techniques on a regular basis, whereas other families need constant instruction and support to even modify feeding, dressing, or daily care routines.

Fourth, although there is no prescribed method to ensure successful teaching, methods of instruction include demonstration, written programs, verbal instructions, repetition, and continual support. The intensity of instruction and a need to adhere to a systematic teaching method will vary from family to family. The therapist must be able to evaluate the family's resources and vary the style of instruction, as well as goals for the home program, to meet the constantly changing levels of skill, knowledge, and attitudes of the family.

Finally, the individual family's involvement in an intervention program varies. U.S. laws passed to assist children with disabilities, Public Law 94-142, Public Law 99-457, and Public Law 102-119, have mandated the family's participation in program planning and emphasize the essential role of families in facilitating the development of their children with disabilities. Nevertheless, the extent that any individual family participates in the process may vary based on when they have their initial contact with the intervention program. Parents who have a young baby with suspected CNS dysfunction may not initially see the infant as different from other babies. All babies need to be dressed, bathed, diapered, and loved. The parents, therefore, may not see the need to change their method of caring for their infant, particularly if the child is comfortable in the present interaction and protests with imposition of new positions and movements. On the other hand, parents who first begin therapy with an 18-month-old child diagnosed with CP may be quite anxious to have a role in deciding which activities to do at home to "help their child walk" or achieve some other obviously delayed motor milestone.

The family's involvement with the intervention program varies with the age of the child too. Babies, toddlers, and preschool children generally spend a great deal of time with their own parents and are usually assisted with daily care routines. A number of early-intervention studies have reported that parents' participation might have a greater impact on outcomes for children younger than 3 years of age than for older children.[155] In this preschool age group, parents have the opportunity to provide continued input for facilitating activities involving dressing, feeding, and self-care, as well as functional motor skills. A school-aged child has a greater need for independence and may refuse assistance from a parent once the child has discovered some way to accomplish the task independently. At this point, the parents may be more involved with transporting the child to after-school activities and assisting with homework, and, in their need to be parents, are realistically less involved with therapeutic intervention. This does not mean their role is any less significant, and they continue to advocate for their child. Programs for preteens and teenagers often involve instructing the child to carry out mobilizing techniques independent of adult assistance or stressing recreational activities that encourage mobility and reinforce functional movement. Older teens, headed to college or independent living, must become self-reliant not only in carrying out their physical activities and daily exercises but in recognizing and seeking medical and therapeutic help as needed. They need to be comfortable in calling and scheduling their own appointments and transporting themselves to the appointment and understanding their own medical insurance reimbursement plan. Many children with CP will never achieve this level of independence or assume full responsibility for their lives. However, to the extent possible, this practice should be followed. A child who cannot feed or dress herself can select food and clothes and experience a sense of control in these daily tasks. The family-centered program does not decrease as the child grows older; however, the goals and activities must change and the responsibility for the program shifts from the parents to the child if it is to remain an effective method of intervention.

Adaptive Equipment

Adaptive equipment to increase functional skills has become an integral part of therapeutic, educational, and home management programs for children with CP. Adaptive equipment provides independence from adults for mobility, play, and social interactions and allows the child to discover and test the effects they can have on people and their environment.

Adaptive equipment is frequently used to meet the following goals:

1. To properly position the child so that the child feels secure and motivated to practice newly acquired skills; with such positioning, many children are able to participate in feeding, toileting, grooming, or other self-help skills that would otherwise be impossible.
2. To reduce primary impairment by providing a greater variety of movement experiences and to prevent habit patterns that limit the development of more normal variations of posture and movement.
3. To prevent secondary impairment such as contractures and deformities by positioning a child to prevent the deforming influence.
4. To reinforce normal movement components, providing an opportunity for more normal alignment, weight shift, and postural adjustment during functional movement.
5. To increase the child's opportunity to participate in social interaction and educational programs.
6. To provide mobility and encourage exploration. This is often the goal of providing adapted standard or electric wheelchairs for children who have no other means of mobility or whose movements are so slow that the effort is not worth the goal toward which the movement is directed.

Appropriate equipment provides enough support so that children can direct their energies toward participation in the educational or social environment rather than exclusively toward maintaining posture. This reason alone may warrant the use of adaptive equipment for children with severe disabilities. These children are often unable to experience any degree of interaction or independence in school, recreation centers, or shopping areas without the assistance of adaptive chairs or mobility devices.

Attempts have been made to document changes in posture or function in children using adaptive equipment, particularly mobility aids and seating devices. Several studies have implicated proper seating as an important factor contributing to motor function and voluntary control of the upper extremities in children with CP.[123, 156] Additional studies have shown the importance of sitting erect with the pelvis stable and with the seat horizontal or tilted forward in order to gain postural control or optimal arm and hand function, or both.[157–163] Cristarella also found a more vertical pelvis with normal spinal curves and improved hip and knee position if a child was positioned straddled on a bolster rather than seated on a small chair.[157]

Hulme and colleagues reported on the results of a survey constructed to assess the benefits of adaptive equipment used in the homes of clients who were primarily nonambulatory and multiply handicapped, ranging from 1 to 68 years of age.[164] Adaptive chairs were the most consistently used types of equipment. Significant improvement was noted in social interactions and motor coordination.

Several studies have evaluated the impact of walker design on the mobility of children with CP. These studies compared ambulation abilities of children with CP using standard forward walkers and reverse posture control walkers.[61–63] All three studies found that the use of posterior walkers produced a more upright posture during walking and improved gait characteristics than when using anterior walkers. According to Greiner and colleagues, parents reported that when using the posterior walker their children walked more normally with increased stability and interacted more easily with other children.[63]

Adaptive equipment and mobility aids must meet the needs of the children as they grow, gain better control of their posture and movement, and develop educational and daily living skills (Figs. 2–4 and 2–5). Appropriately selected adaptive equipment allows movement and encourages the children to make postural adaptations necessary in any given situation. It should not restrict the children's movements but rather increase the children's possibilities to practice and use the functional movements that they are developing. It is important to reevaluate the goals for the use of any equipment at regular intervals to make certain the child still needs the equipment to meet the goal and that it is properly adjusted or replaced as the child grows and develops.

Tests for assessing functional changes in children who are using special equipment are now available. The Sitting Assessment for Children with Neuromotor Dysfunction is an observational rating scale that was developed by Reid to assess the quality of sitting at rest and during upper extremity movement.[123, 165, 166] This test consists of two modules, the rest module and the reach module. The items on the rest module assess postural tone, proximal stability, postural alignment, and balance. Items on the reach module assess four components of reaching during sitting. The Seated Postural Control Measure was developed by Fife and colleagues for use with children requiring adaptive seating systems.[167] It is an observational scale of 22 seated postural alignment items and 12 functional movement items, each scored on a four-point, criterion-referenced scale. The Sitting Assessment Scale was developed by Myhr and von Wendt and rates the postural control of the head, trunk, and feet as well as obtaining functional performance measures in a variety of reaching and grasping tasks.[168] These ratings have been shown to be useful in longitudinal assessment of changes produced by seating systems. The Supported Walker Ambulation Performance Scale was developed to measure changes in the locomotor status of children who do not yet walk independently.[169] It consists of four dimensions: support, posture, the quality of steps, and the quantity of steps. The four dimensions are weighted so that support is worth 40 percent and the other three dimensions 20 percent each. Each dimension is scored on a four-point Likert scale. Although this test was not developed with standardization procedures for the use of

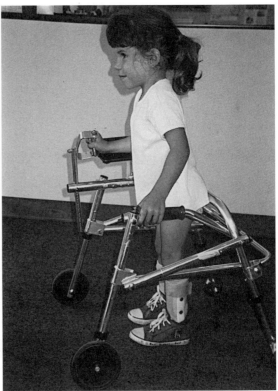

FIGURE 2–4. Stephanie uses a posture control walker to walk at school and in her community. She rarely uses it at home because of space restrictions and the presence of siblings. She uses a forearm support on the right because she is not able to maintain her grasp with her elbow extended when she is walking fast or is excited. She can get into and out of her walker from the floor and walks independently on all terrains. The walker gives her the freedom to keep up with her peers and participate more fully in family outings. A lack of balance in standing prevents her from walking independently from support.

support, it could serve as a tool to assess changes in locomotor status of children who use walkers or crutches even when they do not become independent from support. Finally, the modification scale of the PEDI can also be used to assess the frequency of use of special equipment to promote function.[78]

Casting and Orthoses

Lower extremity orthoses, including tone-reducing plaster casts and polypropylene ankle-foot orthoses (AFOs), are used to reduce primary impairments of abnormal joint motions

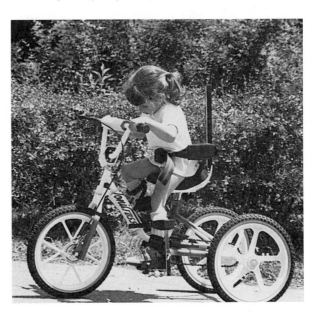

FIGURE 2–5. Stephanie has begun to use a therapeutic tricycle at school to build strength and endurance. The wide base of support, chain drive, and hand brake make it possible for her to do this independently. She cannot get on or off the tricycle by herself, but she is very proud of being able to ride a cycle as her friends do.

including dynamic equinus and abnormal muscle timing to prevent secondary impairment of muscle contracture, and to facilitate function, specifically changing the temporal-distance characteristics of walking and alignment in standing.[120, 170, 171] Short-leg tone-inhibiting casts are designed to maintain normal alignment of the foot and ankle while inhibiting toe grasp and plantar flexion as a habitual or compensatory stabilizing effort.[171–173] Tone-inhibiting casts are used as an adjunct in therapy and during selected intervals of treatment and management at home and school. They are an inexpensive alternative to AFOs and are primarily used with very young children who are first learning to stand and walk. Cusick has written extensively about the use of tone-reducing casts and developed specific criteria for patient selection and use.[174] Casts were implemented when the passive foot and ankle range was complete and only during a closely supervised program of positioning and movement training, when it was be-lieved that gains in movement control could be made faster or sooner if the foot was stabilized in good alignment. Several authors have recommended that inhibitive casts should be replaced by polypropylene inhibitive AFOs when the child with CP begins ambulating.[170, 175, 176]

AFOs are used extensively in children with spastic CP. Many varieties are available and can be constructed based on the biomechanical and functional needs of the child. Solid-ankle orthoses are used if the restriction of ankle motion benefits movement at more proximal joints. Bilateral solid-ankle orthoses are used primarily to develop stability in standing as it is very difficult for a child to develop ambulation with limited motion at the ankles. Hinged-ankle orthoses are usually designed to permit dorsiflexion while inhibiting plantar flexion (Figs. 2–6 and 2–7). Hinged AFOs have been found to produce a reduction in energy expenditure and promote a more natural ankle motion during the stance phase, greater symmetry of lower extremity motion, and more normal knee motion than do solid-ankle orthoses.[177, 178] Wilson and colleagues evaluated the effect of articulating and solid AFOs on the transitional movement of sitting to standing in children with spastic CP.[179] They found that children with uncontrolled dynamic equinus benefited from the use of articulating AFOs because this allowed the children to shift their body weight forward over their feet when rising to stand, which is a necessary movement component in producing this transition.

The use of orthoses in the treatment of children with CP is well accepted but must fit into the overall treatment and assessment plan. The therapist needs to evaluate the specific need for an orthotic device and determine its effectiveness with the same attention to functional goals as any other aspect of the treatment plan. The therapist

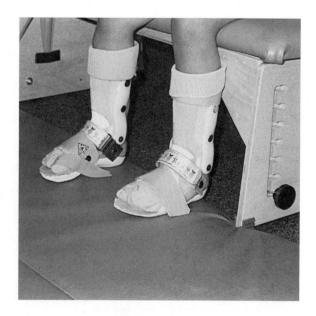

FIGURE 2–6. Stephanie is currently wearing total con-tact hinged ankle-foot orthoses to improve the align-ment of her feet and ankles. Because they restrict floor play and crawling, the decision was made not to use the orthoses at home where her environment is more suited to crawling and floor sitting, but to use them during the school day when she sits on a chair and uses her walker for ambulation.

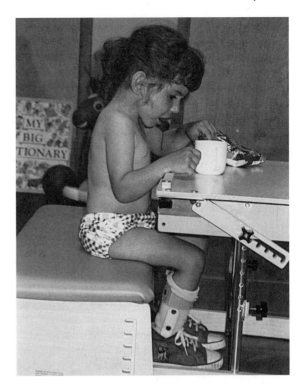

FIGURE 2-7. Stephanie's ankle-foot orthoses provide her with increased stability in sitting and are useful when she is required to use her hands for feeding herself or during preschool activities. In addition, she is better able to rise to standing from a seated position because her orthoses control plantar flexion and maintain the foot and ankle in good alignment.

must know why the orthosis was included in the plan of care and the functions that will change as a result of its use.

Noncompliance regarding the use of orthoses is a common problem. Families who do not understand the rationale for the appliance and do not see any functional difference find the orthoses burdensome. Some equipment is also difficult or costly to maintain or repair. Custom-made total-contact orthoses are outgrown regularly by growing children, and frequent trips to the orthotist can be expensive and time-consuming for working parents. Orthotic devices simply increase their need to attend to those aspects of special care needed by their child. If attentional or financial costs are higher than the motor benefit to the child, the device will not be used. Older children must be consulted before orthoses are considered for inclusion in their program. School-aged children often will not wear appliances to school because they see this as making them different from their peers. The social and psychologic aspects of any treatment method are as important as the therapeutic aspects, which will only be effective if the family and child accept them.

Specialized Treatment

Medical Management

Various drugs have been used over the years to reduce spasticity or control involuntary movement in the child with CP. The objective has been to find substances that normalize the threshold for activation and the input-output relations of the abnormal and generally excessive reflex responses.[180] This is achieved by pharmacologic agents that activate receptors at different sites along the reflex arc to dampen effects of afferent inputs, inhibit or block the excitation of intraspinal neurons, reduce motoneuron output, or lessen muscle contraction. All these drugs have had limited success because of their side effects, which often include sedation and attention and behavioral problems.

More recently, botulinum toxin type A (Botox) and baclofen have been used to control spasticity through reducing muscle or motoneuron activation, respectively. Corry and colleagues reported on a double-blind trial of botulinum toxin type A in the upper limb of children with hemiplegia.[181] They were able to show increased active movement and reduced tone with minimal functional changes in the hand. Several other investigators have injected botulinum toxin type A into the gastrocnemius muscle of children with CP and found positive changes in several parameters of gait, including the stance-phase dorsiflexion range, the step length, and other gait kinematics.[182, 183, 183a] In addition, Koman[184] reported that the use of botulinum toxin type A delayed or prevented orthopedic surgery for heel-cord contracture. The drawbacks to this therapy include repeated painful injections, the cost of the procedure, and variability in gaining the desired effect. Botulinum toxin type A has the advantage of producing a localized muscle effect that can last several months, so it is especially effective for use during periods of training or growth or for preoperative evaluation. Repeated injections can be done on the same muscle group without any apparent side effects.

Baclofen has been shown to be useful in the control of spasticity in children with CP by inhibiting the activation of motoneurons in the spinal cord. Initially baclofen was given orally to reduce spasticity and improve active movement.[102, 185–188] In all studies, side effects of sedation, enuresis, and deterioration in behavior and concentration were reported. Since then, baclofen has been given intrathecally (continuous intrathecal baclofen infusion [CIBI]) with better results and fewer side effects. An intrathecal catheter is typically placed at the level of T12–L1 and connected to a pump placed in a subcutaneous pocket in the abdominal area. CIBI can be titrated for the desired clinical response. Reports have shown decreased upper and lower extremity muscle tone and an increased speed of movement with improvements in self-care skills in children with CP.[103, 189, 190] In another study, Albright and colleagues reported on the use of intrathecal baclofen in children with dystonic CP and found that CIBI reduces generalized dystonia that interfered with care and activities of daily living in these patients.[191] Other investigators reporting on children with severe spastic quadriplegic CP also describe decreased coactivation of antagonist muscles during baclofen administration, decreased spasticity, and greater ease in achieving short-term gains in daily living skills.[103, 190, 192] Almeida and colleagues reported on a 1- and 2-year follow-up on an 11-year-old boy with spastic diplegia.[103] They found that after 2 years, lower extremity ROM was worse than at baseline but that single-joint movement control and independence improved and spasticity decreased. Although this procedure has been clearly shown to reduce spasticity associated with CP, it has not been extensively used, and the long-term gains are unclear. The drawbacks of CIBI include its high cost, extended hospitalization for initial screening procedures, and a high incidence of complications.[192]

Orthopedic Surgery

Orthopedic surgery is an important aspect of the management of the child with CP. The literature describes both soft tissue and bony procedures for the upper extremities, spine, and lower extremities.[49, 119, 193] Soft tissue procedures include muscle lengthening or transfers and tendon lengthening or tenotomies to equalize the effective strength of agonist and antagonist muscles in order to improve the function of the muscle groups around a joint and prevent limitation of movement resulting from neuromuscular impairment.[194, 195] Bony procedures are done to prevent or correct deformities resulting from musculoskeletal impairments and include various procedures to correct malrotation, subluxation, dislocation, or joint instability. General agreement exists that the outcome of surgical treatment of patients with spasticity is more predictable than in children with other types of CP.

Children with hemiplegic CP make up the great majority of children for whom upper extremity surgery is indicated. Age and IQ are not significant factors in surgical decisions as long as the child is old enough to cooperate with the program. Goals for upper extremity surgery include improved functional position of the hand, improved grip strength and dexterity, new functional skills related to everyday activities, and better cosmesis and hygiene.[196–198, 198a]

Surgical management of scoliosis in children with CP is generally considered to be the most difficult problem facing the orthopedic surgeon. Because of the many other problems of CP, scoliosis treatment by conventional means is difficult and presents many postoperative management problems.[193] A report by Dias and colleagues describes the correction of spinal deformities using a unit rod.[199] They found that this method gave the best correction; however, postoperative complications were described as a problem. Harrington rod instrumentation requires prolonged postoperative management in a body cast, a treatment difficult for the child with CP to tolerate.[200, 201] Dwyer instrumentation and anterior fusion are associated with pseudoarthrosis and broken cables.[200] Managing children in body jackets presents many problems including pressure sores. Allen and Ferguson reported on L-rod instrumentation in which L-shaped rods were secured by a sublaminar wire at each vertebra.[202] The advantage of this procedure is that the wire fixation was sufficiently secure so that there was generally no need for a child to wear a postoperative plaster cast or orthosis.

Most orthopedic surgical management involves the lower extremities and ranges from tenotomies, muscle lengthening, and muscle transplants to osteotomies, neurectomies, and fusions. Most procedures are done on children with spastic diplegia. Goals for soft tissue procedures almost always include improving walking and reducing the effects of spasticity at one or more joints to improve or maintain function and prevent secondary deformities. The reported results of various procedures are extremely variable. Truscelli and colleagues suggest that the variation in long-term results depends on differences in underlying pathophysiology rather than differences in surgical techniques.[203] They suggest that there may be a reduction in the number or length of muscle sarcomeres in CP, resulting in varied outcomes after muscle lengthening and immobilization. Castle and associates suggest that abnormalities in the muscle may contribute to variations in the surgical outcome.[204] They demonstrated various degrees and combinations of types I and II muscle fiber atrophy and hypertrophy in children with CP. In order to understand the short- and long-term effects of soft-tissue surgery, it is necessary to understand the mechanics and biology of muscle as well as neural control and the responses of muscles to the various types of procedures.

Neurosurgery

Various neurosurgical procedures have been tried over the years to reduce spasticity in children with CP. In the mid 1970s, Cooper and associates introduced chronic electric stimulation of the cerebellum with the aim of reducing spasticity and improving motor function.[205] Numerous articles have been written on the technique, but controversy over its effectiveness remains.[206, 207] Double-blind studies have produced little support for the stated effects of cerebellar stimulation.[208, 209]

More recently, Peacock and associates introduced selective dorsal rhizotomy (SDR) as a neurosurgical method to permanently reduce spasticity in children with CP.[210, 211] This procedure has now become a viable option for children with spasticity that affects primarily the lower extremities. The goal is to reduce stiffness at the muscle level by reducing the sensory input to the spinal cord from dorsal root afferents. Selective division of dorsal spinal nerve rootlets is believed to balance afferent input against the decrease of normal supraspinal and segmental influences on the motoneuron present in CP. As spasticity is reduced, it is easier for the child to move and improve motor functions. Diminished inhibition of afferent input to motoneurons, however, is not the only effect of the upper motoneuron lesion in CP. Weakness, poor balance and postural control, and impaired selective motor control remain after surgical reduction of spasticity and continue to affect motor function.

Many studies have noted functional improvements in children who have undergone SDR, including improvements in trunk stability, sitting ability, and function of the upper limbs.[211–216] Most recently Yang and colleagues showed significant improvement in static and dynamic sitting stability in 17 children with spastic CP when evaluated 3 months postoperatively.[216a] Gait analysis has shown an increased ROM at the hip, knee, and ankle and increased velocity and stride length.[217–220] Thomas and colleagues evaluated children at 1 and 2 years postoperatively.[217] They demonstrated significant changes in gait kinematics at all three joints with the greatest improvements in the knee and ankle. Similar findings were reported by Boscarino and associates.[221] Thomas and colleagues did not find that changes in joint motion correlate well with changes in the electromyographic response. This may be attributed to continued problems with motor control that prohibit the proper sequencing of muscle action.[222] Problems related to decreased muscle power and sensory changes have been reported but appear to be transient in most children. Green and coworkers reported problems of hip instability after this procedure,[223] but this has not been confirmed by other investigators.[224–227]

The effects of SDR appear to be similar to those produced by CIBI, but the two approaches have different advantages and disadvantages. Albright and colleagues compared the effects of SDR and CIBI on spasticity and concluded that SDR has a more definitive but permanent effect whereas CIBI can be discontinued if results are poor and the drug dosage can be titrated for more selective tone reduction.[228, 229] At the present time, CIBI is much more costly than SDR and appears to have many more postoperative complications related to the delivery pump and need for follow-up.[192]

Therapeutic Electrical Stimulation

Electrical stimulation is receiving renewed attention as a method of treatment to improve muscle power and gait. Therapeutic electrical stimulation (TES) employs a low-intensity stimulation, delivered just above sensory threshold, and does not produce a muscle contraction. It is applied at home during sleep. The recommended treatment is done over a period of 1 to 2 years. This treatment is directed toward improving the growth and thus strength of nonspastic muscles. Pape and Kirsch describe muscle growth as measured by magnetic resonance imaging and hypothesize that the effect of TES is actually mediated by changes in regional blood flow.[230] Most studies describe the use of TES in children with diplegic or hemiplegic CP.[231, 232] In addition, this procedure has been used to treat weakness in children with diplegia after rhizotomy.[233] Functional changes, including changes measured with the GMFM, and improvements in strength and gait parameters are reported.[231–233] Further study is needed to document claims of changes in gait or strength.

EVALUATION OF OUTCOMES

Evaluating treatment outcomes presents a dilemma to those involved in treating children with CP. The dilemma exists because, on the one hand, therapists hold a strong belief that early intervention is essential and effective, but, on the other hand, documenting effectiveness is difficult because of the complex problems characterizing the population. The dilemma is heightened by the fact that the state of the art of patient examination is not far advanced and results of clinical studies present confusing and sometimes contradictory results.[234] The confusion is partly caused by differences among studies in the subject selection, sample size, criteria for diagnosis, rigorousness of experimental design, and methods of evaluating and documenting change. The Gross Motor Function Classification System proposed by Palisano and colleagues will help with the comparability of subject selection in future research.[51] As therapists become more familiar with the HOAC model they will become comfortable hypothesizing which aspects of the child's limitations and impairments they believe will change. Additionally, clear statements of goals, specific methods or tactics, and outcome measures to support their hypotheses set in a realistic time frame will provide objective, reliable information.

Parents and consumer groups as well as funding agencies, however, increasingly demand accountability. Although it may not yet be possible to rigidly apply scales and measurements to quantify program results, efforts must be made to document and compare various strategies of intervention. Numerous measurements of effectiveness have been used to determine the long-term effect of treatment. These measurements include assessment of general motor development,[235, 236] standardized developmental scales,[237] maturation of developmental reflexes,[238, 239] increase in passive joint ROM,[238, 240] the age of onset of walking and the quality of gait,[240] improvements in home management,[241] and changes in functional abilities.[238, 240] Many studies have used multiple measures because it is not clear in which realms changes can be expected.

Reports of Clinical Case Series

The rate of achievement of motor milestones after intervention in children with CP has been reported in the literature.[242] Individual case histories and case review series have been used to evaluate the effectiveness of therapy. Paine presents a case review follow-up study of 117 patients comparing treated and nontreated children from 1930 to 1950.[240] The groups were comparable as to type, the severity of involvement, and intelligence. Outcome assessments included gait, hand use, the presence of contracture, and the frequency of orthopedic surgery. The data presented suggest that intensive physical therapy of the type available from 1930 to 1950 had its chief effect on the patient with moderately severe spastic hemiparesis or quadriparesis, who developed a better gait and had fewer contractures if treated. Among the athetoid patients, no difference in gait or hand function was found. Some data suggested that children with spastic CP who began treatment before 2 years of age had a better outcome.

Köng performed clinical case reviews of 96 children receiving a specific therapeutic approach (Bobath) for at least 1 year.[243] The degree of involvement at the end of the treatment period provided the only basis for comparison, but the degree of involvement before treatment was not described. After 1 to 4 years of treatment, 53 (75 percent) had a normal gait and showed only minimal neurologic signs. No specific tests of outcome were described and no controls were used.

Kanda and associates evaluated the changes in an early-treated versus late-treated group in which the Vojta method of treatment was used.[244] They demonstrated that children treated before 9 months of age walked an average of 8 months earlier than children treated after 9 months of age and had better postural stability during walking. Sixty-three percent of the early-treated group could walk steadily for 30 minutes, compared with 33 percent of the late-treated group. There was no untreated control group. They postulated that early treatment was more effective because it prevented the development of abnormal postures that were otherwise retained when these children learned to walk. This study was notable for attempting to link impairment with functional performance.

Sharkey also reported on the effects of early intervention with respect to the age the child is referred for treatment.[245] Sixty-three children were referred before 9 months of age and were compared with 63 children referred between 9 and 25 months of age. The earlier-referred group showed a faster rate of development in the acquisition of gross motor skills. The rate of development in the areas of self-care and fine motor, cognitive, language, and social-emotional skills favored the early group, but not at a statistically significant level. The intervention was based on NDT and a home program.

Group Comparison Studies of Development and Function

Several attempts have been made to use a more well controlled study design involving a control group. Hochleitner compared groups of children with and without Bobath therapy.[246] Direct matching of the two groups was not attempted; the diagnoses varied, as did the severity and associated disabilities. Results demonstrated a significant reduction in the degree of disability among the treated children in comparison with the control group, but specific outcome measurements were not described.

Wright and Nicholson studied 47 children with spasticity under 6 years of age assigned to immediate-treatment, delayed-treatment, or no-treatment groups.[239] This study showed no evidence after 1 year that physical therapy affected the range of dorsiflexion of the ankle or abduction of the hip or that it had any effect on the retention or loss of primitive reflexes.

Scherzer and colleagues used a double-blind design to study the effects of physical therapy on 22 children with CP who were younger than 18 months of age.[241] The treatment group received a combination of several modalities of NDT physical therapy, and the control group received passive ROM exercises. Assignment to groups was random. The NDT group showed significantly greater improvement in all areas evaluated, including motor development, social maturity, and the ease of home management, than the group receiving ROM exercises.

Some investigators have compared the effects of different methods of providing physical therapy. Ottenbacher and colleagues reported on nine studies that demonstrated a modest gain relative to controls in children who had received NDT either in isolation or in combination with other developmental therapies.[242] Their analysis revealed that the children who received NDT performed slightly better than the control-comparison subjects who did not receive the intervention. Palmer and associates demonstrated that in children with spastic diplegia, intervention after 1 year of age in the form of 6 months of parental training in the facilitation of multiple aspects of development followed by 6 months of NDT was more effective than 12 months of NDT only.[247] Sommerfeld and associates compared the effects of two methods of physical therapy services in 19 students with severe mental impairment and CP.[238] In a school setting, the students were paired by the severity of motor problems and assigned to either a direct therapy group or a supervised therapy management group. A group of 10 students from a school in which there was no physical therapy available served as a control comparison. The results of this study showed no significant differences in the maturity of developmental reflexes, gross motor skills, or passive joint ROM among students placed in direct therapy, supervised management, or comparison groups.

Several studies have attempted to compare the effectiveness of one method of intervention with another. Sparrow and Zigler used three groups, each with 15 institutionalized children with profound mental retardation, to evaluate a modification of the sensorimotor patterning treatment (developed at the Institutes for the Achievement of Human Potential).[237] The treatment group received a program developed after the Institutes for the Achievement of Human Potential method; a matched group participated in motivational activities with the same duration and intensity. A no-treatment group received the standard care of the institution. A wide variety of behavioral measurements were used. On the majority of outcome measurements, no differences in posttest performance among the three groups were found. All three groups showed some improvement in performance between the beginning and the end of the study.

D'Avignon and colleagues studied three groups of children who showed early signs of CNS dysfunction before 6 months of age in order to compare the effectiveness of early physical therapy according to Bobath or Vojta versus development in a control group.[248] Of the total group of 30 children, an evaluation at 33 months to 6 years of age showed 15 children with CP and 15 who were considered normal. Vojta's criteria for "complicated" CP (with sensory problems, seizures, or mental retardation) and "uncomplicated" CP were used for comparison of the outcome severity among the three experimental groups. The number of children with uncomplicated CP was higher in the Vojta group; however, the difference among groups was not significant. The intervention for the treated groups is not clearly described, and the control group received "a less strictly performed and combined form of physiotherapy."

Abdel-Salam and colleagues compared the effects of physical therapy on seven children with infantile spastic CP with those on seven children with postencephalitic spastic paralysis.[249] Both groups received the same therapeutic intervention. After 4 months, the group with infantile spastic CP showed significant improvement in function, as measured by a decreased time to begin a movement and increased tempo of the movement, as well as improvement in activities of daily living and perceptual motor performance (as measured by tests devised by the researchers) relative to the group with postencephalitic spastic paralysis.

Bower and associates reported changes in 44 children with quadriplegic CP who were randomized into four treatment groups.[128] The intensity of physical therapy was varied as well as the specificity of measurable goals. Changes in motor skills were measured with the GMFM. Eighty-two percent of the children improved. Over a 2-week period, intensive 1-hour-daily physical therapy produced a slightly greater effect than conventional physical therapy, 1 to 3 hours per week. The factor more strongly associated with increased motor skill acquisition, however, was the use of specific measurable goals.

Single-Case Studies

Single-case research designs and case reports have been used to evaluate both long-term and immediate effects of intervention. Horn and associates used a single-subject design that combined behavioral analysis to address "how to teach" with NDT to address "what to teach."[131] This study reported a positive outcome in the motor skills of four children with CP treated in an educational setting. The children demonstrated the movement component addressed in treatment both in a treated skill and in a generalized skill. This work is particularly important because the model demanding an assessment strategy to show the generalization of treatment effects to a functional outcome is an important innovation. In addition, all four children improved with an NDT approach using this goal-setting and generalization strategy. This study is a significant step in demonstrating positive outcomes with a specific therapeutic approach (NDT) and generalization of treatment effects to changes in functional skills.

Jonsdottir and colleagues investigated the effect of two different treatment interventions, NDT and practice, on postural control of children with CP during a reaching task.[250] The eight children were treated daily for 5 days with NDT and 5 days with practice. Postural displacement during reaching and postural alignment were evaluated using the Posture Assessment Scale. No difference in postural displacement was noted for either treatment condition; however, there was a significant improvement in postural alignment after NDT.

Using a single-case study design, Watube and associates used serial photographs to document changes in posture and gait in a child with spastic diplegic CP during the course of a single treatment session.[251] Palisano, using a single-case experimental design, used surface electrode electromyographic recording to demonstrate changes in the phasing of muscle activity during the walking of a 10-year-old child with spastic diplegia after a 1-hour treatment session using neurodevelopmental techniques (Bobath).[252] In both these studies, changes in gait could be identified immediately after therapy.

Almeida and colleagues published a case report of an 11-year-old boy with spastic diplegia that used multiple measures, including the GMFM, before and after the implantation of an indwelling system for intrathecally administered baclofen.[103] After 1 and 2 years on CIBI, GMFM scores were higher than at baseline, and single-joint movement control and functional independence improved. The ROM, however, was worse than at baseline.

Studies of Strength and Fitness

Interest in the importance of fitness in children and adolescents with CP has produced studies evaluating strength-training programs and associated functional changes in CP. Parker and colleagues reported on a study to determine whether performance on the GMFM was related to the physiologic fitness of 15 boys and girls between the ages of 7 and 14 years.[70] They found a good relationship between the standing and walking and the running and jumping dimension scores and anaerobic performance of the legs. MacPhail and Kramer investigated changes in knee extensor and flexor strength of 17 adolescents with mild CP in response to an 8-week strength-training program.[253] Peak torque and work were used as strength outcome measures. Strength gains of 25 percent were observed and were similar to those reported for able-bodied individuals undergoing strength training. The walking velocity and efficiency were unchanged. Damiano and associates reported on changes in strength in 14 ambulatory children with spastic diplegic CP who participated in a strengthening program to decrease knee crouch during walking.[117] A normal comparison group of 25 children was tested under identical conditions. When the program began, the children with CP were significantly weaker in the quadriceps and hamstrings muscle groups than the controls. At the end of the program the strength gains in the children with CP did not differ statistically from normal and the stride length improved.

Although the evidence is still not strong, research studies that have been published since the early 1990s point directly to positive outcomes related to physical therapy intervention. The need to document changes in children as a function of a specified intervention still exists in order to distinguish what changes therapies make in children beyond the effects of maturation, to measure the effects of alternative treatments directed at the same problems, and to compare standard intervention with new approaches.[95] Palisano and colleagues suggest that the identification of appropriate outcome variables, defined with reliable and valid measures that link impairment, functional limitations, and disability in daily life, is needed.[130] The results of studies using multidimensional assessment, such as the case report by Almeida and associates, which employed variables from these three dimensions of disability, could answer questions of efficacy and effectiveness of physical therapy in improving the quality of life of children with CP and their families.

LOOKING TO THE FUTURE

The treatment of the child with CP presents an ongoing challenge to the physical therapist. First, intensive care of newborn infants is changing this population and their presenting symptoms. Second, exciting work by Prechtl and coworkers allows earlier identification of infants who might profit from treatment,[24] and clearer classification systems like the one described by Palisano and colleagues[51] allows the recognition of varied levels of motor impairment and function to promote the ease of comparison of outcomes among various studies. Third, better understanding of motor development, motor control, and motor learning has expanded our basis for developing testable theories. Fourth, disability models such as the one described by the National Center for Medical Rehabilitation Research can serve as a framework to describe disability, functional limitations, and underlying neuromuscular and musculoskeletal impairments. Finally, a conceptual model such as the HOAC places greater responsibility on the physical therapist to base examination and treatment planning on sound decision theory. Nevertheless, a lack of systematic, longitudinal data on the development of children with disabilities, a lack of clear documentation of research outcomes, and a lack of defined strategies to measure developmental changes related to programming limit the ability of therapists to engage in evidence-based practice. Therapists should accept the following challenges as we look to a new decade and the new millennium:

1. Clearly define in functional terms the outcomes that we expect.
2. Identify the processes by which we improve function, describing both what we do and how we do it.
3. Recognize and separate what we *know* from what we *believe* without being overcommitted to either one.
4. Communicate thoughtfully with parents, physicians, health care providers, and other professionals, making clear distinctions about what we believe and what we know.
5. Accept the challenge presented by new theories and integrate these new ideas with current standards of practice.
6. Question openly, without judgment, new ideas, theories, and strategies, recognizing that we don't yet have all the answers.
7. Submit what we believe is true to the rigors of experimental research.
8. Abandon adherence to one method, strategy, or approach and broaden our intervention base.
9. Question and test, formally and informally, our beliefs that treatment is making a meaningful change.

10. Listen carefully to what families and children "who have been there" say in regard to what made a difference in their lives.
11. Respect the priorities and values of children and their families living with disabilities.

Therapists who believe that intervention is effective and essential must assume the professional responsibility to document treatment methodology and resulting changes in motor outcomes. Only through objectively documenting these changes will the treatment of children with CP advance. As caring professionals, we have ahead of us the important task of documenting support for our strong commitment to the improvement of function of children with physical disabilities

REFERENCES

1. Bax MC: Terminology and classification of cerebral palsy. Dev Med Child Neurol 6:295, 1964.
2. Campbell SK: Therapy programs for children that last a lifetime. Phys Occup Ther Pediatr 17(1):1, 1997.
3. Baroff GS: Developmental Disabilities. Psychosocial Aspects. Pro-Ed, Austin, Tex, 1991.
4. Olney SJ, Wright MJ: Cerebral palsy. *In* Campbell SK, Vander Linden DW, Palisano RJ (eds): Physical Therapy for Children. WB Saunders, Philadelphia, 1994, p 489.
5. Pape K, Wigglesworth J: Haemorrhage, Ischaemia and the Perinatal Brain. Clinics in Developmental Medicine 69/70. JB Lippincott, Philadelphia, 1979.
6. Vulpe JJ: Neurology of the Newborn, 3rd ed. WB Saunders, Philadelphia, 1995.
7. Capute AJ, Accardo PJ: Developmental Disabilities in Infancy and Childhood. Paul H Brookes, Baltimore, 1991.
8. Hagberg B, Hagberg G, Olow I, von Wendt L: The changing panorama of cerebral palsy in Sweden. The birth year period 1979–82. Acta Paediatr Scand 78:283, 1989.
9. Meberg A, Broch H: A changing pattern of cerebral palsy: Declining trends for incidence of cerebral palsy in the 20 year period 1970–89. J Prenatal Med 23:395, 1995.
10. Nottidge VC, Okogbom ME: Cerebral palsy in Ibadan, Nigeria. Dev Med Child Neurol 33:241, 1991.
11. Forfar JO: Low birthweight and disability. Scand J Rehabil 2:163, 1996.
12. Hagberg B, Hagberg G: The origins of cerebral palsy. *In* David TJ (ed): Recent Advances in Pediatrics. Churchill Livingstone, New York, 1993.
13. Pharoah POD, Cooke T, Cooke RWI, Rosenbloom L: Birthweight trends in cerebral palsy. Arch Dis Child 65:602, 1990.
14. Zupan V, Gonzalez P, Lacaze-Masmonteil T, et al: Periventricular leukomalacia: Risk factors revisited. Dev Med Child Neurol 38:1061, 1996.
15. Kuban KCK, Leviton A: Cerebral palsy. N Engl J Med 330:188, 1994.
16. Okumura A, Hayakawa F, Kato K, et al: MRI findings in patients with spastic cerebral palsy: Correlation with gestational age at birth. Dev Med Child Neurol 39:363, 1997.
17. Campbell S, Wilhelm I: Development of infants at risk for central nervous system dysfunction: Progress report. *In* Slaton DS, Wilson JM (eds): Caring for Special Babies. Division of Physical Therapy, University of North Carolina at Chapel Hill, Chapel Hill, NC, 1983, p 96.
18. Roth SC, Baudin J, Pezzani-Goldsmith M, et al: Relation between neurodevelopmental status of very preterm infants at one and eight years. Dev Med Child Neurol 36:1049, 1994.
19. Hadders-Algra M, Klip-Vanden Nieuwendijk A, Martijn A, van Eyhern LA: Assessment of general movements: Towards a better understanding of a sensitive method to evaluate brain function in young infants. Dev Med Child Neurol 39:89, 1997.
20. Kahn-D'Angelo L: The special care nursery. *In* Campbell SK, Vander Linden DW, Palisano RJ (ed): Physical Therapy for Children. WB Saunders, Philadelphia, 1994, p 787.
21. Piper MC, Darrah J: Motor Assessment of the Developing Infant. WB Saunders, Philadelphia, 1994.
22. Chandler L, Andrews M, Swanson M: Movement Assessment of Infants. Infant Movement Research, Rolling Bay, Wash, 1980.
23. Prechtl HFR: Qualitative changes in spontaneous movements in fetus and preterm infants are a marker of neurological dysfunction. Early Hum Dev 23:151, 1990.
24. Prechtl HFR, Einspieler C, Cioni G, et al: An early marker for neurological deficits after perinatal brain lesions. Lancet 349:1361, 1997.
25. Ellenberg J, Nelson K: Early recognition of infants at high risk for cerebral palsy: Examination at age four months. Dev Med Child Neurol 23:705, 1981.
26. Nelson KB, Ellenberg J: Neonatal signs as predictors of cerebral palsy. Pediatrics 64:225, 1979.

27. Dubowitz LMS, Dubowitz V, Palmer PG, et al: Correlation of neurologic assessment in the preterm newborn infant with outcome at 1 year. J Pediatr 105:452, 1984.
28. Allen MC, Capute AJ: Neonatal neurodevelopmental examination as a predictor of neuromotor outcome in premature infants. Pediatrics 83:498, 1989.
29. Allen MC, Alexander GR: Using motor milestones as a multistep process to screen preterm infants for cerebral palsy. Dev Med Child Neurol 39:12, 1997.
30. Harris SR: Early detection of cerebral palsy: Sensitivity and specificity of two motor assessment tools. J Perinatol 7:11, 1987.
31. Sparling JW, Kolobe THA, Ezzelle L: Family-centered intervention. *In* Campbell SK, Vander Linden DW, Palisano RJ (eds): Physical Therapy for Children. WB Saunders, Philadelphia, 1994, p 823.
32. Minear WI: A classification of cerebral palsy. Pediatrics 18:841, 1956.
33. Feldman RG, Young RR, Koella WP: Spasticity: Disordered Motor Control. Year Book Medical, Chicago, 1980.
34. Campbell SK: Central nervous system dysfunction in children. *In* Campbell SK (ed): Pediatric Neurologic Physical Therapy, 2nd ed. Churchill Livingstone, New York, 1991, p 1.
35. Forssberg H, Hirschfeld (eds): Movement Disorders in Children. Karger, Basel, 1992.
36. Krageloh-Mann I, Hagberg G, Meisner C, et al: Bilateral spastic cerebral palsy—A comparative study between south-west Germany and western Sweden. II: Epidemiology. Dev Med Child Neurol 36:473, 1994.
37. Torner JC: Designing outcome studies in cerebral palsy. *In* Sussman MD (ed): The Diplegic Child. American Academy of Orthopedic Surgeons, Rosemont, Ill, 1992, p 117.
38. Okumura A, Kato T, Kuno K, et al: MRI findings in patients with spastic cerebral palsy. II: Correlation with type of cerebral palsy. Dev Med Child Neurol 39:369, 1997.
39. Fletcher NA, Marsden CD: Dyskinetic cerebral palsy: A clinical and genetic study. Dev Med Child Neurol 38:873, 1996.
40. Yokochi K, Shimabukurok S, Kodama M, et al: Motor function of infants with athetoid cerebral palsy. Dev Med Child Neurol 35:909, 1993.
41. Foley J: The athetoid syndrome. A review of a personal series. J Neurol Neurosurg Psychiatr 46:289, 1983.
42. Foley J: Dyskinetic and dystonic cerebral palsy and birth. Acta Paediatr Scand 81:57, 1992.
43. Yokochi K, Aiba K, Kodama M, Fujimoto S: Magnetic resonance imaging in athetotic cerebral palsied children. Acta Paediatr Scand 80:818, 1991.
44. Cote L, Crucher MD: The basal ganglia. *In* Kandel E, Schwartz JH, Jessell TM (eds): Principles of Neuroscience, 3rd ed. Elsevier, New York, 1991, p 647.
45. Guyton AC, Hall JE: The cerebellum, the basal ganglia, and overall motor control. *In* Textbook of Medical Physiology, 9th ed. WB Saunders, Philadelphia, 1996, p 715.
46. Esscher E, Lodmark O, Hagberg G, Hagberg B: Non-progressive ataxia: Origins, brain pathology and impairments in 78 Swedish children. Dev Med Child Neurol 38: 285, 1996.
47. Shumway-Cook A, Woollacott M: Physiology of motor control. *In* Motor Control, Theory and Practical Applications. Williams & Wilkins, Baltimore, 1995, p 45.
48. Lesny IA: Follow-up study of hypotonic forms of cerebral palsy. Brain Dev 1:87, 1979.
49. Bleck EE: Orthopedic Management in Cerebral Palsy. Clinics in Developmental Medicine 99/100. JB Lippincott, Philadelphia, 1987.
50. Jarvis S, Hey E: Measuring disability and handicap due to cerebral palsy. *In* Stanley F, Alberman E (eds): The Epidemiology of the Cerebral Palsies. Clinics in Developmental Medicine 87. JB Lippincott, Philadelphia, 1984.
51. Palisano R, Rosenbaum P, Walter S, et al: The development and reliability of a system to classify gross motor function in children with cerebral palsy. Dev Med Child Neurol 39:214, 1997.
52. Keshner EA: How theoretical framework biases evaluation and treatment. *In* Lister MJ (ed): Contemporary Management of Motor Control Problems. Proceedings of the II Step Conference. Foundation for Physical Therapy, Alexandria, Va, 1991, p 37.
53. Horak FB: Assumptions underlying motor control for neurologic rehabilitation. *In* Lister MJ (ed): Contemporary Management of Motor Control Problems. Proceedings of the II Step Conference. Foundation for Physical Therapy, Alexandria, Va, 1991, p 11.
54. Heriza C: Motor development: Traditional and contemporary theories. In Lister MJ (ed): Contemporary Management of Motor Control Problems. Proceedings of the II Step Conference. Foundation for Physical Therapy, Alexandria, Va, 1991, p 99.
55. Thelen E, Kelso JAS, Fogel A: Self-organizing systems and infant motor development. Dev Rev 7:39, 1987.
56. Campbell S: The child's development of functional movement. *In* Campbell SK, Vander

Linden DW, Palisano RJ (eds): Physical Therapy for Children. WB Saunders, Philadelphia, 1994, p 3.

57. Bly L: Motor Skills Acquisition in the First Year. An Illustrated Guide to Normal Development. Therapy Skill Builders, Tucson, Ariz, 1994.

58. McClenaghan BA, Thombs L, Milner M: Effects of seat surface inclination on postural stability and function of the upper extremity of children with cerebral palsy. Dev Med Child Neurol 34:40, 1992.

59. Seeger BR, Caudrey DS, O'Mara NA: Hand function in cerebral palsy: The effect of hip-flexion angle. Dev Med Child Neurol 26:601, 1984.

60. Carlson SJ, Ramsey C: Assistive Technology. *In* Campbell SK, Vander Linden DW, Palisano RJ (eds): Physical Therapy for Children. WB Saunders, Philadelphia, 1994, p 621.

61. Logan L, Byers-Hinley K, Ciccone C: Anterior vs posterior walkers for children with cerebral palsy: A gait analysis study. Dev Med Child Neurol 32:1044, 1990.

62. Levangie P, Chimera M, Johnston M, et al: Effects of posture control walker versus standard rolling walker on gait characteristics of children with spastic cerebral palsy. Phys Occup Ther Pediatr 9(4):1, 1989.

63. Greiner BM, Czerniecki JM, Deitz JC: Gait parameters of children with spastic diplegia: A comparison of effects of posterior and anterior walkers. Arch Phys Med Rehabil 74:381, 1993.

64. Guiliani C: Theories of motor control: New concepts for physical therapy. In Lister MJ (ed): Contemporary Management of Motor Control Problems. II Step Conference. Foundation for Physical Therapy, Alexandria, Va, 1991, p 29.

65. Bobath B: Motor development: Its effect on general development and application to the treatment of cerebral palsy. Physiotherapy 57:526, 1971.

66. Bobath K: A neurological basis for the treatment of cerebral palsy. Clinics in Developmental Medicine 75. JB Lippincott, Philadelphia, 1980.

67. Massery MH, Moerchen V: Coordinating transitional movements and breathing in patients with neuromotor dysfunction. NDTA Network Nov/Dec:1, 1996.

68. Stout JL: Physical fitness during childhood and adolescence. *In* Campbell SK, Vander Linden DW, Palisano RJ (eds): Physical Therapy for Children. WB Saunders, Philadelphia, 1994, p 127.

69. Duffy CM, Hill AE, Cosgrove AP, et al: Energy consumption in children with spina bifida and cerebral palsy: A comparative study. Dev Med Child Neurol 38:238, 1996.

70. Parker DF, Carriere L, Hehestreit H, et al: Muscle performance and gross motor function of children with spastic cerebral palsy. Dev Med Child Neurol 35:17, 1993.

71. Vulpe S: Vulpe Assessment Battery: Developmental Assessment, Performance Analysis, Individualized Programming for the Atypical Child. National Institute on Mental Retardation, Toronto, Ontario, 1977.

72. Bradley N: Motor control: Developmental aspects of motor control in skill acquisition. *In* Campbell SK, Vander Linden DW, Palisano RJ (eds): Physical Therapy for Children. WB Saunders, Philadelphia, 1994, p 39.

73. Prechtl HFR, Nolte R: Motor behavior of preterm infants. *In* Prechtl HFR (ed): Continuity of Neural Functions from Prenatal to Postnatal Life. Clinics in Developmental Medicine 94. JB Lippincott, Philadelphia, 1984, p 79.

74. Rothstein JM, Echternoch JL: Hypothesis-oriented algorithm for clinicians: A method for evaluation and treatment planning. Phys Ther 66:1388, 1986.

75. Russell D, Rosenbaum P, Gowland C, et al: Gross Motor Function Measure Manual, 2nd ed. McMaster University, Hamilton, Ontario, 1993.

76. Boyce C, Gowland PL, Rosenbaum M, et al: The Gross Motor Performance Measure: Validity and responsivity of a measure of quality of movement. Phys Ther 75:603, 1995.

77. Russell D, Rosenbaum P, Codman D, et al: The Gross Motor Function Measure: A means to evaluate the effects of physical therapy. Dev Med Child Neurol 31:341, 1989.

78. Haley SM, Coster WJ, Ludlow LH, et al: The Pediatric Evaluation of Disability Inventory: Development Standardization and Administration Manual. New England Medical Center, Boston, 1992.

79. Feldman AB, Haley SM, Coryell J: Concurrent and construct validity of the Pediatric Evaluation of Disability Inventory. Phys Ther 76:602, 1990.

80. Wright FV, Boschen KA: The Pediatric Evaluation of Disability Inventory (PEDI): Validation of a new functional assessment outcome instrument. Can J Rehabil 7:41, 1993.

81. Nichols DS, Case-Smith J: Reliability and validity of the Pediatric Evaluation of Disability Inventory. Pediatr Phys Ther 8:15, 1996.

82. Bailey DB, Worley MR: Teaching Infants and Preschoolers with Handicaps. Charles E Merrill, Columbus, Ohio, 1984.

83. Johnson-Martin N, Jens KG, Attermeier SM: The Carolina Curriculum for Handicapped Infants and Infants at Risk. Paul H Brookes, Baltimore, 1986.

84. Johnson-Martin N, Attermeier SM, Hacker B: The Carolina Curriculum for Preschoolers with Special Needs. Paul H Brookes, Baltimore, 1990.

85. Nashner LM, Shumway-Cook A, Marin O: Stance posture control in select groups of children with cerebral palsy: Deficits in sensory organization and muscular coordination. Exp Brain Res 49:393, 1983.

86. Tscharnuter I: A new therapy approach to movement organization. Phys Occup Ther Pediatr 13(2):19, 1993.

87. Bobath K, Bobath B: The neuro-developmental treatment. *In* Scrutton D (ed): Management of the Motor Disorders of Children with Cerebral Palsy. Clinics in Developmental Medicine 90. JB Lippincott, Philadelphia, 1984, p 6.

88. Saint-Anne Dargassies S: Neurological Development in the Full-term and Premature Neonate. Excerpta Medica, New York, 1977.

89. Amiel-Tison C: Neurological evaluation of the maturity of newborn infants. Arch Dis Child 43:89, 1968.

90. McKinly JC, Berkowitz NJ: Quantitative studies on human muscle tonus: A description of methods. Arch Neurol Psychol 19:1036, 1982.

91. Stillwell DM, Gersten JW: Effect of ischemia and curare on spasticity. Arch Phys Med 37:533, 1956.

92. Prechtl H: The Neurological Examination of the Full-Term Newborn Infant, 2nd ed. Clinics in Developmental Medicine 63. JB Lippincott, Philadelphia, 1977.

93. Dubowitz L, Dubowitz V: The Neurological Assessment of the Preterm and Full-term Newborn Infant. Clinics in Developmental Medicine 79. JB Lippincott, Philadelphia, 1981.

94. Bohannon RW, Smith MB: Interrater reliability of a modified Ashworth scale of muscle spasticity. Phys Ther 67:206, 1987.

95. Campbell SK: Quantifying the effects of interventions for movement disorders resulting from cerebral palsy. J Child Neurol 11(suppl 1):S61, 1996.

96. Shepherd RB: Physiotherapy in Paediatrics, 2nd ed. Heinemann, London, 1980.

97. Chan SWY: Motor and sensory deficits following a stroke: Relevance to a comprehensive evaluation. Physiother Can 38:29, 1986.

98. Brunnstrom S: Movement Therapy in Hemiplegia—A Neurophysiological Approach. Harper & Row, Hagerstown, Md, 1970.

99. Corcos DM, Gottlieb GL, Penn RD, et al: Movement deficits caused by hyperexcitable stretch reflexes in spastic humans. Brain 109:1043, 1986.

100. Sahrmann SA, Norton BJ: The relationship of voluntary movement to spasticity in the upper motor neuron syndromes. Ann Neurol 2:460, 1977.

101. Bohannon RW, Andrew AW: Correlation of knee extensor muscle torque and spasticity with gait seen in patients with stroke. Arch Phys Med Rehabil 71:330, 1990.

102. McLellan DL: Co-contraction and stretch reflex in spasticity during treatment with baclofen. Neurol Neurosurg Psychiatry 40:30, 1973.

103. Almeida GL, Campbell SK, Girolami GL, et al: Multi-dimensional assessment of motor function in a child with cerebral palsy following intrathecal administration of baclofen. Phys Ther 77:751, 1997.

104. Knutsson E, Martensson A: Dynamic motor capacity in spastic paresis and its relation to prime mover dysfunction, spastic reflexes and antagonist co-activation. Scand J Rehabil Med 12:93, 1980.

105. Leonard CT, Moritani T, Hirschfeld H, Forssberg H: Deficits in reciprocal inhibition of children with cerebral palsy as revealed by H reflex testing. Dev Med Child Neurol 32:974, 1990.

106. Molnar G: Motor deficit of retarded infants and young children. Arch Phys Med 55:393, 1974.

107. Barnes M, Crutchfield C, Heriza C: The Neurophysiological Basis of Patient Treatment. Reflexes in Motor Development. Stokesville, Morgantown, W Va, 1978.

108. Capute AJ, Accardo PJ, Vining EP, et al: Primitive Reflex Profile. University Park, Baltimore, 1978.

109. Fetters L: Cerebral palsy: Contemporary treatment concepts. In Lister MJ (ed): Contemporary Management of Motor Control Problems. Proceedings of the II Step Conference. Foundation for Physical Therapy, Alexandria, Va, 1991, p 219.

110. Horak F, Shupert C: The role of the vestibular system in postural control. In Herdman S (ed): Vestibular Rehabilitation. FA Davis, Philadelphia, 1994, p 72.

111. Nashner LM: Sensory, neuromuscular, and biomechanical contributions to human balance.

In Duncan P (ed): Balance: Proceedings of the APTA Forum. American Physical Therapy Assoc, Alexandria, Va, 1989, p 5.

112. Lee DN, Aronson E: Visual proprioceptive control of standing in human infants. Percept Psychophysiol 15:529, 1974.

113. Jouen F: Early visual-vestibular interactions and postural development. *In* Block H, Bertenthal BI (eds): Sensory-motor Organizations and Development in Infancy and Early Childhood. Kluwer, Dordrecht, 1990, p 199.

114. Butterworth G, Hicks L: Visual proprioception and postural stability in infancy. Perception 6:255, 1978.

115. Bohannon RW: Hand-held compared with isokinetic dynamometry for measurement of static knee extension torque. Clin Physiol Measure 11:217, 1990.

116. Goskings GP, Bhat US, Dubowitz V, Edwards RHT: Measurements of muscle strength and performance in children with normal and diseased muscle. Arch Dis Child 51:957, 1976.

117. Damiano D, Vaughan CL, Abel MF: Muscle response to heavy resistance exercise in children with spastic cerebral palsy. Dev Med Child Neurol 37:731, 1995.

118. Campbell SK, Gardner HG, Ramakrishnan V: Correlates of physician's decisions to refer children with cerebral palsy to physical therapy. Dev Med Child Neurol 37:1062, 1995.

119. Samilson R (ed): Orthopaedic Aspects of Cerebral Palsy. Clinics in Developmental Medicine 52/53. JB Lippincott, Philadephia, 1975.

120. Radtka S, Skinner SR, Dixon DM, Johanson ME: A comparison of gait with solid, dynamic and no ankle-foot orthoses in children with spastic cerebral palsy. Phys Ther 77:4, 1997.

121. Hainsworth F, Harrison MJ, Sheldon TA, et al: A preliminary evaluation of ankle orthoses in the management of children with cerebral palsy. Dev Med Child Neurol 39:243, 1997.

122. Berry E, McLauren SE, Sparling JW: Parent/caregiver perspectives on the use of power wheelchairs. Pediatr Phys Ther 8:146, 1996.

123. Reid DL: The effect of the saddle seat on seated postural control and upper extremity movement in children with cerebral palsy. Dev Med Child Neurol 38:805, 1996.

124. Pellegrion L: Cerebral palsy: A paradigm for developmental disabilities. Dev Med Child Neurol 37:834, 1995.

125. McCuaig M, Frank G: The able self: Adaptive patterns and choices in independent living for a person with cerebral palsy. Am J Occup Ther 45:224, 1992.

126. Stevenson CJ, Pharoah POD, Stevenson R: Cerebral palsy—The transition from youth to adulthood. Dev Med Child Neurol 39:336, 1997.

127. Effgen SK: The educational environment. *In* Campbell SK, Vander Linden DW, Palisano RJ (eds): Physical Therapy for Children. WB Saunders, Philadelphia, 1994, p 847.

128. Bower E, McLellan DL, Arney J, Campbell MJ: A randomized controlled treatment of different intensities of physiotherapy and different goal-setting procedures in 44 children with cerebral palsy. Dev Med Child Neurol 38:226, 1996.

129. Embrey DG, Yates L, Nirider B, et al: Recommendations for pediatric physical therapists: Making clinical decisions for children with cerebral palsy. Pediatr Phys Ther 8:165, 1996.

130. Palisano RJ, Campbell SK, Harris SR: Clinical decision making in pediatric physical therapy. *In* Campbell SK, Vander Linden DW, Palisano RJ (eds): Physical Therapy for Children. WB Saunders, Philadelphia, 1994, p 183.

131. Horn EM, Warren SF, Jones HA: An experimental analysis of a neurobehavioral motor intervention. Dev Med Child Neurol 37:697, 1995.

132. Campbell S, Wilson J: Planning infant learning programs. Phys Ther 56:1347, 1976.

133. Redman-Bentley D: Parent expectations for professionals providing services to their handicapped children. Phys Occup Ther Pediatr 2(1):13, 1982.

134. Gajdosik CG: Issues of parent compliance: What the clinician and researcher should know. Phys Occup Ther Pediatr 11(2):73, 1991.

135. Schaefer E: Evaluating intervention effects on children, parents and professionals. *In* Wilson J (ed): Planning and Evaluating Developmental Programs, 2nd ed. Division of Physical Therapy, University of North Carolina at Chapel Hill, Chapel Hill, NC, 1979, p 85.

136. Scherzer A, Tscharnuter I: Early Diagnosis and Therapy in Cerebral Palsy, 2nd ed., Vol 6: Pediatric Habilitation. Marcel Dekker, New York, 1990.

137. Etaugh C: Effects of maternal employment on children: A review of recent research. Merrill-Palmer Q Behav Dev 20:71, 1974.

138. Kolobe THA: Family-focused early intervention. *In* Campbell SK (ed): Pediatric Neurologic Physical Therapy, 2nd ed. Churchill Livingstone, New York, 1991, p 397.

139. King GA, King SM, Rosenbaum PL: How mothers and fathers view professional caregiving for children with disabilities. Dev Med Child Neurol 38:397, 1996.

140. Bricker D: Early Intervention for At-Risk and Handicapped Infants, Toddlers and Preschool Children, 2nd ed. VORT, Palo Alto, Calif, 1989.

141. Lonsdale G: Family life with a handicapped child: The parents speak. Child Care Health Dev 4:99, 1978.

142. Floyd FJ, Zmich DE: Marriage and the parenting partnership: Perceptions and interactions of parents with mentally retarded and typically developing children. Child Dev 62:1434, 1991.

143. McMichael J: Handicap: A Study of Physically Handicapped Children and Their Families. Staples, London, 1971.

144. Butler N, Gill R, Pomeroy D, et al: Handicapped Children—Their Homes and Life Styles. Department of Child Health, University of Bristol, Bristol, 1978.

145. Burden RL: Measuring the effects of stress on the mothers of handicapped infants. Must depression always follow? Child Care Health Dev 6:111, 1980.

146. Dunlap WR, Hollingsworth JS: How does a handicapped child affect the family? Implications for practitioners. Fam Coord 26(3):286, 1977.

147. Wishart MC, Bidder RT, Gray OP: Parents' report of family life with a developmentally delayed child. Child Care Health Dev 7:267, 1981.

148. Gath A: The impact of an abnormal child upon the parents. Br J Psychiatry 130:405, 1977.

149. Taanila A, Kokkonen J, Jarvelin MR: The long term effects of children's early-onset disability on marital relationships. Dev Med Child Neurol 38:567, 1996.

150. Simeonsson RJ, McHale SM: Review: Research on handicapped children: Sibling relationships. Child Care Health Dev 7:153, 1981.

151. Stoneman Z, Berman PW (eds): The Effects of Mental Retardation, Disability, and Illness on Sibling Relationships: Research Issues and Challenges. Paul H Brookes, Baltimore, 1993.

152. Tew B, Laurence KM: Mothers, brothers and sisters of patients with spina bifida. Dev Med Child Neurol 15:69, 1973.

153. Caldwell BM, Guze SB: A study of the adjustment of parents and siblings of institutionalized and non-institutionalized retarded children. Am J Ment Defic 64:845, 1960.

154. Grossmann FK: Brothers and Sisters of Retarded Children: An Exploratory Study. Syracuse University Press, Syracuse, NY, 1972.

155. Shankoff JP, Hausen-Cram P: Early intervention for disabled infants and their families: A quantitative analysis. Pediatrics 80:650, 1987.

156. Sochaniwskyj AE, Koheil R, Bablich K, et al: Dynamic monitoring for sitting posture for children with spastic cerebral palsy. Clin Biomech 6:161, 1991.

157. Cristarella M: Comparison of straddling and sitting apparatus for the spastic cerebral-palsied child. Am J Occup Ther 29:273, 1975.

158. Carlson J, Winter R: The "Gillette" sitting support orthosis for nonambulatory children with severe cerebral palsy or advanced muscular dystrophy. Minn Med 61:469, 1978.

159. Sugar BR, Caudrey DJ, O'Mara NA: Hand function in cerebral palsy: The effect of hip-flexion angle. Dev Med Child Neurol 26:601, 1984.

160. Nwaobi OM, Burbaker CE, Cusick B, et al: Electromyographic investigation of extensor activity in cerebral palsied children in different seating positions. Dev Med Child Neurol 25:175, 1983.

161. Myhr U, von Wendt L: Influence of different sitting positions and abduction orthoses on leg muscle activity in children with cerebral palsy. Dev Med Child Neurol 35:890, 1993.

162. Mulcahy CM, Pountney TE, Nedham RL, et al: Adaptive seating for motor handicap: Problems, a solution, assessment and prescription. Br J Occup Ther 51:347, 1988.

163. Myhr U, von Wendt L: Reducing spasticity and enhancing postural control for the creation of a functional sitting position in children with cerebral palsy—A pilot study. Physiother Pract 6:65, 1990.

164. Hulme JB, Poor R, Schillein M, et al: Perceived behavioral changes observed with adaptive seating devices and training programs for multihandicapped, developmentally disabled individuals. Phys Ther 63:204, 1983.

165. Reid DT: The Sitting Assessment for Children with Neuromotor Dysfunction (SACND) Administration and Scoring Manual. Research Version. Department of Occupational Therapy, University of Toronto, Toronto, Ontario, 1994.

166. Reid DT: Development and preliminary validation of an instrument to assess quality of sitting of children with neuromotor dysfunction. Phys Occup Ther Pediatr 15(1):53, 1995.

167. Fife SE, Roxborough LA, Harris SR, et al: Development of a clinical measure of postural control for assessment of adaptive seating in children with neuromotor disabilities. Phys Ther 71:981, 1991.

168. Myhr U, von Wendt L: Improvement of functional sitting position for children with cerebral palsy. Dev Med Child Neurol 33:246, 1991.

169. Malouin F, Richards CL, Menier C, et al: Supported Walker Ambulation Performance Scale (SWAPS): Development of an outcome measure of locomotor status in children with cerebral palsy. Pediatr Phys Ther 9:48, 1997.

170. Sussman M, Cusick B: Preliminary report: The role of short-leg, tone reducing casts as an adjunct to physical therapy of patients with cerebral palsy. Johns Hopkins Med J 145:112, 1979.
171. Knutson L, Clark D: Orthotic devices for ambulation in children with cerebral palsy and myelomeningocele. Phys Ther 71:947, 1991.
172. Carlson S: A neurophysiological analysis of inhibitory casting. Phys Occup Ther Pediatr 4(4):31, 1984.
173. Duncan W, Mott D: Foot reflexes and the use of inhibiting casts. Foot Ankle 4:145, 1983.
174. Cusick BD: Progressive Casting and Splinting for Lower Extremity Deformities in Children with Neuromotor Dysfunction. Therapy Skill Builders, Tucson, 1990.
175. Harris S, Riffle K: Effects of inhibitive ankle-foot orthoses on standing balance in a child with cerebral palsy. Phys Ther 66:663, 1986.
176. Sussman M: Casting as an adjunct to neurodevelopmental therapy for cerebral palsy. Dev Med Child Neurol 25:804, 1983.
177. Mossberg K, Linton K, Friske K: Ankle-foot orthoses: Effects on energy expenditure of gait in spastic diplegic children. Arch Phys Med Rehabil 71:490, 1990.
178. Middleton E, Hurley G, McIlwain J: The role of rigid and hinged polypropylene ankle-foot orthoses in the management of cerebral palsy: A case study. Prosthet Orthot Int 12:129, 1988.
179. Wilson H, Haideri N, Song K, et al: Ankle-foot orthoses for preambulatory children with spastic diplegia. J Pediatr Orthop 17:370, 1997.
180. Blackman JS, Reed MD, Roberts CD: Muscle relaxant drugs for children with cerebral palsy. In Sussman MD (ed): The Diplegic Child. American Academy of Orthopedic Surgeons, Rosemont, Ill, 1992, p 229.
181. Corry IS, Cosgrove AP, Walsh EG, et al: Botulinum toxin A in the hemiplegic upper limb: A double blind trial. Dev Med Child Neurol 39:185, 1997.
182. Sutherland DH, Kaufman KR, Wyatt MP, Mubarak SJ: Effects of botulinum toxin on gait of patients with cerebral palsy: Preliminary results. Abstract. Dev Med Child Neurol suppl 70 (36):11, 1994.
183. Cosgrove AP, Corry IS, Graham HK: Botulinum toxin in the management of the lower limb in cerebral palsy. Dev Med Child Neurol 36:386, 1994.
183a. Thompson NS, Baker RJ, Cosgrove AP, et al: Musculoskeletal modelling in determining the effect of botulinum toxin on the hamstrings of patients with crouch gait. Dev Med Child Neurol 40:622, 1998.
184. Koman LA, Mooney JD, Mulvaney T, et al: Further evaluation of botulinum-A toxin in the management of cerebral palsy. Abstract. Dev Med Child Neurol suppl 69 (35):29, 1993.
185. Milla PT, Jackson ADM: A controlled trial of baclofen in children with cerebral palsy. J Int Med Res 5:398, 1977.
186. McKinlay I, Hyde E, Gordon N: Baclofen—A team approach to drug evaluation of spasticity in childhood. Scott Med J 1(suppl):526, 1980.
187. Young JA: Clinical experience in the use of baclofen in children with spastic cerebral palsy: A further report. Scott Med J 1(suppl):523, 1980.
188. Minford A, Brown JK, Minns RA, et al: The effect of baclofen on the gait of hemiplegic children assessed by means of polarized light goniometry. Scott Med J 1(suppl):529, 1980.
189. Albright AL, Cervi A, Singletary J: Intrathecal baclofen for spasticity in cerebral palsy. JAMA 265:1418, 1991.
190. Steinbok P, Armstrong R, Farrell K, et al: Intrathecal baclofen for treatment of spasticity in children: Report of nine cases. Can J Neurol Sci 18:232, 1991.
191. Albright AL, Barry MJ, Painter MJ, Schultz BL: Continuous intrathecal baclofen infusion for symptomatic generalized dystonia. Neurosurgery 38:934, 1996.
192. Steinbok P, Daneshvar H, Evans D, Kestle JRW: Cost analysis of continuous intrathecal baclofen versus selective functional posterior rhizotomy in the treatment of spastic quadriplegia associated with cerebral palsy. Pediatr Neurosurg 22:225, 1995.
193. Samilson R (ed): Orthopaedic Aspects of Cerebral Palsy. Clinics in Developmental Medicine 52/53. JB Lippincott, Philadelphia, 1975.
194. Massagli TL: Spasticity and its management in children. Phys Med Rehabil Clin North Am 2:867, 1991.
195. Moseley CF: Physiologic effects of soft tissue surgery. In Sussman MD (ed): The Diplegic Child. American Academy of Orthopedic Surgeons, Rosemont Ill, 1992, p 259.
196. House JH, Gwathmey FW, Fidler MO: A dynamic approach to thumb-in-palm deformity in cerebral palsy. Evaluation and results in 56 patients. J Bone Joint Surg Am 63:216, 1981.
197. Goldner LJ: The upper extremity in cerebral palsy. In Samison RL (ed): Orthopaedic Aspects of Cerebral Palsy. Clinics in Developmental Medicine 52/53. JB Lippincott, Philadelphia, 1975.

198. Zancolli EA, Zancolli ER: Surgical management of the hemiplegic spastic hand in cerebral palsy. Surg Clin North Am 61:2, 1981.

198a. Eliasson AC, Ekholm C, Carlstedt T: Hand function in children with cerebral palsy after upper-limb tendon transfer and muscle release. Dev Med Child Neurol 40:612, 1998.

199. Dias RC, Miller F, Dabney K, et al: Surgical correction of spinal deformity using a unit rod in children with cerebral palsy. J Pediatr Orthop 16:734, 1996.

200. Bonnett C, Brown JC, Grow T: Thoracolumbar scoliosis in cerebral palsy. Results of surgical treatment. J Bone Joint Surg 58:328, 1976.

201. MacEwen GD: Operative treatment of scoliosis in cerebral palsy. Reconstr Surg Traumatol 13:58, 1972.

202. Allen BL, Ferguson RL: L-rod instrumentation for scoliosis in cerebral palsy. J Pediatr Orthop 2:87, 1982.

203. Truscelli D, Pespargot A, Tardieu G: Variation on the long-term effects of elongation of the tendo Achillis in children with cerebral palsy. J Bone Joint Surg Br 61:466, 1979.

204. Castle ME, Reyman TA, Schneider M: Pathology of spastic muscle in cerebral palsy. Clin Orthop 142:223, 1979.

205. Cooper IS, Riklan M, Amin I, et al: Chronic electrical cerebellar stimulation in cerebral palsy. Neurology 26:744, 1976.

206. Ivan LP, Ventureyra EC: Chronic cerebellar stimulation in cerebral palsy. Childs Brain 9:121, 1982.

207. Wong PKH, Hoffman HJ, Froese AB, et al: Cerebellar stimulation in the management of cerebral palsy: Clinical and physiological studies. J Neurosurg 5:217, 1979.

208. Penn RD, Myklebust BM, Gottlieb GL, et al: Chronic cerebellar stimulation for cerebral palsy. Prospective and double-blind studies: J Neurosurg 53:160, 1980.

209. Gahm NH, Russman BS, Cerciello RL, et al: Chronic cerebellar stimulation for cerebral palsy: A double-blind study. Neurology 31:87, 1981.

210. Oppenheim WL, Staudt LA, Peacock JW: The rationale for rhizotomy. *In* Sussman MD (ed): The Diplegic Child. American Academy of Orthopedic Surgeons, Rosemont, Ill, 1992, p 271.

211. Peacock WJ, Staudt L: Selective dorsal rhizotomy: History and results. *In* Park TS, Philipps LH, Peacock WJ (eds): Neurosurgery: State of the Arts Reviews 4(2). Hanley & Belfus, Philadelphia, 1989, p 403.

212. Peacock WJ, Staudt LA: Functional outcomes following selective posterior rhizotomy in children with cerebral palsy. J Neurosurg 74:380, 1991.

213. Steinbok P, Reiner A, Beauchamp RD, et al: Selective functional posterior rhizotomy for the treatment of spastic cerebral palsy in children. Pediatr Neurosurg 18:34, 1992.

214. Arens LJ, Peacock WJ, Peter J: Selective dorsal rhizotomy: A long-term follow-up study. Childs Nerv Syst 5:148, 1989.

215. Berman B, Vaughan CL, Peacock WJ: The effect of rhizotomy on movement in patients with cerebral palsy. Am J Occup Ther 44:511, 1990.

216. Steinbok P, Reiner AM, Beauchamp R, et al: A randomized clinical trial to compare selective posterior rhizotomy plus physiotherapy with physiotherapy alone in children with spastic diplegic cerebral palsy. Dev Med Child Neurol 39:178, 1997.

216a. Yang TF, Chan RC, Wong TT, et al: Quantitative measurement of improvement in sitting balance in children with spastic cerebral palsy after selective posterior rhizotomy. Am J Phys Med Rehabil 75:348, 1996.

217. Thomas S, Aiona MD, Buckon CE: Does gait continue to improve two years following selective dorsal rhizotomy? J Pediatr Orthop 17:387, 1997.

218. Vaughan CL, Berman B, Peacock WJ: Cerebral palsy and rhizotomy. A three year follow-up evaluation with gait analysis. J Neurosurg 74:178, 1991.

219. Thomas SS, Aiona MD, Pierce R, Piatt HJ: Gait changes in children with spastic diplegia after selective dorsal rhizotomy. J Pediatr Orthop 16:747, 1996.

220. Cahan L, Adams J, Perry J, et al: Instrumented gait analysis following selective posterior rhizotomy. Dev Med Child Neurol 32:1037, 1990.

221. Boscarino LF, Ounpuu S, Davis RB: Effects of selective dorsal rhizotomy on gait in children with cerebral palsy. J Pediatr Orthop 13:174, 1993.

222. Guiliani CA: Dorsal rhizotomy for children with cerebral palsy. Phys Ther 71:80, 1991.

223. Green WB, Dietz FR, Goldberg MJ, et al: Rapid progression of hip subluxation in cerebral palsy after selective posterior rhizotomy. J Pediatr Orthop 11:494, 1991.

224. Hiem RC, Park TS, Volger GP, et al: Changes in hip migration after selective dorsal rhizotomy for spastic quadriplegia in cerebral palsy. J Neurosurg 82:567, 1995.

225. Gaebler-Spira DJ, Stempien L, Marty G, Dias L: Hip anatomy in children with cerebral palsy following selective posterior rhizotomy. Abstract. Dev Med Child Neurol suppl. 69(35):29, 1993.

226. Dales MC, Baum D, Bjornson KF, McLaughlin JF: The effect of selective dorsal rhizotomy on hip status in cerebral palsy. Abstract. Dev Med Child Neurol suppl 74 (38):27, 1996.

227. Aiona MD, Piatt JH: Hip stability after selective dorsal rhizotomy in patients with cerebral palsy. Abstract. Dev Med Child Neurol suppl 74(38):28, 1996.

228. Albright LA: Neurosurgical treatment of spasticity: Selective posterior rhizotomy and intrathecal baclofen. Stereotact Funct Neurosurg 58:3, 1992.

229. Albright LA, Barry MJ, Fasick MP, Janosky J: Effects of continuous intrathecal baclofen infusion and selective posterior rhizotomy on upper extremity spasticity. Pediatr Neurosurg 23:82, 1995.

230. Pape KE, Kirsch SE: Technology-assisted self-care in the treatment of spastic diplegia. *In* Sussman MD (ed): The Diplegic Child. American Academy of Orthopedic Surgeons, Rosemont, Ill, 1992, p 241.

231. Hazlewood ME, Brown JK, Rowe PJ, Salter PM: The use of therapeutic electrical stimulation in the treatment of hemiplegic cerebral palsy. Dev Med Child Neurol 36:661, 1994.

232. Reiner A, Steinbok P, Kestle JRW: The relationship of baseline motor skills to functional outcome in a study of therapeutic electrical stimulation. Abstract. Dev Med Child Neurol suppl 74(38):23, 1996.

233. Steinbok P, Reiner AM, Kestle JR, et al: Therapeutic electrical stimulation (TES) following selective posterior rhizotomy in children with spastic diplegia due to cerebral palsy: A randomized clinical trial. Childs Nerv Syst 11:550, 1995.

234. Simeonsson RJ, Cooper DH, Scheiner AP: A review and analysis of the effectiveness of early intervention programs. Pediatrics 69:635, 1982.

235. Ingram AJ, Withers E, Speltz E: Role of intensive physical and occupational therapy in the treatment of cerebral palsy: Testing and results. Arch Phys Med Rehabil 40:429, 1959.

236. Piper MC: Efficacy of physical therapy: Rate of motor development in children with cerebral palsy. Pediatr Phys Ther 2:126, 1990.

237. Sparrow S, Zigler E: Evaluation of a patterning treatment for retarded children. Pediatrics 62:137, 1978.

238. Sommerfeld D, Fraser B, Hensinger RN, et al: Evaluation of physical therapy service for severely mentally impaired students with cerebral palsy. Phys Ther 61:338, 1981.

239. Wright T, Nicholson J: Physiotherapy for the spastic child: An evaluation. Dev Med Child Neurol 15:146, 1973.

240. Paine R: On the treatment of cerebral palsy—The outcome of 177 patients, 74 totally untreated. Pediatrics 29:605, 1962.

241. Scherzer A, Mike V, Ilson J: Physical therapy as a determinant of change in the cerebral palsied infant. Pediatrics 58:47: 1976.

242. Ottenbacher KJ, Biocca Z, DeCremer G, et al: Quantitative analysis of the effectiveness of pediatric therapy: Emphasis on the neurodevelopmental treatment approach. Phys Ther 66: 1095, 1986.

243. Köng E: Very early treatment of cerebral palsy. Dev Med Child Neurol 8:198, 1966.

244. Kanda T, Yuge M, Yamari Y, et al: Early physiotherapy in the treatment of spastic diplegia. Dev Med Child Neurol 26:438, 1984.

245. Sharkey MA: Age of referral to early intervention as a dependent factor in the acquisition of gross motor skills. NDTA Network Jan/Feb:1, 1996.

246. Hochleitner M: Vergleichende Untersuchung von Konder mit zerebraler Bewegungsstörung, mit und ohne neurophysiologischer Fruhtherapie. Oesterr Aertz 32:1108, 1977.

247. Palmer FB, Shapiro BK, Wachtel RC, et al: The effects of physical therapy on cerebral palsy: A controlled trial in infants with spastic cerebral palsy. N Engl J Med 318:803, 1988.

248. D'Avignon M, Noren L, Arman T: Early physiotherapy ad modum Vojta or Bobath in infants with suspected neuromotor disturbance. Neuropaediatrics 12:232, 1981.

249. Abdel-Salam E, Maraghi S, Tawfik M: Evaluation of physical therapy techniques in the management of cerebral palsy. J Egypt Med Assoc 61:531, 1978.

250. Jonsdottir J, Fetters L, Kluzik J: Effects of physical therapy on postural control in children with cerebral palsy. Pediatr Phys Ther 9:68, 1997.

251. Watube S, Otabe T, Kii K, et al: Improving the walking patterns of a spastic diplegic child. Totline 7(1):14, 1981.

252. Palisano RJ: Investigation of Electromyographic Gait Analysis as a Method of Evaluating the Effects of Neurodevelopmental Treatment in a Child With Cerebral Palsy. Unpublished master's thesis. Division of Physical Therapy, School of Medicine, University of North Carolina at Chapel Hill, Chapel Hill, NC, 1981.

253. MacPhail HEA, Kramer JF: Effects of isokinetic strength training on functional ability and walking efficiency in adolescents with cerebral palsy. Dev Med Child Neurol 37:763, 1995.

Traumatic Brain Injury

Jocelyn Blaskey, MS, PT
Maureen C. Jennings, MPT

Traumatic injuries are the major cause of death in children, with brain injury the most common source.[1-3] Of the more than 1 million children who suffer a traumatic brain injury (TBI) each year, an estimated 165,000 require hospitalization.[4] The incidence is highest in males between the ages of 15 and 20 years, followed by children between the ages of 6 and 10 years.[5, 6] Reported mortality rates from severe head injury vary from 6 to 59 percent.[7-19] The highest mortality rates occur in children younger than 2 years and older than 15 years.[20] The cause of death is seldom the primary brain damage but rather intracranial or extracranial secondary complications of the brain damage or concomitant injuries.[18, 21-23] The majority of severe head injuries, 70 to 98 percent, result from motor vehicle accidents, although falls and assaults are common causes. Motor vehicle accidents, more prevalent in older children, often result in severe cranial injuries with focal deficits and long-lasting neurologic problems. Blunt trauma due to falls from trees, swings, or jungle gyms to grass or concrete, typical of midchildhood, often results in skull fractures and more generalized cerebral injury. Falls and nonaccidental trauma are most frequent in children younger than 1 year.[8-22]

The median direct cost of acute and rehabilitative care following mild, moderate, or severe TBI is estimated at $823, $16,553, and $73,433, respectively (1997 dollars). Direct costs following severe injury range from $6905 to $465,920 (1997 dollars). Forty-five percent of the total cost for severe head injury is rehabilitation costs.[23]

Epidemiologic studies identify that children who die from traumatic injuries were often unrestrained in a car (or seated in the front passenger seat), were not wearing helmets when riding a bicycle, or were not well supervised.[23, 24] Preventive efforts include the education of families during routine medical visits and community-based education on avoiding risky behaviors and using preventive equipment. Legislation requiring the use of automobile restraint systems and helmets has been shown to reduce the incidence of deaths.[2, 24] For further review, see Boswell and associates,[24] Finney and coworkers,[2] Hazinski and colleagues,[25] and Kraus and McArthur.[26]

Throughout recovery, physical, cognitive, and behavioral impairments improve. The children's abilities and disabilities are influenced by their impairments, their age, their previous functional status and cognitive level, and the resources available to them. After closed head injury of a child, intervention by the physical therapist and the rehabilitation team is guided by the cognitive and functional abilities of the child; the potential for recovery; and the family's or caregivers' understanding of the child's injury, expected outcome, and long-term needs for care. The caregiver will be primarily responsible for managing the child's health care, education, and developmental needs. A primary goal for the health care team is educating the caregiver about the child's injury, recovery process, likely secondary complications as the child matures, and how to access appropriate community resources. Education empowers the family to negotiate the complex health care and educational systems as well as community services in order to meet the child's expected future needs.

A current literature review regarding brain injury pathology, recovery, and expected outcomes is presented in this chapter. Complications associated with trauma and subsequent brain injury, including an impaired level of consciousness and cognition, poor motor control, musculoskeletal limitations, swallowing dysfunction, and abnormal physiologic responses, are also discussed. Three case studies illustrate the issues involved. Physical therapy goal establishment, examination, and intervention are discussed, followed by the presentation of a detailed case report highlighting different points in the continuum of care. The case study illustrates the decision-making processes involved in establishing an appropriate plan of care for a child with a TBI.

PATHOLOGY

Injuries resulting from head trauma include scalp and cranial injuries, contusions, concussions, extraparenchymal or intracranial hematomas, cranial nerve injuries, and herniations caused by edema.[20, 27–30] Head injuries can be classified according to how they are inflicted, including acceleration-deceleration injuries (closed head injuries), crush injuries, and penetration injuries. Acceleration-deceleration injuries, the most common form of trauma, result when the head hits an immobile object or a mobile object hits an immobile head.

Cerebral injury may include diffuse, focal, or hypoxic-ischemic injuries, or all of these. Focal injuries (usually frontal and temporal) evidenced on computed tomography (CT) scan result in contusions and hematomas. Berney and associates found subdural hematomas more common in children aged zero to 3 years, and extradural hematomas more common in children aged 9 years and older.[20]

Diffuse axonal injury (DAI) due to shearing forces (usually involving the brainstem and corpus callosum) is apparent on magnetic resonance imaging.[14, 31–34] Through experimental TBI in animal models, researchers have identified a series of events leading to cellular-level changes that are related to the degree and extent of behavioral changes. Early work by Gennarelli and colleagues found that recovery, the extent of DAI, the length of coma, and the resulting disability were related to the direction of acceleration in monkeys (lateral greater than oblique, greater than sagittal).[32] Focal and diffuse edema, increased intracranial pressure, and diffuse axonal deafferentation accompanied by denervation hypersensitivity and ingrowth of spared axonal input follow DAI. A similar series of changes has been confirmed in human head injury.[35] Elucidating the components of the biochemical-neurometabolic cascade following brain injury allows research into the use of hypothermia and pharmacologic management to interrupt the process or enhance the recovery of neuronal function. See Povlishok and Christman,[35] McIntosh,[36] Faden,[37] and Clifton[38] for further information.

Secondary brain damage, usually resulting from hypoxia or ischemia, can be caused by intracranial factors such as mass lesions or cerebral edema, or extracranial factors such as hypoxemia or hypotension.[22, 30, 31, 39] Early ischemia and hypotension (systolic blood pressure <90 mm Hg), present in about 30 percent of the cases, are correlated with a poor outcome and a high mortality.[22, 39] (See Bouma and Muizelaur[39] for a summary of research into the causes of ischemia.)

Compared with the adult cerebral cortex, children at 2 years of age have a greater number of synapses. Over the next 10 years of normal growth and development, the number of synapses is reduced. During the same time period, neurotransmitter modifications change synapse sensitivity to enhance long-term potentiation. These normal differences make the child's brain particularly vulnerable to hypoxia, ischemia, and other insults.[22, 40, 41] (See Johnston[40] and Sharples and coworkers[41] for a further review of pathologic processes unique to the developing brain.)

RECOVERY

Recovery of function after a brain injury is dependent on the extent of primary and secondary injury and on the neuroplasticity of the residual areas. Gains in function after injury can be attributed to mechanisms of restitution, substitution, sparing, and compensation.[34, 35, 42] Restitution involves resolution of cellular toxicity, metabolic dysfunction, diaschisis, edema, and absorption of blood products, allowing recovery of the neural network and return of function. Pharmacologic management attempts to limit the primary and secondary neural injury and enhance recovery.[20–22, 27, 30–33, 35–43] Early physical therapy is limited to interventions that would not exacerbate the pathologic processes or interfere with resolution. Before and during interventions the therapist closely monitors the child's physiologic responses to stay within safe guidelines as determined by the physician.

Substitution involves adaptation at the neuronal level or within the neural network to access spared portions of the network. This process can be influenced by rehabilitation therapies.[42, 43] Neuronal changes (which may be enhanced by pharmacologic management) include synaptic sprouting, axonal and dendritic regeneration, remyelination, changes in the number of receptors, ion channel changes, changes in actions of neurotransmitters and neuromodulators, changes in the uptake and release of neurotransmitter, and increased neuronal responsiveness resulting from denervation hypersensitivity. Unfortunately, in severe injury, maladaptive or disordered reorganization is consistent with residual morbidity.[35, 42, 43]

Goal-oriented therapeutic activities may result in activity-dependent "unmasking" of previously ineffective synapses, and activity-dependent changes in synaptic strength (tied to memory and learning). Functional neuroimaging has helped to reveal how enhancement of activity in partially spared pathways, expansion of representational maps, recruitment of parallel neuronal pathways, or dependence on task-specific cues can enhance a return of function.[42–45] Knowledge about neuroplasticity continues to expand through research at both the molecular and the neural network levels. Understanding developmental neurobiology, neural control of complex functions, and mechanisms of learning in both the injured and the uninjured brain will allow rehabilitation specialists to identify and test appropriate and efficient therapeutic strategies to enhance function. The use of functional neuroimaging will assist researchers and clinicians to elucidate the effect of interventions on neural reorganization and identify the sequence and timing of interventions to optimally and efficiently enhance function.[42, 43, 46] Further discussion of mechanisms responsible for a loss of consciousness and recovery is offered by Berney and colleagues,[20] Carlsson and associates,[21] Gennarelli and coworkers,[30, 32] Dimitrijevic,[33] Povlishok and Christman,[35] McIntosh,[36] and Dobkin.[42, 43]

PROGNOSIS

Although the recovery of consciousness and preinjury functional status is usually complete within 3 weeks, behavioral difficulties, a shortened attention span, and irritability may persist.[7–18, 29, 33, 34, 42, 47, 50] An estimated 5 to 30 percent of those hospitalized manifest neurologic or psychologic sequelae, or both, 6 months or more after injury.[17, 47, 48, 51–61] The interplay between the neurologic and psychologic sequelae, as well as the effect of the child's preinjury functional and cognitive status,[9] the family support and interaction,[49] and the availability of appropriate professional and nonprofessional intervention support systems, determines the ultimate reintegration of the child into society.[3, 12, 13, 15, 48–50, 52, 58] Physical and mental improvement is evident 2, 3, and even 7 years after the injury;[8, 52, 53, 57] however, it is generally agreed that the greatest change occurs by the first 6 to 12 months after injury.[8, 47, 56, 61, 62]

Much research attempts to expand the confidence with which physicians can predict the ultimate outcome from the patient's status within the first few hours. Established outcome categories, reviewed by Jennett and associates[50, 63] and referred to as the Glasgow Outcome Scale in many reports,[9, 15, 18, 50, 59] are as follows:

1. Death
2. Persistent vegetative state
3. Severe disability
4. Moderate disability
5. Good recovery

More current outcome measures that further define moderate disability and good recovery include the Pediatric Evaluation of Disability Inventory (PEDI),[64] the Functional Independence Measure (FIM),[65] and the Functional Independence Measure for Children

(WeeFIM).[66] These are further defined in the section Physical Therapy Examination and Intervention.

The Glasgow Coma Scale (GCS), devised by Teasdale and Jennett,[67] is an international assessment that measures the acute depth and duration of impaired consciousness and coma. It was conceived as a graded measurement of three aspects of behavior: motor responsiveness, verbal performance, and eye opening (Table 3–1). The best response for each behavior is noted, and the sum of the grades is recorded. The sum is an indication of the depth of coma, ranging from 3 to 15.[67] Injury severity is often classified as mild (GCS score 13 to 15), moderate (GCS score 9 to 12), or severe (GCS score 3 to 8).

An initial GCS score of 4 portends a poor outcome, often death.[3, 7, 16, 17, 19, 59] Young and associates[59] and Kraus and colleagues[3] report that when the GCS score is 5 to 7, outcomes are equally distributed across outcome categories; with scores greater than 7, there is 95 percent good to moderate recovery. A slow response time and difficulties with short-term memory are major residual abnormalities with an initial GCS score of 5 to 8.[50, 63] Changes in the GCS score during the first 24 hours improve the precision of prediction of outcome.[59] Mamelek and coworkers found age and the GCS motor score at 24 hours to be the best independent predictors of survival (93 percent survival rate for children with a GCS motor score ≥3 at 24 hours after injury).[19] At 5 to 7 years after severe brain injury (GCS score 3 to 8), the Glasgow Outcome Scale was reported as good recovery (27 percent), moderate disability (55 percent), severe disability (15 percent), and death (3 percent; one patient).[68] By FIM criteria, 64 percent were independent in all mobility items, 70 percent were independent in self-care, and 24 percent were independent in all cognitive items. After mild brain injury (GCS score 9 to 15) all children scored within the average range for age on the PEDI at 1 and 6 months after injury.[47] The perceived impact of the injury on the family, however, was related to the amount of caregiver assistance needed (PEDI ratings) and the number of behavior problems noted.[47] After severe brain injury, the duration of coma may be a better predictor of the outcome and the presence of impairments than the initial GCS score.[15, 62, 69] Brink and associates reported that a good or moderate outcome is expected if coma does not exceed 6 weeks;[69] Eiben and colleagues reported that no patient with coma exceeding 1 month had a good outcome;[15] and Massagli and coworkers found a median length of coma to be 1 day for a good outcome, 6 days for moderate disability, and 62 days for severe disability.[70] After severe brain injury, compared with adults, children

Glasgow Coma Scale

TABLE 3–1

Behavior	Score	Response
Motor behavior	1	No motor response to pressure
	2	Decerebrate posturing
	3	Decorticate posturing
	4	Pulls part of body away with pressure
	5	Pulls examiner's hand away
	6	Follows simple commands
Verbal performance	1	Makes no noise
	2	Makes sounds
	3	Talks so that examiner can decipher words but makes no sense
	4	Is confused or disoriented
	5	Converses and states where he or she is, who he or she is, months, and year
Eye opening	1	Does not open eyes to pain
	2	Opens eyes to pressure
	3	Opens eyes when asked in loud voice
	4	Opens eyes on own

Adapted from Teasdale G, Jennett B: Assessment of coma and impaired consciousness. Lancet 2:81, 1974. Copyright © 1981 by Oxford University Press, Inc. Used by permission of Oxford University Press, Inc.

(younger than 16 years) had higher average FIM scores at discharge and a higher number of discharges to the home.[56] We will further identify outcomes associated with specific impairments. (See Coster and associates[47] and Massagli and colleagues[70] for a review of the literature on outcomes in young children, and see Bruce and associates,[9] Gilchrist and Wilkinson,[12] Cartlidge and Shaw,[10] Klonoff and coworkers,[52, 53] Filley and associates,[60] Eiben and colleagues,[15] Kraus and associates,[3] Humphreys,[16] Wagstyll and coworkers,[17] Massagli and colleagues,[70, 71] Michaud and associates,[68] Mayer and coworkers,[11, 72, 73] and Whitlock and Hamilton[56] for detailed reviews of outcomes.)

IMPAIRMENTS ASSOCIATED WITH BRAIN INJURY

Many impairments may be associated with TBI. Discussion here is limited to those that may influence the child's ability to perform effective and efficient functional movements. A brief synopsis of the associated impairments in cognition and behavior, motor control, and postural control; and musculoskeletal complications (including orthopedic problems, "spasticity," range-of-motion [ROM] limitations, and heterotopic ossification [HO]) based on a review of the current literature is presented. Discussion of assessment and intervention related to limitations in functional mobility and feeding and associated impairments is presented in the Physical Therapy Examination and Intervention section. Three abbreviated case reports are used to illustrate the concepts presented in the following sections (Table 3–2).

CASE STUDY

Consider the GCS score and length-of-coma information (see Table 3–2) in light of the review of the literature on prognosis. One might expect Carl to have a good outcome with residual memory and response-time deficits, whereas Rick and Anne are likely to have moderate to severe disability.

Cognitive and Psychologic Complications

Psychologic sequelae may be present even after only "minor" injuries.[47, 49, 53] Changes in personality and behavior often include hyperactivity, distractibility, a low tolerance for frustration, poor social judgment, a lack of impulse control, and aggression.[18, 21, 55, 58, 60, 70, 71] Anxiety and depression are common in adults who were injured when they were children.[53] These problems are often reflective of a diffuse injury. Persistent deficits in learning and memory may be severe for the child with a brain injury and affect educational and vocational potential.[47, 49, 51–53, 60, 70] More profound effects on intellectual performance are found in children who were injured at earlier ages. Additionally, the intelligence quotient (IQ) 1 year after injury has been found to be directly related to the length of coma.[8, 53] Intellectual deficits and personality changes that persist are difficult for the family to manage and often require special school placement.[55, 70] During adolescence, children in poorly functioning families may show deterioration rather than continued improvement.[49] By the time the child reaches adolescence, poor judgment and difficulties with problem solving may seriously hinder the achievement of future vocational potential and financial independence.[13, 48, 51, 52, 55, 58, 70, 74]

Studies of psychologic testing in children with TBI have identified a significant slowing of the response time, a reduction in the performance IQ compared with the preinjury state, and difficulty with auditory and visual perception.[53, 55, 57] These impairments have been found to markedly limit school performance. Only 30 percent of children with severe brain injuries ($n = 300$) were found to have normal intelligence; 64 percent were found to benefit from a special educational program.[75] On long-term follow-up (6 to 133 months, mean 34 months) children younger than 7 years showed a poorer outcome in measures of social and school abilities than older children. After severe brain injury, 50 percent of children injured at preschool age and 29 percent of

Initial Examination Results of Selected Case Reports

TABLE 3–2

Area of Interest	Anne	Carl	Rick
Preinjury status	12 years old Reportedly in 6th grade; school records indicated learning difficulties Foster home placement, precipitating reasons unknown	12.5 years old Prior medical history significant for asthma Reportedly had "learning problems," hyperactivity (took methylphenidate [Ritalin]) Previous school records indicated "questionable" supervision in the home; reportedly, Carl's parents withdrew him from school 4 months earlier because of an argument with school personnel Hobbies: fishing	18 months old Reported age-appropriate performance of functional skills and cognition
Cause of injury	Struck in pedestrian vs. auto accident	Struck by car while riding his bicycle at 11 PM; he was not wearing a helmet	Struck in pedestrian vs. auto accident
Initial acute assessment	Multiple skull fractures including depressed skull fracture with cerebral contusion, intracerebral hemorrhage into right parietal area, basal ganglial contusion Intrapulmonary hemorrhage, large right pneumothorax	Bicortical shearing; right cerebral peduncle shearing with contusion, left cortical shearing Laceration to left anterior lower leg with sutures, right obturator ring fracture	Basilar brainstem contusion, hemorrhage and edema in cerebellar area Third day after onset, right middle cerebral artery infarct
Glasgow Coma Scale (GCS); length of coma	GCS scores not available Duration of coma, 3.5 mo Length of time since onset, 4 mo	Initial GCS, 5; GCS at 24 hr, 8 Duration of coma, 4 days Length of time since onset of injury, 1 wk	Initial GCS, 3–4 GCS at 24 hr, 7–8 Duration of coma, 3 wk Length of time since onset, 4 wk
Family involvement	Foster home care before injury; mother infrequently present	Family infrequently present; only one documented visit, day *after* injury, over 5 mo	Supportive intact family
Previous therapy reports	Therapy reports, if any, were not included in transfer summary	Physical therapy intervention consisted of "balance activities, supported sitting, transfer training"	Eats one-half jar of baby food; turns when his name is called
Other relevant information from acute care setting	Acute surgical intervention: débridement of brain tissues, ventriculostomy, ventriculoperitoneal shunt; chest tube placement, tracheostomy tube placement with mechanical ventilation (ventilation was discontinued before transfer to rehabilitation hospital)	Combative with nursing staff at acute hospital High elopement risk	Skull fracture Right femur fracture (initially treated with traction, subsequently placed in cast brace at 5 wk after injury)
Family's goals	Family not present for consultation, unable to determine family's goals Anne's goal: to dress herself	Family's goal: "for Carl to eat real food"	Family's goal: to take their child home

(continued)

(continued) **Initial Examination Results of Selected Case Reports**

TABLE 3-2

Area of Interest	Anne	Carl	Rick
Length of time since injury	4 mo	1 wk	4 wk
Cognition and level of consciousness	Rancho adult level VII; alert and oriented to place and name, followed 1- to 2-step commands, communicated with gestures	Rancho adult level VI; confused appropriate	Rancho pediatric level III; localized response to stimuli (focused on bright objects, withdrew from noxious stimuli)
Functional abilities	Required moderate assistance for rolling and coming to sit in bed Moderate assistance needed for maintaining supported sitting on edge of bed Required maximal assistance for transfers to and from bed; otherwise dependent in all other transfers	Independent with rolling, but required minimal assistance for coming to sit Minimal to moderate assistance for transfers to and from bed and toilet Unable in all ambulation	Unable with all self-care, play, and functional mobility
Motor control	Able to move joints of right upper extremity selectively; all communication performed through gestures of this, her most "functional" extremity Right lower extremity demonstrated selective control with movements performed against gravity (fair); left lower extremity predominated by patterned movement, extensor > flexor muscles Muscle stiffness severe in left upper extremity, flexor > extensor muscles (Ashworth Scale 3) Moderate left lower extremity (Ashworth Scale 2)	Able to selectively move all joints in response to command MMT: poor minus hip extension and abduction as well as knee flexors and extensors and ankle plantar flexors Ataxia noted at left hand Mild spasticity noted in bilateral ankle plantar flexors (Ashworth Scale 1+)	Spontaneous flexion of bilateral lower extremities (R > L) No movement of left upper extremity Muscle stiffness noted in left shoulder, wrist, and finger flexors, forearm pronators, and bilateral ankle plantar flexors (Ashworth Scale 1+)
Somatosensory	Diminished light touch sensation throughout left extremities Unable to formally assess proprioception	Grossly intact to light touch	Tactile sensation grossly intact throughout although appeared hypersensitive to touch (responded with crying and squirming) Unable to formally assess proprioception
Postural control	Moderate to maximal assistance to maintain her trunk and head aligned over her base of support; severely delayed (nonfunctional) protective extension responses to perturbations in balance in all directions while standing or seated	Poor static and dynamic control of trunk in sitting (needed to prop with arms to maintain sitting position) Good static and dynamic head control in sitting and standing	Poor head and trunk control Absent balance reactions to perturbations

(continued)

TABLE 3–2 *(continued)* **Initial Examination Results of Selected Case Reports**

Area of Interest	Anne	Carl	Rick
Musculoskeletal status	Unable to open left hand (specific measurements unknown) to place on flat surface; left hip flexion contracture, 30°; otherwise no ROM constraints throughout remaining extremities	No PROM limitations noted with exception of right ankle dorsiflexion (with knee extended) 0°	PROM: bilateral ankle dorsiflexion (with knee extended) 0°
Physiologic response	Adaptive physiologic response to activity	Adaptive physiologic response to activity	Adaptive physiologic response to activity
Dysphagia and feeding	Reported left facial numbness, unable to manage saliva (as noted by copious drooling); able to close jaw and approximate teeth, but unable to close lips Poor coordination of tongue movements Unable to initiate saliva swallow on command	Audible swallow and "raspy" voice after swallow with solids and puree and thickened liquids, but able to spontaneously clear throat	Eats half jar of baby food when fed; incoordination when drinking liquids Left muscle weakness (cranial nerves VI and VII)

MMT, manual muscle testing; ROM, range of motion; PROM, passive range of motion.

children injured at elementary school age required special educational arrangements. After moderate brain injury, the percentages were 25 and 11 percent, respectively.[51] In all children tested using the revised Wechsler Intelligence Scale for Children, the performance IQ was more affected than the verbal IQ initially; both scores improved and equalized but did not return to estimated premorbid levels. Refer to Klonoff and colleagues,[52, 53] Fay and coworkers,[55] Coster and associates,[47] Rivara and colleagues,[49] Telzrow,[58] and Ewing-Cobbs and Fletcher[48] for reviews of incidence of behavioral and cognitive deficits and a discussion of measurement tools and methods of intervention for the management of significant residual behavioral and cognitive deficits.

Recovery of Consciousness and Cognition

Documentation of depth of coma and the level of consciousness permits ongoing assessment of progressive changes in consciousness and provides a means to monitor recovery. Brink and associates[8, 69] and Cartlidge and Shaw[10] adapted Ommaya's original classifications of five levels of consciousness[76] to evaluate the depth and duration of coma and the return to consciousness. Brink and associates further classified the level of pediatric consciousness by three age groups:[8, 69, 77] infants (6 months to 2 years); preschool-aged children (2 to 5 years); and school-aged children (5 years and older) (Table 3–3). These scales will be referred to as the *Rancho pediatric levels*. The levels on each of these scales range from V (no response to stimuli) to I (oriented). The behavioral expectations at each of the pediatric levels are variable depending on the age group.

Cognitive function of children 12 years of age and older can be assessed using the Rancho Levels of Cognitive Functioning (this will be referred to as the *Rancho adult levels*).[76] This scale is reversed in order compared with the Rancho pediatric scale and further delineates adult cognitive functioning into eight levels (Table 3–4). Note that Rancho adult levels I, II, and III are the same as Rancho pediatric levels V, IV, and III, respectively.

Rancho Pediatric Levels of Consciousness (Infants, Preschool, and School-Age)

TABLE 3-3

Rancho Pediatric Level	Infants: 6 Mo to 2 Yr	Preschool: 2–5 Yr	School-age: 5 Yr and Older
I	Interacts with environment a. Shows active interest in toys; manipulates or examines before mouthing or discarding b. Watches other children at play; may move toward them purposefully c. Initiates social contact with adults; enjoys socializing d. Shows active interest in bottle e. Reaches or moves toward person or object	Oriented to self and surroundings a. Provides accurate information about self b. Knows he or she is away from home c. Knows where toys, clothes, etc., are kept d. Actively participates in treatment program e. Recognizes own room, knows way to bathroom, nursing station, etc. f. Is potty trained g. Initiates social contact with adult; enjoys socializing	Oriented to time and place; records ongoing events a. Provides accurate, detailed information about self and present situation b. Knows way to and from daily activities c. Knows sequence of daily routine d. Knows way around unit; recognizes own room e. Finds own bed; knows where personal belongings are kept f. Is bowel and bladder trained
II	Demonstrates awareness of environment a. Responds to name b. Recognizes mother or other family members c. Enjoys imitative vocal play d. Giggles or smiles when talked to or played with e. Fussing is quieted by soft voice or touch	Is responsive to environment a. Follows simple commands b. Refuses to follow commands by shaking head or saying "no" c. Imitates examiner's gestures or facial expressions d. Responds to name e. Recognizes mother or other family members f. Enjoys imitative vocal play	Is responsive to environment a. Follows simple verbal or gestured requests b. Initiates purposeful activity c. Actively participates in therapy program d. Refuses to follow request by shaking head or saying "no" e. Imitates examiner's gestures or facial expressions
III	Gives localized response to sensory stimuli a. Blinks when strong light crosses field of vision b. Follows moving object passed within visual field c. Turns toward or away from loud sound d. Gives localized response to painful stimuli	Gives localized response to sensory stimuli a. Blinks when strong light crosses field of vision b. Follows moving object passed within visual field c. Turns toward or away from loud sound d. Gives localized response to painful stimuli	Gives localized response to sensory stimuli a. Blinks when strong light crosses field of vision b. Follows moving object passed within visual field c. Turns toward or away from loud sound d. Gives localized response to painful stimuli
IV	Gives generalized response to sensory stimuli a. Gives generalized startle to loud sound b. Responds to repeated auditory stimulation with increased or decreased activity c. Gives generalized reflex response to painful stimuli	Gives generalized response to sensory stimuli a. Gives generalized startle to loud sound b. Responds to repeated auditory stimulation with increased or decreased activity c. Gives generalized reflex response to painful stimuli	Gives generalized response to sensory stimuli a. Gives generalized startle to loud sound b. Responds to repeated auditory stimulation with increased or decreased activity c. Gives generalized reflex response to painful stimuli
V	No response to stimuli a. Complete absence of observable change in behavior to visual, auditory, or painful stimuli	No response to stimuli a. Complete absence of observable change in behavior to visual, auditory, or painful stimuli	No response to stimuli a. Complete absence of observable change in behavior to visual, auditory, or painful stimuli

From Rehabilitation of the Head Injured Child and Adult: Pediatric Levels of Consciousness, Selected Problems, pp 5–7. Professional Staff Association of Rancho Los Amigos Hospital, Inc., 1982, with permission from Rancho Los Amigos Medical Center, Pediatric Brain Injury Service and Los Amigos Research and Education Institute, Inc., Downey, Calif.

Rancho Levels of Cognitive Functioning*

TABLE 3–4

Rancho Adult Level		
I	No response	Completely unresponsive to any stimuli
II	Generalized response	Inconsistent and nonpurposeful response to stimuli
III	Localized response	Specific yet inconsistent response to stimuli; response is related to type of stimuli (turning head toward sound)
IV	Confused-agitated	Heightened state of activity Demonstrates bizarre and nonpurposeful behaviors relative to the environment
V	Confused-inappropriate	Inconsistently follows simple commands Shows gross attention to environment, but easily distractible and lacks ability to focus attention on specific task Memory is severely impaired, new information very difficult to learn
VI	Confused-appropriate	Goal-directed behavior Appropriate responses to environment Can consistently follow simple commands and demonstrates carryover of *relearned* tasks Dependent on external cues for direction Shows little carryover to independent performance of *newly* learned tasks
VII	Automatic-appropriate	Appears appropriate and oriented to self and environment Participates in automatic daily routines Recent memory is impaired resulting in shallow recall of activities and decreased rate of learning new information
VIII	Purposeful-appropriate	Recalls and integrates past and recent events Adapts responses to environment Demonstrates carryover of new learning and does not require supervision once an activity is learned Deficits remain in abstract reasoning, tolerance to stress and judgment in emergencies

Adapted from Malkmus D, Booth BJ, Kodimer C: Levels of Cognitive Functioning. *In* Rehabilitation of the Head Injured Adult: Comprehensive Cognitive Management. Downey, Calif., 1980, p 2. With permission from Los Amigos Research and Education Institute, Inc.

*The Rancho Levels of Cognitive Functioning, referred to here as Rancho Adult Levels, have been revised and expanded to 10 levels by Chris Hagan, PhD. The Revised Rancho Levels of Cognitive Functioning, copyright Chris Hagan, PhD, 1998, are available from Rancho Los Amigos National Rehabilitation Center, Department of Communication Disorders, Harriman Building, 7601 E. Imperial Highway, Downey, Calif., 90242.

CASE STUDY

As an example of the use of the cognitive functioning levels, refer to the three case examples in Table 3–2. Anne and Carl are 12 years old, so a Rancho adult level is assigned. Rick, however, is only 18 months old and is assessed according to the Rancho pediatric levels (6 months to 2 years).

Finally, the Coma/Near-Coma[79] and Western Neurological scales[80] were designed to measure small clinical changes in patients slow to recover consciousness (Rancho pediatric levels V to III or Rancho adult levels I to III). Refer to Dobkin[29] for discussion of additional scales used to measure changes in patients with minimal responsiveness.

Functional Abilities and Motor Control

The ability to produce functional movements reflects the complex interaction of many factors and systems, which include cognition and the level of consciousness; behavior; sensation; sensorimotor integration; supraspinal regulation; and the state of the musculoskeletal and physiologic systems. Children with TBI may have any or all of these systems affected. After a severe brain injury, the frequency and severity of velocity-dependent muscle stiffness (i.e., "spasticity"),[69] ataxia,[62, 69] contractures,[62] paralysis,[62] and speech impairments[62] increase as the length of coma increases. The incidence of spasticity and ataxia in children with severe brain injuries is approximately 65 and 50 percent, respectively, with a 35 percent incidence of combined ataxia and spasticity.[8, 69, 75] In adults (aged 16 to 88 years), Wong and colleagues found the probability of impairments in individuals who were in coma for 2 days or more to be the following: ataxia, 23.5 percent; contractures, 13 percent; paralysis, 60 percent; and speech impairment, 53.5 percent.[62] The probability of ataxia and contractures increases to 40 percent after a person is in coma for 30 days and 15 days, respectively.[62] The probability of impairments relative to coma length has not been reported in the pediatric population; however, paralysis would likely follow a similar pattern. A follow-up study of 53 children (≤18 years old) with severe closed head injury found an increased duration of coma and an increased frequency of a GCS score of 2 or less in those children with a combination of diffuse and focal injuries. The presence of residual motor signs was equally distributed among those with diffuse and focal injuries.[60] Chaplin and coworkers found deficits in the speed of motor performance (as measured by the Bruininks Test of Motor Proficiency) in children (aged 5 to 15 years, GCS score 3 to 10) 1 to 4 years after injury.[57] Persistent deficits in gross motor complex skills indirectly affected fitness and self-perception. Systematic follow-up of motor abilities, fitness, and persistent impairments may suggest appropriate interventions to maximize motor performance.

Influence of Cognitive Impairments on the Production of Functional Movement

It is often difficult to determine the extent to which cognitive impairments influence the child's ability to perform a task after a brain injury. A classic example is the child who was able to catch a ball yet unable to lift his arms when asked. The child responded automatically to the ball coming toward him by reaching up and catching it. When a command was given to raise his arms, however, the child did not demonstrate the motor response. It is apparent that the child's visual perception, sensorimotor system, and musculoskeletal system were adequate for the motor response. Dobkin identifies common cognitive and language impairments associated with TBI that may account for the lack of response to the verbal commands.[29] Cognitive and language impairments that may influence functional motor abilities include attention (alertness, sound mental processing, selective attention, and sustained attention); perception (visual, auditory, and visual-spatial); executive function (planning, initiation, and maintenance and monitoring of goal orientation); problem solving; abstract reasoning; memory (immediate, delayed, cued, visual and verbal learning); and language (receptive and expressive).

Motor Control Impairments

Velocity-dependent muscle stiffness ("spasticity") is a common sequela of upper moto-neuron injury. It has been found to peak at 2 to 3 months, then gradually decrease, sometimes over 2 years.[75] Bilateral moderate to severe spasticity is most common in individuals with coma lasting more than 4 weeks.[8]

Ataxia and spasticity, common after severe brain injury, may interfere with a child's functional abilities.[8, 18, 60, 69] Ataxia may result from damage to the sensory or motor systems related to either central or peripheral nervous systems.[81] Specifically, damage to the cerebellum often results in ataxic movements associated with voluntary limb movement (possibly high-amplitude tremor with movement) and gait. If damage is unilateral, ataxia may be manifested on the side ipsilateral to the lesion. The extent to which ataxia influences these movements is dependent on the location, size, and extent of the lesion.[49] It is thought that ataxia is due partially to an inability to "coordinate the relative activity of multiple muscles at a given joint for the effects of other moving joints."[49] Hypotonicity, fatigability, and weakness are also associated with cerebellar dysfunction.[82]

CASE STUDY

Spasticity and muscle weakness were present in all three children (see Table 3–2). Ataxia was noted in Carl; however, ataxia was also likely in Rick and Anne based on the reported areas of brain injury.

Somatosensory Systems and Postural Control

The sensory processes involved with postural control, that is, somatosensory complexes (joint, tactile, and proprioceptive systems), visual systems, and vestibular systems, may be affected after a brain injury. Interactions among these systems are critical for the production of effective functional movements, including adequate postural control. Postural control has been defined as a person's ability to maintain the center of mass in relation to the base of support during the completion of functional movements.[83] Both static and dynamic balance are critical in the successful performance of functional movements.

The effect of perceptual deficits on a child's postural control may vary with the child's age and stage of postural development. Typically, postural stability develops in a cephalocaudal manner. Children younger than 4 years have a greater reliance than older children on visual input for postural control. Adult-like patterns may not be present until 7 to 10 years of age, after a transitional period from 4 to 6 years, when timing and the selection of patterns are less well coordinated than before or after.[83, 84]

CASE STUDY

At 12 years of age, Anne and Carl (see Table 3–2) would have adult-like postural responses. Rick, however, is only 18 months old and would typically be dependent on visual information for balance. If his vision is affected, he will not substitute as easily with somatosensory information as would Anne or Carl.

The child's behavioral goals, the task demands, and the environmental conditions influence the selection of postural strategies. Constraints within the child's postural control system may limit the choice of strategies. In children with TBI, the level of consciousness and cognition affect the awareness of the task and the perception of its demands. Postural orientation problems may result from internal constraints such as sensation impairments (e.g., hemianopsia, diplopia, impaired proprioception, or impaired tactile sensation) or central abnormalities resulting in an inability to coordinate normal sensory inputs from vestibular, visual, or somatosensory systems. The postural response latency, the muscle force used, and the spatiotemporal coordination, which are typically adapted to the task demands, may be affected by neurologic impairments or biomechanical constraints (common after brain injury).[84–86]

Individuals with ataxia commonly demonstrate a use of greater force than normal and, occasionally, an increased latency of the normal spatiotemporal coordination of postural responses. A delayed onset of muscle activity is also seen with a delay in control processing. Abnormal spatiotemporal coordination after head injury is postulated to result from erosion in the creation of the synergies and from abnormal sensorimotor or biomechanical restraints.[87]

Musculoskeletal Complications

Orthopedic problems associated with TBI may include spinal cord injury; brachial plexus injury; fractures and dislocations resulting from concomitant trauma to limbs and spine; contractures related to spasticity; pressure sores; HO; scoliosis; and limb-length discrepancies.[61, 62, 75, 88] Muscle atrophy and weakness (predominately type II fibers), is typical of prolonged bed rest and may be complicated by poor neural control of muscle recruitment.[42]

The extent of musculoskeletal injuries is often difficult to assess in the unconscious and cognitively impaired child. Using bone scans on admission to rehabilitation, Sobus and colleagues identified previously undetected sites of fracture, soft tissue damage, and HO in 63 percent of the children ($n = 60$, ages 6 to 19 years).[88] The undetected sites were found to interfere with the production of functional activities in 25 percent of the children. Generally, the therapist suspects undiagnosed injury when the child resists joint movement or seems to be in pain during functional activities. The therapist then alerts the physician to areas of suspected injury and incorporates appropriate precautions into the therapy program.

Orthopedic Impairments

ROM constraints, common especially after severe brain injury, may be associated with prolonged posturing and persistent spasticity.[75, 89–91] Blasier and Letts reviewed the onset of occurrence of orthopedic deformities in children with severe brain injuries and spasticity.[89] The average time of deformity onset after injury was as follows: plantar flexion contractures, 5.3 months; scoliosis, 22 months; hip adduction contractures, 31 months; pes valgus, 35 months; and knee flexion contractures, 37 months.

HO of soft tissues occurs in some patients with prolonged unconsciousness, typically 2 to 4 months after the injury. The most commonly involved sites include the shoulder, elbow, hip, and knee. In children, ectopic bone is often spontaneously resorbed. As a result, surgical resection of bone to improve function is frequently delayed. Recurrence of the bone growth may follow surgical excision.[75]

Cardiopulmonary Impairments

Hypertension with systolic pressures between 160 and 180 mm Hg and diastolic pressures between 100 and 140 mm Hg are not uncommon after TBI.[75] Systolic blood pressure greater than 130 mm Hg and diastolic pressure greater than 100 mm Hg, persisting for more than 6 weeks after injury, however, are associated with a decreased chance of significant neurologic recovery.[22, 43, 69, 75] A return of blood pressure to normal levels coincides with neurologic improvement.[75] A decreased heart rate variability due to abnormal autonomic control of cardiac tone is common after injury and improves with neurologic recovery.[54]

Once the child demonstrates mobility within the environment, endurance limitations and maladaptive responses to physical activity may become evident. Impaired circulatory and ventilatory efficiency and responses to exercise have been found in young adults with TBI (compared with normal individuals). Specifically, these factors include reduced vital capacity, inspiratory capacity, total lung capacity, and forced expiratory volumes at 1 second (FEV_1). Inefficiencies were suggested to be related to inherent brainstem disturbances, resulting in deficient automatic motor performances that contribute to the development of secondary deconditioning.[91–93]

PHYSICAL THERAPY EXAMINATION AND INTERVENTION

Physical therapy examination and subsequent intervention are variable for the child with a TBI. The needs of the child and the family dictate the establishment of goals; examination procedures; and the treatment plan. The severity of the injury and the length of time since its onset also direct the course of intervention. The unpredictable and varied rate of recovery and the complex mechanisms of recovery necessitate continual assessment and modification of therapeutic intervention in order to appropriately enhance recovery and function.

The processes of data gathering, goal establishment, clinical examination, and intervention related to children with TBI are discussed. Specific discussion related to every level of severity of injury and age group is beyond the scope of this chapter. Rather, general concepts and special considerations specifically related to TBI are presented. Finally, a detailed case report of a 3.5-year-old child with a severe brain injury is discussed to further illustrate the decision-making processes throughout the continuum of care of this child in terms of the Hypothesis-Oriented Algorithm for Clinicians (HOAC) framework (see Chapter 1).[94]

Data Gathering and Goal Establishment

A complete and thorough review of the medical record and a focused family interview provide the therapist with valuable information regarding the child's prior functional abilities and cognitive level. This information is crucial for the establishment of relevant, functional, and appropriate goals. Interpretation of the data based on knowledge of the current literature can provide the therapist with hypotheses regarding possible impairments and a prognosis for recovery. A summary of recommended areas for focused review, with rationale and implications, is presented in Table 3–5.

Establishment of goals for a child with a TBI is often more complex than that for an adult because the child will continue to mature and refine cognitive and functional abilities. Optimally, long-term goals include the attainment of age-appropriate function, communicative skills, and self-care skills with eventual successful employment as an adult. Persistent residual physical or cognitive deficits, or both, may, however, impair the child's ability to achieve these ideal goals. Goal establishment should reflect the child's and family's needs and concerns. The child should be integrated into goal setting if motivated and cognitively able to participate in the process. Frequent and effective communication between the child and family and the team members is invaluable for the achievement of established goals and maximization of recovery. The cause and severity of the injury and the length of time since it occurred also contribute to the prediction of the extent of recovery and the establishment of realistic expectations.

Rancho Pediatric Levels V to III and Rancho Adult Levels I to III

In our experience, expectations for a child with persistent cognitive deficits functioning at Rancho pediatric levels V to III or Rancho adult levels I to III generally include

Data Gathering Rationale and Implications

TABLE 3–5

Area of Inquiry	Rationale and Implications
Preinjury status	
Age	
Preinjury functional status	Information regarding prior functional status provides baseline for assessment of motor abilities and identification of preinjury "problem" areas
Prior behavior and cognitive level	Prior behavior and cognitive abilities may be identified from school performance records and through family interview
Interests, favorite play activities	Knowledge of favorite play and recreational activities aids in designing treatment activities of interest to child
Cause of injury	Cause may suggest location and extent of cerebral injury
	Circumstances of injury alert therapist to possible concomitant injuries and necessary precautions before initiation of examination
Acute neurologic assessment	Neuroimaging and radiographic reports indicate location and extent of injuries
Glasgow Coma Scale; length of coma	Coma score at onset and changes during first 24–48 hr are key prognosticators
	Duration of coma and time course of recovery of consciousness indicate severity of injury and expected outcome
Family involvement and goals	Involvement during acute hospitalization may be indicative of expected level of involvement during rehabilitation and subsequent discharge
	Goals must be established based on family needs and desires
Previous therapy reports	Therapy reports before transfer provide information regarding functional abilities, responsiveness to therapy, and progress since injury
Other pertinent information	Additional information may provide insight for goal establishment and intervention strategies

dependence in all functional mobility, self-care, and social interactions. The caregivers must, therefore, be instructed in how to safely and effectively perform all self-care, feedings, and dependent transfers. Family members can perform or continue with interventions such as ROM exercises for contracture prevention and the maintenance of optimal skin integrity. Therapeutic intervention at these levels focuses on increasing periods of alertness and reducing a delay in response to specific stimulation. The efficacy of prolonged sensory stimulation programs is controversial.[29, 95] At these levels, children do not usually benefit from the 3 hours of daily intensive therapy from two or more disciplines (PT, OT, speech) required for acute rehabilitation funding.[96] Walker reviews the pros and cons of different levels of care,[96] including extended care facilities, which may find it challenging to have adequate numbers of staff and staff appropriately trained to meet the medical and behavioral needs of these children.

Rancho Pediatric Level II and Rancho Adult Levels IV and V

A child functioning at Rancho pediatric level II or Rancho adult level IV or V with only minimal physical limitations is typically able to perform previously well-learned activities such as rolling, sitting up, crawling, and walking. Despite these abilities, impaired judgment and problem solving necessitate constant supervision and assistance to prevent injury. In contrast, when physical constraints are moderate to severe for the child functioning at the same Rancho pediatric or adult level, it is difficult for the child to implement compensatory strategies in the performance of functional mobility activities. After many repetitions of a novel task the child may be able to learn the task using procedural memory.[29] Learning to use mobility aids such as crutches or a wheelchair may not be successful for the child at this level possibly because of poor memory and sequencing abilities. Because procedural memory is generally better preserved than declarative memory after brain injury, the child may not recall learning to use a walker or demonstrate on request the sequence of walking with an assistive device but can learn and use the skill through observation and much practice. The skill may not, however, be generalized to other task demands or environmental constraints.

Rancho Pediatric Level I or Rancho Adult Levels VI to VIII

The expected outcome for a child functioning at Rancho pediatric level I or Rancho adult levels VI to VIII with only minimal physical limitations may include independence with functional mobility and self-care activities. Supervision in the community may be necessary as a result of an impaired frustration tolerance, problem-solving abilities, judgment, and impulse control.

Interdisciplinary team goals for patient and family education include the caregivers' and the child's understanding of the injuries to the child's brain, short-term and long-term expectations for the child's recovery, the child's expected future needs, and how to access available and necessary resources for ongoing care (including educational services). Long-term goals include the child's understanding of the injury and his or her abilities, disabilities, and individual rights, and empowering the child to participate in informed decision making regarding care needs as an adult.

Physical Therapy Examination

General Considerations

A systematic and accurate examination provides the basis to establish a hypothesis regarding realistic functional goals and the extent to which impairments are constraining function. It also provides the therapist with knowledge regarding current functional abilities and the state of the systems that control and regulate movement.

Examination procedures should be appropriately selective and thorough, based on the previously identified needs of the child and family, established functional goals, and a review of clinical records. Assessment includes testing functional skills as well as the measurement of impairments. Indications for the examination of cognition, motor control, postural control, and somatosensory and musculoskeletal impairments are discussed later (with recognition of the interrelationships and interdependence of these factors). Additional areas of assessment focus include the child's goals and motivations; identification of the family's or the caregiver's involvement; the family's or the caregiver's understanding of the injury and the child's return to function; family and community resources; and the discharge destination. Examinations performed by other team members (e.g., those involved with communication disorders, occupational therapy, psychology, social work, and nursing) assist in gathering this information. A summary of the rationale for functional and impairment assessments is presented in Table 3–6.

Cognitive and Behavioral Factors Associated with Assessment

Behavioral, cognitive, and psychologic impairments are frequently present and problematic for the child with TBI. Decreased consciousness, maladaptive behaviors, and impaired cognition often interfere with the child's ability to participate in the assessment. Although the speech pathologist and psychologist perform specific examinations of these areas, the physical therapist can grossly determine the child's level of consciousness (with reference to the Rancho pediatric or adult scales) and cognitive ability to participate

Examination Procedures and Rationale for Inspection

TABLE 3-6

Functional Goals	Rationale	Testing Procedures
Age-appropriate cognitive skills	*Cognition* and level of consciousness play critical role in degree of alertness, desire to move and interact in environment, and ability to learn new skills	GCS Rancho Pediatric Level (infants–2 yr; preschool [2–5 yr]; school age [5 yr and older]) Rancho adult level (12 yr and older)
Functional skills related to mobility and self-care	*Functional abilities:* assessment of child's functional abilities and comparison to age-expected skills	PEDI WeeFIM FIM
	Motor control: creation of adequate muscle torque in appropriate timing relationships is required to meet task demands and environmental constraints; ability to access appropriate motor control can be influenced by somatosensory processing, presence of ataxia, available ROM, and muscle stiffness	Palpation of muscle activity (spontaneous or voluntary) Clinical observation of quality of movements, including notation regarding ability to move against force of gravity, postural control in response to tactile and positional stimulation; observation of movements made spontaneously or in response to stimuli (stimuli may include verbal or tactile input)
	Sensory processing: postural control, functional movements and learning are conditional on adequate perception and processing of somatosensory (visual, tactile, proprioceptive) and vestibular information	Manual muscle testing; torque testing Upright motor control test
	Postural control: assessment of child's ability to control center of body mass over base of support during functional movements; adequate postural stability is required to perform all mobility skills; must also meet demands of task and overcome environmental constraints	Responsiveness of head and trunk to planned and unexpected perturbations in balance during functional activities; information can be derived from performance of functional activities (as measured during functional assessments) Choice of motor strategies used in response to disturbances in balance should be noted (i.e., arm and leg counterbalancing vs. stepping strategy)
	Musculoskeletal status: selective examination based on data gathered regarding concomitant injuries, history of trauma, "posturing," prolonged bed rest; these factors may be indicative of expected ROM limitations or increased velocity-dependent muscle stiffness, or both	Passive joint ROM and muscle-length assessment by goniometry (measured in supine) Velocity-dependent muscle stiffness (spasticity) Fast ROM assessment (measured in upright) Ashworth Scale
	Knowledge of potential limitations guides plan for preventative measures to minimize problems resulting from joint malalignment (e.g., abnormal biomechanical forces, skin breakdown)	
	Physiologic response and endurance	Heart rate, blood pressure, respiratory rate (at rest and with activities), dyspnea level
Consumption of age-appropriate diet by mouth	*Dysphagia:* presence or absence of voluntary or reflexive saliva swallow, reflexes (gag, cough), cognitive impairments, sensory deficits, weakness, or apraxia of oral or pharyngeal structures, or both, all influence ability to safely consume nutrition by mouth	Observation of spontaneous saliva swallow Assessment of perioral and oral sensation by response to tactile, thermal, and gustatory input Observation of intraoral control and swallow response when presented with small (1–3 mL) bolus of water and "simple" foods (pureed fruits or vegetables) if indicated (see text)

ROM, range of motion; GCS, Glasgow Coma Score; PEDI, Pediatric Evaluation of Disability Inventory; FIM, Functional Independence Measure; WeeFIM, Functional Independence Measure for Children.

in testing. Physical therapy examination procedures must be modified to best elicit the child's motor performance.

A child with severe cognitive impairments functioning at Rancho pediatric level III or IV or Rancho adult level II or III such as Rick (see Table 3–2) would be unable to follow commands. Examination of his motor abilities, therefore, would focus on observation of spontaneous or stimulus-induced movements and passive manipulation rather than response to commands.

CASE STUDY

Rick could not follow commands, but he would focus on a bright light and withdraw his arm or leg from a noxious stimulus. We could observe his spontaneous movements and movements elicited by withdrawal to determine relative muscle strengths and ROM impairments interfering with movement (see Table 3–2).

A child functioning at Rancho pediatric level II or Rancho adult level IV or V is able to follow simple one-step commands with structure and cueing; however, distractibility, a limited attention span, and memory impairments may preclude the accurate completion of standard tests. This is especially evident when multiple commands are given or prolonged attention and understanding of the task are required such as in manual muscle testing (MMT). Elicitation of automatic activities (e.g., having the child catch a ball rather than asking child to lift the arms) is more useful in assessing purposeful and functional motor control in the child with cognitive limitations. Generally the "best" responses are evoked when the child is the most alert and attentive, so multiple short examination periods are ideal.

CASE STUDY

Carl was able to participate in MMT procedures. In each test position the motion was demonstrated, and a period of delay was allowed for processing the request and initiation of the motion. Multiple attempts were allowed before the grade was determined. Essentially, the MMT was presented as a series of one-step commands rather than multiple commands presented at once. Simple commands such as "Let's see you sit here on the edge of the bed" and "Let's go for a walk" elicited spontaneous well-coordinated movements in rolling, coming to a sitting position, and standing, although he required assistance to complete these transitional activities and maintain postural control. He was able to tolerate 15-minute testing sessions before fatiguing (see Table 3–2).

The confused-agitated child at Rancho adult level IV is in a heightened state of activity and may demonstrate bizarre and nonpurposeful behaviors. For the child at this level, the therapist must recall that the child is responding to cerebral irritation and internal confusion as he or she attempts to interact with and understand the environment. A calm environment with structured stimuli may facilitate the child's ability to follow commands for a short period of time. Increased sensory input, such as tactile input, or a request for difficult or complex movements may result in frustration and agitation. It has been our experience, however, that children often demonstrate their "best" functional motor abilities when agitated. At these times, the therapist should perform careful observation of purposeful movements, which will provide information regarding functional abilities, the available ROM, sensation, and motor and postural control.

The child functioning at Rancho pediatric level I or Rancho adult level VII or VIII is oriented to self, time, and place, although distractibility, a limited attention span, and memory impairments may remain. At these levels cognition does not interfere with the use of traditional assessment tools for short periods of time. However, behaviors such as aggression, a lack of self-initiation, a low frustration tolerance, emotional lability, or withdrawal, may be present, limit the length of therapy sessions, and necessitate a structured environment. We have found that a quiet environment with minimal distractions enhances the accuracy and reproducibility of motor control examination for a child functioning at any of the impaired levels of consciousness. It is important for the therapist to note, however, that the child's inability to perform activities in the presence of typical distractions may elucidate functional impairments related to cognitive status that have important implications for a successful return to home and community.

CASE STUDY

Anne participated in testing procedures for 30 minutes at one time. She was able to understand typical MMT procedures without modification. She became frustrated, however, when the task was difficult for her to perform (see Table 3–2).

Functional Assessments

A complete examination of functional abilities includes assessment of age-appropriate cognition and function. Many functional assessment tools are available to the practitioner, so the selection should be based on the child's age and the ability of the measure to establish a baseline of abilities and track functional recovery. The PEDI,[64] the FIM,[65] and the WeeFIM[66] are nationally recognized standardized tests that are frequently used for the previously mentioned purposes. Because these measures are relatively new, the impact of the severity of injury and the presence of impairments on the outcome is yet to be elucidated.

The FIM[65] and the WeeFIM[66] measure 18 items related to independence in daily functions including self-care, sphincter control, mobility, locomotion, communication, and social cognition. Each item is scored by indicating the amount of assistance needed to complete the activity. The WeeFIM was designed for use with children 6 months to 7 years of age, the FIM for adults and children 7 years of age and older. Interrater reliability of the FIM has been found to be good.[97] The PEDI[64] was designed for the functional assessment of children between the ages of 6 months and 7 years, but it may be used for older children whose functional abilities are below that expected of a 7-year-old. The PEDI measures a child's capability and functional performance in self-care, mobility, and social function. The PEDI yields normative and scaled scores that may be used to compare the child's performance with that of age-matched peers or to track a child's performance over time, respectively. Each of these functional tests may provide documentation of motor control, postural control, and somatosensory function as related to the "successful" production of functional movements as measured by the assessment.

Some of these measures, however, may not be sensitive to the functional abilities or progression of changes in motor performance in the severely injured child who is unable to interact with the environment or to capture the acquisition of skills beyond walking. Other functional assessments that are more sensitive to small, yet important, motor changes, such as the Alberta Infant Motor Scale,[98] Movement Assessment of Infants,[99] Gross Motor Function Measure (GMFM),[100] Bruininks-Oseretsky Test of Motor Proficiency (BOTM),[101] or Peabody Developmental Motor Scales (PDMS)[102] may, depending on the child's age and functional motor level, provide the therapist with needed objective information to clarify the child's progress, identify the child's impairments, or plan intervention. It is important to note that such measures were not developed for, nor standardized on, children with brain injuries; therefore, the interpretation of findings needs further development with this population. For further information regarding current motor development theories and functional measures see Westcott and coworkers.[83]

Examination of Impairments That Constrain Function: Motor Control

Initially, the quality of movement is assessed in general terms. A lack of spontaneous or stimulus-induced movement may indicate the level of consciousness or the presence of a neglect syndrome (due to sensory deficits). If the child is able to perform only stimulus-induced movements, the therapist must carefully observe the timing, force, duration, direction, and location of movement in response to controlled stimulation. This provides valuable information regarding the status of sensory, motor, and sensorimotor integrative aspects of movement.

The level of consciousness dictates whether movement is random or purposeful. For the child who is functioning at least at Rancho pediatric level II or adult level IV (responds to the environment), the therapist can observe the variability of movements available to perform a given motor task by manipulating the task demands. For example, in the task of kicking a ball, is the child able to move the limbs and joints in variable movements (selective control) or are movements limited to a few abnormal stereotypic patterns (patterned movements)? As recovery occurs, the child is generally able to move the limbs and joints selectively, complexly, adjusting balance and postural demands according to the demands of the task and the environment (e.g., demonstrate greater selective control). The therapist must recognize that many factors may influence these abilities, including cognition and behavior, postural control, spasticity, sensorimotor integration deficits (e.g., apraxia or impaired visual discrimination), ROM, ataxia, sensation (particularly proprioception), and visual perceptual deficits. The influence of individual factors and the relationships among multiple impairments must be considered when the therapist performs an examination and hypothesizes about the constraints limiting function. Assessments by a speech pathologist and an occupational therapist identify the presence of cognitive, visual perceptual, and sensorimotor integration deficits. Once these impairments are identified, the physical therapist can consider their impact on functional limitations.

Careful observation of the production of functional movements may assist the therapist in the identification of the child's skill in coordinating movement. Movements should be observed in variable situations: in opposition to gravity and in gravity-eliminated positions, in upright (sitting or standing) positions, statically and dynamically, and with variable task demands. These movements provide information regarding the relative strength of muscle groups and possible peripheral nerve injuries. Dynamometry and MMT is useful in the assessment of muscle strength in children as young as 3 years.[103–107] Cognitive level and motor control problems affect the child's ability to generate a maximal voluntary contraction. Plantar flexion strength is best assessed with the child in the standing position with 20 heel rises indicating normal strength for older children.[103, 105] The ability to lift body weight or weighted items may provide even more information about the relative function, control, and strength of selected muscle groups. More important, however, is the child's ability to move between postures and subsequently maintain the new position while performing variable motor activities to meet the demands of the environment or the task at hand.[83]

Examination of control in the standing position indicates the child's ability to use available motor control dynamically. The Upright Motor Control Test assesses the ability to quickly flex the hip, knee, and ankle as well as the ability to control the hip, knee, and ankle in single-limb stance.[103] Control of each joint in flexion and extension is graded on a three-point scale. This motor control scale can be used for children as well as adults as long as they are able to cognitively participate. See Hislop and Montgomery[103] for the test procedure.

Ataxia of the limbs and trunk is observed during functional activities, such as self-care, feeding, or walking. The intensity, magnitude, and effect of ataxic tremors and their influence on functional activity is documented by clinical observation. Ataxia may be distinguished as sensory or cerebellar in origin. Differentiation between the two types is made by observing the child perform an activity with and without the eyes closed. Sensory ataxia is defined as an increase in ataxia when movements are performed with the eyes closed. Hypermetria (overshooting a target) may also be present in the child with ataxia. See Bastian for a further discussion of ataxic mechanisms.[81]

Examination of Postural Control

Examination of postural control may be directed at the impairment or the functional limitation level. Shumway-Cook and Horak describe a test to differentiate impairments in sensory integration that may interfere with balance in standing.[108] This test is appropriate when the child is older than 8 years, can follow simple commands, and does not have musculoskeletal problems.[108, 109] Typically, however, therapists use "nonstandardized observations" of a child's response to induced disturbances to the child's center of gravity.[83] There is a need to increase the objectivity of such measures. The Pediatric Clinical Test of Sensory Interaction for Balance[110, 111] is a quantitative test that assists in the identification of impairments in motor responses in variable sensory environments for children 4 to 9 years of age.[110–113] Its validity in discriminating children with learning disabilities has been demonstrated.[114] Further research that identifies its validity for use with children after brain injury is needed.

Many different reliable and valid measures may serve a dual function to assess functional abilities as well as postural control. Many of the tests examine balance as related to gross motor skills and activities of daily living. Such tests include the functional measures previously discussed (PEDI, FIM or WeeFIM, GMFM, PDMS, or BOTM), the "timed Up & Go" and the Functional Reach Test.[83] See Westcott and associates for a current detailed review of the reliability and validity, as well as recommendations for use, of measurement tools related to balance.[83] Further research is needed to determine the validity of these tools with children after brain injury.

The child's performance of functional mobility activities on such tests implies the child's adequate ability to maintain the location of the center of mass in relation to the base of support. Until better quantitative measures of impairments are available, assessment of functional abilities provides the needed qualitative information on postural control. The child's choice of balance "strategy" can also be documented. For example, a child may choose a "hip strategy" or a "dorsiflexion strategy" when the center of mass is displaced posteriorly (e.g., forward flexion at the hips rather than dorsiflexion at the ankle is used to maintain balance). Notation of the child's choice of compensatory strategy reflects the influence of constraining factors affecting functional mobility (such as limited dorsiflexion ROM).[109] It is also important that the therapist note the child's ability to respond appropriately to vestibular, visual, and proprioceptive information in the maintenance of postural stability during functional activities.

CASE STUDY

Initially all three children demonstrated poor postural control in the sitting position (see Table 3–2).

Carl was able to maintain the sitting position using his upper extremities for support and had good static and dynamic head control. The presence of selective limb motion, the absence of contractures, and minimal spasticity in his plantar flexor muscles suggest that his impaired postural control and functional abilities were related to muscle weakness (disuse), possible impairments in sensorimotor integration, or ataxia (noted in his hand). Motor-planning impairments and peripheral sensory deficits were not noted during the observation of functional movements.

In contrast, Rick's complete lack of postural control responses in sitting were consistent with his limited ability to recognize and respond to external stimuli (Rancho pediatric level II). Limited movements of his left extremities compared with the right suggest limitations in sensory and motor abilities on his left side and a need to compensate for deficits in function.

Anne's poor postural control may be influenced by impaired sensation, limited variability in movement patterns, and increased muscle stiffness on her left side. Her severely delayed protective responses suggest impairments in somatosensory systems as well.

Musculoskeletal Impairments

Range-of-Motion Limitations

ROM limitations may be associated with one or a combination of different causes such as prolonged abnormal positioning due to immobility, pain, peripheral nerve injury, or spasticity.[75, 90] Regardless of the precipitating factors, ROM limitations are measured by clinical observation and goniometry.[115, 116] Accurate examination can provide information regarding the current ROM status and potential limitations that may provide constraints to functional mobility.

Measurement reliability is problematic in children, especially after brain injury. Attention to external conditions and retesting by the same examiner may reduce the variability of measures.[116] A child who is agitated, confused, or unable to follow commands may resist ranging and cry in response to pain. Observation of the ROM used during spontaneous movements and functional activities provides the therapist with information regarding joint motions and possible limitations. Joint capsule tightness, shortened muscle length, and HO are other sources of ROM limitations. A warm and painful joint motion is associated with HO. Any associated ROM limitations, however, must be measured and subsequently minimized with treatment.

CASE STUDY

Anne's hip flexion contracture would be treated too if ambulation is a goal (see Table 3–2).

Muscle Stiffness (Spasticity)

The Modified Ashworth Scale is a quick, simple and reliable method for the examination of muscle response to passive stretch.[117] The scale is based on an ordinal scale: zero (no increase in muscle stiffness) to 4 (rigid in flexion or extension) (Table 3–7). The predictability of functional performance or recovery from Ashworth Scale scores has yet to be determined, however.

Another consideration when assessing muscle stiffness is the position of the child (e.g., sitting or standing versus supine). Examination of the fast ROM performed with the patient in a functional position such as standing can provide information about the child's ability to use available movement during upright functional activities. Clinical

Modified Ashworth Scale for Grading of Spasticity

TABLE 3–7

Grade	Description
0	No change in muscle response to movement into flexion or extension
1	Slight increase in muscle response to movement (into flexion or extension), visible by *catch and release* or by only minimal resistance at end of range of motion
1+	Slight increase in muscle resistance to movement into flexion or *extension followed by* only *minimal* resistance throughout the remainder (less than half) of range
2	Notable increase in muscle resistance *throughout most* of range of motion, but joint is easily moved
3	Marked increase in muscle resistance, passive movement is difficult into flexion or extension
4	Affected part or parts are rigid into flexion or extension when passively moved

Adapted from Bohannon RW, Smith MB: Interrater reliability of a Modified Ashworth Scale of muscle spasticity. Phys Ther 67:206, 1987, with permission of the American Physical Therapy Association.

observation of muscle stiffness and performance of functional activities provides the therapist with hypotheses about the influence of spasticity, but no studies are available to validate these postulations. If the child is able to cognitively and physically participate in the process, response of the adjacent muscles to fast passive stretch or fast passive joint ROM is assessed by supporting the child in a single-leg standing position on a block while the test leg is non–weight bearing. A selected joint is *passively* placed through selected movements *quickly,* and the specific point at which muscle stiffness limits further movement is noted (the fast ROM response is noted as a range such as zero to 30 degrees). Movements that are typically assessed (because of their relationship to ambulation) include dorsiflexion, knee flexion and extension, hip flexion, and straight-leg raising. This test was developed in part to consider the need to achieve a ROM quickly during functional activities. In our experience, the amount of dorsiflexion actually achieved in stance and of knee flexion in swing is often similar to the amount of "fast range" tested at these joints. This type of testing that considers the influence of position and muscle stiffness on the available ROM may be more indicative of the effect of these constraints on functional performance than ROM measurements performed with the patient in the supine position. For example, passive dorsiflexion ROM assessed with the patient in the supine position may be zero to 10 degrees, but a fast ROM assessed in the upright position may be lacking 10 degrees. Further research is needed to discern the validity of these proposed relationships.

Somatosensory Examination

Response to a specific sensory stimulus is variable, depending on the child's level of consciousness. Stimulation of auditory, visual, olfactory, gustatory, and pain pathways will evoke a response in the child at all levels of consciousness except Rancho pediatric level V (no response to stimuli). Table 3–8 indicates the expected "localized responses" at Rancho pediatric level III or Rancho adult level III.

Specific sensory testing is limited by the child's age and cognition. Once the child initiates purposeful movement in the environment (Rancho pediatric level II), a *gross observational* examination of proprioception can be performed. Precise assessment of light touch, proprioception, sharp-dull and two-point discrimination testing require memory, the ability to process information, and the ability to follow complex commands. As a result these specific tests are difficult to assess accurately in the child with a brain injury. Total body, perioral, and oral hypersensitivity are often present in the child with a brain injury. Hypersensitivity is hypothesized to result from a prolonged lack of stimulation after injury.

Accurate measurement of somatosensory deficits can also provide the therapist

Localized Responses to Sensory Stimulus

TABLE 3–8	Sensory Tract	Stimulus	Response
	Auditory	Voice	Opens eye
		Bell	Looks toward stimulus
		Hand clapping	Turns head toward or away from stimulus
	Visual	Threat near eyes	Blinks
		Bright object	Focuses and tracks
		Familiar toy	
		Familiar person	
	Olfactory	Ammonia	Grimaces or turns away
	Gustatory	Sugar	Smiles
		Lemon	Grimaces
	Pain	Squeezed muscle belly	Pulls extremity away
		Squeezed nail bed	Looks toward pain stimulus
		Pin prick	

with information regarding the child's ability to perform appropriate postural reactions. The child with a head injury may have visual and visual perceptual problems affecting the selection of motor patterns. Specific sensorimotor processing problems are commonly assessed by an occupational therapist.

CASE STUDY

Although none of the children could follow formal sensory testing procedures, gross sensory examinations were made by observing the child's function and responses to touch (see Table 3–2).

Physiologic Control

Before the initiation of examination of a child with a brain injury the therapist must identify medical precautions and consider the impact of the physiologic response to activity on possibilities for subsequent intervention.[29, 31, 118, 119] Labile physiologic responses may be present even in the child who no longer requires the use of continuous cardiac monitors. Maladaptive changes in the heart rate and rhythm and in blood pressure as well as in the respiratory rate, rhythm, and pattern may be present in response to muscle stretch, pain, activity, or even position changes. Baseline respiratory and cardiovascular parameters should be determined at rest and in response to activity, and the physician should be consulted to determine a safe level of physiologic challenge and the potential influence of medications. Examination of chest expansion, percussion, and auscultation should also be included.[118–120]

Examination of Dysphagia and Feeding

Children with severe head injuries often demonstrate feeding and swallowing problems due to brainstem and cranial nerve involvement. These children often arrive at the rehabilitation hospital with a nasogastric tube in place for nutritional support. It is important to try to resume oral feedings or place a gastrostomy tube (G-tube) as soon as possible because prolonged nasogastric tube feedings result in deprivation of oral sensation and often inhibit the recovery of normal reflex responses for safe and effective swallowing.[121, 122]

Sensory examination of the face, lips, tongue, inner surface of the cheeks, soft palate, and posterior pharyngeal wall may identify areas of hypo- or hypersensitivity to tactile, gustatory, or thermal input. Assessment of the swallowing, gag, and cough reflexes is indicated to provide information regarding the ability to initiate the swallow and protective mechanisms. Movement of the soft palate and posterior pharyngeal wall are assessed to determine the child's ability to propel a bolus in preparation for the swallow. Selective and voluntary control of the lips, tongue, and jaw can be observed in response to tactile stimulation.

Impaired cognition typically interferes with voluntary initiation of the swallow and the ability to control orofacial musculature, monitor the bolus size, and time the initiation of the voluntary portion of the swallow.[122] Even children functioning at Rancho pediatric level III or IV or Rancho adult level IV, III, or II, however, demonstrate rhythmic jaw movements and repeated tongue movements followed by a reflexive swallow.[122] These rhythmic oral motor movements typically follow a yawn or oral stimulation, or occasionally occur as a generalized reaction in response to noxious stimulation.

Indications for the initiation of a feeding trial as described by Zablotny are as follows:[122]

1. Adequate cognition
2. Demonstration of adequate oral motor control for propulsion of a bolus

3. Demonstration of a reflexive swallow with adequate laryngeal excursion on presentation of a small amount of water
4. No active respiratory problems
5. Presence of a gag reflex or weak posterior pharyngeal wall movement (for propulsion of a bolus)
6. No evidence of aspiration (may be confirmed with video swallowing fluoroscopy if indicated)

If coughing or choking is present before, during, or after a swallow, video swallowing fluoroscopy (VSF) may be indicated to confirm the cause of aspiration when a tracheotomy tube is not present. Lazarus and Logemann describe the problems typically seen in adult TBI that are associated with aspiration.[121] Lazarus and Logemann reviewed VSF assessments of swallowing in 53 persons with closed head trauma. Delayed or absent swallowing, reduced tongue control, and impaired pharyngeal peristalsis were the most common problems. Liquids were aspirated when the tongue control was impaired or the swallowing was delayed or absent. Aspiration most often occurred after the swallowing when reduced pharyngeal peristalsis resulted in food left in the valleculae. Lazarus and Logemann report that VSF may be an invaluable tool to identify the presence and cause of aspiration because many patients do not cough after aspiration.[121] If VSF is indicated, the therapist must consider positioning of the head and trunk as well as food and liquid consistency to be used in order to accurately assess possible aspiration.[121] Finally, the ability to maintain adequate static and dynamic postural control of the head when seated also plays a critical role in the child's ability to efficiently perform feeding activities.

CASE STUDY   All three children had difficulty swallowing clear liquids. VSF may identify aspiration if it is present (see Table 3–2).

Assessment of Family Needs and Education

Family support, the family's needs, and available resources should be assessed as soon as the family is available. As mentioned previously, it is critical that the therapist develop goals and approach intervention in collaboration with the child and the family. Ongoing family education is needed as the child recovers to optimize carryover and follow through with work on functional changes. A detailed discussion of the decision-making process related to the assessment of family needs and education is presented in the extended case report at the end of this chapter.

Physical Therapy Intervention

The physical therapy plan of care is determined by the needs and priorities of the child and the family. Continual assessment and modification of intervention are indicated in order to appropriately influence recovery and functional abilities because of the unpredictable rate of improvement. Although hypotheses underlying physical therapy may include functional mobility limited by musculoskeletal constraints, it is likely that the child's functional skills are also limited by cognitive and sensory perceptual deficits. The physical therapist draws on the examination findings of the interdisciplinary team to develop hypotheses regarding the constraints interfering with function. In many cases collaboration among team members results in a coordinated effort at remediation of constraints and reinforcement of new abilities.

It is difficult to determine the extent to which individual impairments and the relationships among these impairments are constraining function. Minimization of musculoskeletal constraints, such as limited ROM, assist the child in finding optimal movement strategies to accomplish the tasks at hand. Additionally, the therapist must design interventions (1) with a view toward the prevention of future musculoskeletal dysfunction (e.g., overuse syndromes, joint deformities) as the child grows and (2) to promote a healthy lifestyle in preparation for adulthood.

A detailed discussion of the progression of care is presented in the case report with regard to specific guidelines and discussion of the decision-making process. General concepts related to the management of the child with a TBI are discussed here.

Intervention as Related to Cognitive Impairments

Persistent severe cognitive limitations (Rancho pediatric levels V to III or adult levels I to III) present a challenge to the treating therapist. At these levels, the child does not attempt to interact with or move within the environment. Intervention, therefore, may be related only to cognitive stimulation, positioning, and the prevention of deformities in preparation for anticipated improvements in the level of consciousness and functional abilities. When the child reaches Rancho pediatric level II or Rancho adult levels IV to VI, intervention is related to the performance of functional mobility activities with varied task demands. As the child begins to initiate interaction with the environment, cognitive impairments become more apparent, including limitations in attention, concentration, visual discrimination, sequencing, categorization, and memory skills. Functional activities can be learned using procedural memory and implicit learning[29] through the repetition of tasks in appropriate contexts with orientation to time, self, and place. Therapeutic activities are designed in light of the child's cognitive limitations. Team members including the nursing staff and family members collaborate to reinforce the development of cognitive and functional skills.

For the child functioning at Rancho pediatric level I or Rancho adult level VII or VIII, physical therapy, in addition to addressing impairments and functional retraining, contributes to the child's cognitive reorganization. Treatment includes activities that focus on improving memory, encourage analysis and synthesis, and promote the use of judgment, problem solving, reasoning, and abstract thinking during functional activities. The therapist needs further assessment of the impact of this training on the child's safety, judgment, and ability to use functional skills in different contexts (e.g., sitting down on a chair versus sitting down on a booth bench) and the impact of attentional deficits on balance in children after brain injury. Observation of performance in actual community situations provides important information regarding the child's functional abilities and identifies factors that would not be evident in the clinical setting. For example, ambulation training practiced in the community incorporates judgment and problem-solving skills (e.g., crossing the street and the interpretation of directional information). "Higher cognitive functions" of decision making, judgment, and problem solving are usually not expected to recover by discharge, and activities demanding these skills typically require close supervision to ensure safety. Family members learn the child's cognitive limitations and strategies to improve or compensate for them, or both. Once discharged from the rehabilitation setting, outpatient services are continued as necessary to maximize independence at school and in the community.

A speech pathologist can provide additional valuable information regarding cognitive processing and language deficits and how the child's level of consciousness will affect the performance of functional skills. The speech therapist can also provide information regarding the amount and complexity of stimulation as well as the rate and duration of presentation the child is able to process.

Intervention to Improve Functional Abilities and Motor Control

Intervention for the child with a TBI should be based on previously established functional goals, hypothesized limitations to function, and motivational interests of the child. The selection of a strategy or combination of approaches should also be based on the age and current cognitive function of the child, as well as on the child's preinjury functional abilities and cognition. In order to encourage maximal participation and carryover of functional abilities, the child should be incorporated into goal setting if motivated and cognitively able to participate.

The therapist must provide opportunities for the child to actively participate and practice meaningful and motivating activities. Functional and relevant skills should be practiced in an efficient manner under a wide variety of task demands and environmental conditions. However, after a TBI, children practicing tasks designed for remediation of perceptual deficits or praxis may show improvements in the practiced tasks, but not transfer of skills into other contexts.[123, 124] Practice in a functional context, errorless learning, or specific training to transfer the new ability, or all of these, may be beneficial.[55, 123, 125] Determining the number of repetitions needed to learn a new task, the ability of the child to do the same task the next day, and the ability to do the task in different contexts provides clues to the child's learning.[124] The therapist has the ability to modify task and environmental variables to adjust the difficulty of the functional activity.[126] The context and parameters with which functional skills are practiced can consequently be easily controlled. For example, ambulation can be practiced outside, at the transition point between different level surfaces (grass to concrete), or in order to place balls in a basketball hoop, using as much repetition as the child and the therapist desire.

It is apparent that the ability to maintain effective static and dynamic postural control plays a critical role in the successful production of functional movement.[83] Because improvements in postural control have been hypothesized to lead to improvements in all movements,[83] it is logical to assume that intervention to improve functional abilities will result in improvements in the child's postural control. To promote such an outcome, the therapist should also consider using interventions that require anticipatory as well as reactive postural responses to perturbations in balance. Interventions must target the components contributing to instability rather than compensatory strategies chosen to maintain balance.[83] (See Horak and coworkers for a current literature review of theories of postural control.[87])

As cognition improves and intentional interaction with the environment occurs with greater frequency, ataxia may become more apparent when the child initiates purposeful movements. Goldberger suggests that spontaneous recovery from cerebellar ataxia is dependent on processing peripheral feedback and is not dependent on training or enhanced training.[127] More recent studies suggest protocols to improve function through training that progressively challenges postural responses in an attempt to scale muscle responses[84, 87] and to reduce hypermetria using training for relaxation and biofeedback.[125] Reduction of the influence of ataxia to improve function may be enhanced by a focus on the reduction of the complexity of the movements through minimization of the number of active moving joints.[81] For example, the child with ataxia may stabilize the upper extremity against a steady surface such as the body or a table to reduce the number of joints moving in order to perform a fine motor task. Further assessment of the efficacy of treatment protocols for children with ataxia after brain injury is needed. Meanwhile, therapists design treatments considering the apparent type of ataxia and other impairments present.[84, 128] Treatment protocols aimed at improving control are preferred over teaching substitution by stabilizing against external surfaces.[84] Follow-up studies of resolution of ataxia and its long-term interference with ambulation as an adult after TBI in childhood are not available.

After a TBI, a child is likely to have multiple cognitive and motor control impairments that interfere with functional tasks. As the child recovers, the cognitive, motor control, and musculoskeletal impairments change. After careful physical therapy examination, therapists consider their findings as well as cognitive and perceptual deficits identified by speech and occupational therapists to hypothesize impairments interfering with function. As treatment progresses, therapists assess changes in impairments and function to challenge or confirm their hypotheses and therefore modify treatment. These children have complex involvement and persistent cognitive and motor control impairments that interfere with the acquisition of new skills.[57] Continued follow-up and intervention by knowledgeable professionals may improve the long-term outcome.

Again, further research is needed to develop and test effective treatment protocols for children after TBI.

Intervention to Reduce Musculoskeletal Impairments

A program to reduce or prevent myostatic and capsular contractures may include positioning, myofascial stretching, joint mobilization, prolonged static stretching, serial casting splints, and electrical stimulation. The program should be designed to minimize, improve, or prevent ROM impairments and should be directed at the hypothesized cause or causes of the limitation (e.g., muscle stiffness, prolonged abnormal positioning). Conservative spasticity management in the child with a TBI may include passive ROM exercises, prolonged static stretching with serial casting or positional splints, or electrical stimulation to antagonistic muscle groups. Electrical "cycling" of antagonistic muscles may assist in attaining an increased ROM.[129–131] Tolerance of electrical stimulation is often low, however, and effects are variable. This modality must, therefore, be used judiciously.[130]

Splints and positioning may assist in the maintenance of available ROM and the prevention of contractures for the child with moderate to severe spasticity.[90, 132] Moseley found the combination of casting and static stretching more effective than static stretching alone for increasing passive dorsiflexion in adults with TBI ($n = 10$ adults at a mean of 72 days after the onset of brain injury).[133] An increase of 13.9 ± 9.3 degrees was found when static stretch and casting were implemented compared with a 1.9 ± 10.2 degree increase when static stretching alone was implemented. Hill also found casting for a 1-month period to be more effective than "traditional" therapy to improve elbow ROM and "clinical indications of spasticity" ($n = 15$, 9 to 48 years old).[134] Additionally, the use of botulinum toxin, injected into the plantar flexors (which were 3 on a Modified Ashworth Scale) was found to improve the gait characteristics in a single-subject case study (19-year-old man 2 years after TBI).[135] Changes in gait characteristics included increased dorsiflexion and knee flexion in stance, especially during the pre-swing, increased velocity and stride length, and a shorter stride time. Further clarification of indications for treatment and efficacious protocols for (as well as the relationship between) changes in the ROM and changes in function is needed. Refer to Dobkin for further review of management of contractures and spasticity.[136]

Positioning typically maintains the ROM by preventing the assumption of prolonged abnormal postures. The primary goals for positioning include the prevention of contractures and minimization of asymmetry. These factors are critical for several reasons; for example, symmetric wheelchair positioning of the pelvis, hips, and trunk may reduce the likelihood of compromise in skin integrity and provide optimal alignment as well as provision of a stable base of support for functional mobility while the child is seated.

Muscle strengthening and endurance improve through increased involvement in functional activities. In addition, strengthening protocols for specific muscle groups and the use of electrical stimulation[130] may promote faster strengthening. It is important to note the controversy surrounding the issue of the relationship between spasticity and function.[136, 137] Many authors argue that decreasing spasticity may not necessarily result in improved functional abilities.[137] In fact, spasticity has been argued to be valuable as a useful adaptation to disability when the force control capacity is impaired. Others argue that spasticity interferes with movement. The therapist can assess the child's function and hypothesize about whether impairments that contribute to difficulty with movement are affecting the child's function. Treatment then is based on this hypothesis. In any case, the therapist must carefully assess the impact of spasticity on the child's functional abilities and minimize problems associated with overuse or musculoskeletal complications that result in pain or decreases in functional abilities as the child grows and develops.

Surgical management may be indicated for the child with severe persistent spasticity and resultant joint malalignment and abnormal biomechanical forces. Surgical intervention may include adductor tenotomies (to prevent subluxation or dislocation of the hips), or phenol block to the musculocutaneous nerve and the motor branches of the median nerve (to counteract severe persistent spasticity of the elbow and finger flexors and allow functional use of the arm, or for hygiene). Later, surgical management may address scoliosis and leg-length discrepancies. Surgery,[75, 89, 92] intrathecal baclofen,[137] and botulinum toxin injection[137] may be used to manage the effects of residual spasticity that interferes with function. (See Hoffer and associates,[90] Meyler and coworkers,[91] and Blasier and Letts[89] for further discussion of acute and long-term orthopedic management.)

ROM limitations associated with HO are the most difficult to manage.[75] Associated pain may interfere with the child's desire to move the affected joint, thereby resulting in the potential for the further development of contractures. Generally, with encouragement, the child will continue to use the extremity within its pain-free range. When the child refuses to use the limb, we have found that immobilization of the joint in a plaster cast may relieve the pain sufficiently to allow the child to incorporate the use of the extremity into functional activities. Often the child must learn to compensate for a limited range due to HO until the bone is reabsorbed or surgical resection is complete. HO is especially problematic because of the frequent recurrence of the bony block even after surgical excision.[75]

Cardiovascular and Respiratory Interventions

In our experience, cardiovascular impairments are typically present when a child has spent even short periods in bed. The therapist must monitor and adhere to acceptable physiologic parameters during therapy sessions. With these factors in mind, the therapist must, nevertheless, challenge the child's endurance limitations.[93, 118, 136] Programs to challenge the child's cardiovascular system consider the persistent impairments.[47, 93] A shuttle walk-run assessment and conditioning program, with good reliability and normative data available, has been designed specifically for the child after TBI.[138, 139] Continued cardiovascular assessment and training may reduce disability and improve the quality of life. Further studies are needed.

In the acutely ill child, chest therapy assists in preventing the complications of atelectasis and pneumonia.[119, 120] Positioning, bronchial drainage, and manual techniques of percussion and vibration assist in mobilizing secretions and increase airflow to the dependent lung.[118–120]

Intervention Regarding Dysphagia and Feeding

The position of the head and trunk may influence the child's ability to perform successful feeding activities. The alignment of the structures of the oropharynx and larynx affect the speed and ease of flow of the liquid or food and, therefore, the motor control required to successfully swallow the bolus. The strength and endurance constraints of the neck and trunk as well as oral and pharyngeal musculature may affect the energy cost of this normally energy-efficient activity, limiting the child's ability to carry out the activity for the length of time required to complete a meal.[121] Silverman and Elfant found that techniques to facilitate efficient eating that appear to improve motor control in response to sensory input include positioning of the head, trunk, and extremities; manually assisted jaw and lip closure; a quick stretch and ice; and resistive exercises to the lips, larynx, and neck musculature.[140]

Hyposensitivity, often present with prolonged nasogastric tube feeding, may interfere with rhythmic oral motor movements. These movements may be so altered that tongue movement ceases before the bolus reaches the pharynx; the reflex swallow may be subsequently delayed, and laryngeal excursion may be incomplete. Perioral sensitization techniques (i.e., thermal, gustatory, or tactile input) may influence the rhythmic motor reflexes of swallowing. Because central control for swallowing exists within the brainstem reticular formation, the general excitatory status of the reticular activating system in the brainstem may increase alertness and consequently assist in completion of the swallow. Additionally, perioral and intraoral hypersensitivity often result in reflexes that interfere with jaw opening and swallowing responses (e.g., tonic bite and hyperactive gag reflex). Desensitization techniques may assist in decreasing the influence of these reflexes and may be necessary before the initiation of any feeding sessions.[121, 122, 140]

Progression of food consistency and liquid viscosity are modified according to the child's motor control abilities, including endurance limitations, and the child's age-appropriate diet. See Table 3–9 for a discussion of considerations regarding food and liquid consistencies.

Cognitive and behavioral impairments often interfere with feeding (especially self-feeding) even after adequate orofacial motor control abilities and endurance are achieved. A shortened attention span and memory impairments often result in distractibility and confusion. The child forgets to swallow or attends to other stimuli in the room but when redirected to the activity can complete the task. The confused child may put too much food in the mouth or forget to swallow, or both. Close supervision and a carefully structured environment for feeding are critical for the child with these types of cognitive impairments. Typically the child must be reminded to swallow after each bite, and the bolus size must be carefully monitored. Self-feeding abilities are often constrained by upper extremity motor control impairments, but when the child begins to initiate purposeful movements in the environment (Rancho pediatric level II or adult level IV, V, or VI), appropriate assistance and supervision for feeding should be implemented to avoid a passive feeding situation.

Family Needs and the Provision of Education

The family or caregivers must be educated regarding the child's injury, expected progression of recovery, and anticipated cognitive and functional level. The family must also be educated regarding rights and advocacy for their child, community resources, and negotiation of the complex medical systems in preparation for discharge. The Brain Injury Association is a national advocacy group and a resource for information on state and community-based services in the United States (The Brain Injury Association, Inc., 105 North Alfred Street, Alexandria, VA 22314. Phone 703-236-6000. Internet site http://www.biusa.org/national.htm)

When available, the family should be incorporated into treatment sessions as much as possible. It is critical for the family to actively participate in order to facilitate carryover of treatment into the daily care routine. The family's inclusion and active participation in decision-making processes have also been found to decrease potential conflicts between the team members and the family during the stressful period after the injury.[141]

Social workers, psychologists, speech pathologists, and psychiatrists may provide family counseling to cope with residual psychologic complications (e.g., hyperactivity, impulsivity, frustration, aggressiveness, and poor social judgment). Assessment of the family support system facilitates assisting family adjustment. Through individual and group media, initial intervention assists the family to cope with the devastating disruption to their lifestyle and the issue of life or death. Education regarding the rehabilitation process and the family's coping strategies attempts to shift them to coping day to day rather than trying to prepare for the long term. As the child recovers, the family responds on an emotional roller coaster of highs as the child lives, wakes up, and progresses—and lows as progress hits plateaus and residual physical, cognitive, and psychologic deficits, as well as behavioral changes, are compared with the preinjury identity. The social worker assists the family to deal with their feelings, anxieties, frustrations, and depression in considering the child's reentry to home and the resultant threat to their lifestyle. As discharge approaches, families are informed of financial, school, mental health, regional center, and voluntary agency resources. The social worker and psychologist also assist other team members in coping with the family's and the child's behaviors. Research is elucidating the effect of the injury on the family[47, 141–146] and the effect of family coping[49] and resources[143, 145] on the child's reintegration into society. Outpatient

Food Consistencies: Properties and Rationale

TABLE 3–9

Consistency	Example	Properties	Clinical Implications and Rationale*
Puree	Strained baby foods; applesauce; puddings, yogurt	*Uniformly* soft, creamy and cohesive texture	Bolus is cohesive; minimizes need for oral manipulation and oral motor endurance
Mechanical soft	Cottage cheese; moist macaroni and cheese; *soft* cooked vegetables; gelatin dessert with pieces of soft fruit; ground meats with sauce or gravy	Cohesive texture; may be mixed with pieces of soft solids	Cohesive texture, greater oral manipulation and endurance demands than pureed textures; provides increased sensory input
Soft	Breads; cakes, cheeses; well-cooked meats	Regular-consistency foods, but texture is soft	Beneficial for those who are unable to adequately masticate hard textures (e.g., when no teeth are present or dentition is compromised)
Regular	Meats; raw fruits and vegetables; potato or corn chips; hard crackers or cookies	Regular consistency, including hard textures; may also include mixed textures (sandwich)	Requires adequate intraoral control to manipulate and masticate complicated bolus; also requires sufficient endurance
Thin liquids	Water, soda, thin juices (apple)	Uniformly thin	Moves quickly in oral cavity and is noncohesive; may not allow sufficient oral transit time to initiate swallow
Thickened liquids	Unstrained fruit juices, milk, milk shakes	May be thickened to nectar, honey, or milk shake consistencies; thickening agents may include commercial thickener, unflavored gelatin, or rice cereal	Proportionate increase in viscosity corresponds with greater oral transport time; may provide needed time to adequately prepare for initiation of swallow; thicker liquids provide more cohesive bolus, thus requiring less oral manipulation

*Additional considerations: increased sensory input of carbonated liquids and thermal variability (warm or cold); cultural preferences; and age of child.

intervention assists the family and the child in dealing with the child's inappropriate social behavior, social isolation, peer rejection, and low self-esteem to assist reintegration into society. The following case study discusses community resources and support groups in more detail.

Families that are empowered with anticipatory guidance about the expected future development or possible impairments can become personally responsible for identification of the need for timely professional consultation. With appropriate education they can also implement much of the treatment plan, thereby reducing the frequency of therapy.

CASE STUDY

The following case report illustrates impairments, functional limitations, and disabilities associated with pediatric TBI. Clinical decision-making processes regarding goal establishment, examination, and intervention are presented in detail with application of the previously presented information. This case presentation focuses on physical therapy management of the child with a brain injury during the inpatient acute rehabilitation, on outpatient follow-up visits, and with recommendations for further care. These processes are outlined in terms of the HOAC[94] model used in conjunction with the systems-based task-oriented strategy for intervention suggested by Shumway-Cook and Woollacott.[147]

INITIAL DATA COLLECTION

History

When Maria was 3 years and 9 months old she suffered a TBI. On admission to our rehabilitation hospital, Maria's family was not present for therapist consultation, and Maria was not able to cognitively participate in the establishment of goals. Initial data collection and goal setting, therefore, were based on information gathered by a thorough review of her acute care hospitalization records. Goals would be revised as needed after consultation with the family. The transfer summary records reflected the following information:

> Maria lived with her mother, father, two younger siblings (2 years old and 7 months old), and other extended family members in a 2-bedroom apartment. Her father worked outside the home, and her mother was a housewife, caring for the home and children. Her parents reported a "normal" developmental history with 3- to 4-word sentences in Spanish, her primary language.
>
> While crossing the street toward an ice cream truck, Maria was hit by a car moving at approximately 35 miles an hour. She was thrown 15 to 20 feet by the force of the impact. Emergency assistance arrived shortly after the injury; at that time Maria's GCS score was 5 with agonal respiration; she responded to stimulation only with generalized withdrawal. She was functioning at Rancho pediatric levels of consciousness IV.
>
> On admission to the acute care facility Maria was intubated and placed on mechanical ventilation. An emergency CT scan revealed right frontal subarachnoid hemorrhage, diffuse cerebral contusion and edema, and a small left intraventricular hemorrhage. Maria was treated with mannitol and the placement of an intracranial pressure monitor. Neurologic examination revealed anisocoria, right greater than left, with the right pupil nonreactive. Occasional "posturing" of the lower extremities was reported. Episodic agitation was treated with medications such as chloral hydrate, lorazepam (Ativan), and methadone. CT scan of the abdomen and an x-ray series revealed other injuries that included a right pulmonary contusion secondary to third, fourth, and fifth posterior rib fractures, a right midshaft femur fracture (100 percent displaced), and right pubic ramus and clavicular fractures (both minimally displaced). Buck's traction was applied to her right femur for 10 days, with excellent reduction of the fracture. Subsequently, an external fixator was placed to stabilize the femur fracture (expected removal was in 6 to 8 weeks). A repeat CT scan showed an enlarged right cerebellar hemorrhagic-contusion, but no hydrocephalus. Ten days after injury she was extubated and the intracranial pressure monitor was removed. An

electroencephalogram revealed diffuse slowing, right greater than left, with no epileptiform activity. Phenytoin (Dilantin) was prescribed for seizure prophylaxis but was discontinued before her transfer to our rehabilitation facility. Approximately 2½ weeks after the onset of injury a G-tube was placed for nutritional support.

Maria remained in a coma for approximately 3½ weeks. After that time she was awake and alert, but functioning only at Rancho pediatric level III. Five weeks after the onset of injury, when medically stable, she was transferred to our rehabilitation hospital. Unfortunately, information regarding previous therapy (if any) was not included in the transfer records.

Analysis of Chart Review

Focused review of the medical records provides the therapist with anticipatory knowledge of possible impairments and the prognosis for recovery. Careful interpretation of this information should be based on a current literature review. Although physical and cognitive recovery is expected to continue for up to 7 years after injury, generally the greatest rate of change occurs within the first 6 months.[8, 58] Maria's coma lasted less than 6 weeks, so a good to moderate outcome was expected.[15, 64, 69] Unresolved hypertension, however, indicated poor neurologic improvement; if not stabilized within the first 6 weeks, continued hypertension decreases the chance for significant neurologic recovery.[69, 75] Unfortunately, the GCS score at 24 hours after injury was not included in the transfer records; these data can also provide predictive information regarding the expected degree of recovery.[59]

The combination of diffuse and focal injuries with loss of consciousness predicted possible residual consequences of slowed response times, short-term memory limitations, and cognitive and behavioral problems.[29] The location of and type of focal injuries, specifically, right cerebellum, left cerebral contusion, and intraventricular hemorrhage, suggested likely ataxia and sensorimotor involvement, particularly of the right extremities.[8, 18, 29] The multiple fractures, history of immobilization, lower extremity "posturing," and bed rest suggested deconditioning, possible peripheral nerve damage, and a decreased ROM, especially of the right lower extremity. We would not expect mature postural response strategies at 3.5 years of age.[79] Her age also indicated that premorbidly she was likely to incorporate the use of somatosensory systems to guide postural control rather than depending predominately on visual information for these activities, as would be expected of a younger child.[148] We expected gradual increases in muscle stiffness as well as the possible presence of HO to occur during her rehabilitation stay (and for the first 4 months after the onset of injury).[8, 62, 69, 75] Respiratory problems, including a decreased vital capacity, were anticipated due to the presence of multiple rib fractures and pulmonary contusion. The location and extent of injuries and cognitive impairment suggested swallowing dysfunction. Furthermore, intubation often results in vocal fold damage. When present, we would expect decreased vocal fold closure during swallowing, thereby reducing the protective mechanism of laryngeal closure to prevent penetration of the laryngeal vestibule or aspiration.

The specific reason for the unavailability of Maria's family was unknown, but absent family is a common occurrence at our rehabilitation hospital. Often families are present throughout the acute hospitalization period, but several weeks later when transfer to a rehabilitation facility occurs, the parents' employers have required them to return to work.[146] An extended hospitalization period (greater than 2 weeks and not discharged home) has been found to result in injury-related financial problems and difficulty maintaining a regular work schedule for the parents of children with severe TBI.[146] For these reasons we anticipated that it would be difficult for Maria's family to be present during business hours, so personnel such as evening shift nurses would be used as our initial link with the family. Emotional stress, stress from the burden of care, depression and anxiety, marital stress, and family role dysfunction may occur soon after the injury and may persist for many years after the injury.[141-144] Specific timelines regarding the onset and progression of emotional symptoms have been debated,[149] but these factors may have been another cause of her family's absence during the initial days after rehabilitation admission.

GOAL ESTABLISHMENT

The process of goal establishment was done in collaboration with the rehabilitation team, including occupational therapy and speech pathology therapists. Goals were based on Maria's previous functional status (physical and cognitive), anticipated family concern for the achievement of maximal age-appropriate functional independence, predictions for recovery, and expected impairments. Collaboration with the family is a critical factor in the establishment of goals and the initiation of treatment, but Maria's family was not present for the first few days after admission to our facility. It was uncertain when they would be available, so the therapists proceeded with goal establishment and examination. Team goals for Maria included the following: (1) to ensure family understanding of Maria's disabilities, her expected future needs, and methods to access available community resources; (2) to ensure that the family demonstrated competence in the provision of appropriate supervision and daily care; and (3) to maximize age-appropriate independence with self-care, mobility, and cognition to a level that would allow the family to safely and effectively care for her at home. Specific functional mobility goals included (1) independence with bed mobility activities (e.g., rolling, scooting, and coming to sit), (2) assisted transfers (e.g., to and from bed, toilet, tub, and floor), and (3) assisted ambulation within the house. The estimated length of stay was 6 to 8 weeks.

It was not anticipated that Maria would attain functional independence during her rehabilitation stay; rather, our goal was to maximize her functional abilities and minimize her disabilities rather than eliminate all limitations (Table 3–10).[150] Further assessment of family or caregiver involvement and their knowledge of the injury; family and community resources; and the discharge destination was indicated when Maria's family was available. A prerequisite for discharge is the establishment of the family's ability to support continued recovery and reintegration into society.

CLINICAL EXAMINATION

General

After the establishment of preliminary goals, the formalized process of clinical assessment was initiated, as suggested by the HOAC.[94] On her admission to our rehabilitation hospital, *disabilities* included a lack of independence for movement in her environment and in performing age-appropriate self-care activities, an inability to consume an age-appropriate diet, and an inability to communicate her needs to her family and peers. Although of obvious importance to the long-term outcome, discussion of disability associated with Maria's cognitive impairments is limited here to concerns related to the physical therapy examination and intervention. *Functional limitations* concerned bed mobility, transfers, and walking. *Impairments* hypothesized to have a causal relationship with these functional limitations were measured with clinical observations, objective test procedures, and standardized functional measures including the PEDI.[64] As suggested by the HOAC,[94] examination procedures were chosen based on their relevance to the previously established functional goals of age-appropriate performance, and anticipated problems based on chart review and Maria's level of cognition (see Table 3–10).

Examination Results

Functional Assessment

Standardized testing procedures such as the PEDI[64] and the GMFM[100] are helpful for tracking functional recovery. Other tools such as the WeeFIM,[66] which measure the "burden of care," would have indicated that Maria had a severe disability, requiring substantial additional time and energy of the caregivers. Functional measures such as these generally require the child to actively initiate movement and interact with the environment. Maria was not making attempts to interact with the environment (cognitively or physically); therefore, these measures would not be sensitive to any of her present abilities or provide any additional information for treatment planning. Such tests are important, however, for the establishment of a baseline of functional abilities, and, when

Functional Goals, Examination Procedures, and Results on Maria's Admission to Acute Rehabilitation (Test 1)

TABLE 3–10

Functional Goals	Examination Procedure	Results
Age-appropriate communication skills	*Level of consciousness:* Rancho pediatric scale (ages 2–5 yr)	Rancho pediatric level III (localized response to stimuli). Inconsistent tracking to midline of toys and faces. Smiled once during assessment. Responded to tactile and positional input with movements localized to area of stimulus.
Independence with bed mobility activities Assisted with transfers Assisted ambulation in home	*Functional assessment:* PEDI	Unable in all functional mobility (see text discussion).
	Motor control and somatosensory: palpation of muscle activity and clinical observation of quality of movements, ability to move against force of gravity, and postural control in response to tactile and positional stimulation	Spontaneous movements were present in response to tactile (e.g., light touch, pressure) stimulation in left extremities, at all joints. Unable to elicit active movements of right arm or ankle. Only minimal movements of right hip and knee were observed, primarily into extension. All extremity movements met demands of force of gravity. No intentional movements noted; therefore, unable to assess ataxia. Unable to perform detailed sensory motor exam due to impaired level of consciousness.
	Ashworth Scale: muscle stiffness in response to passive movement of extremities	Ashworth Scale: 2 (see text discussion of rating scale) in bilateral knee flexor and ankle plantar flexor muscle groups.
	Upright motor control: see text discussion	Unable to assess upright motor control.
	Postural control: observed ability of head and trunk to maintain alignment over base of support during functional movements and in response to imposed perturbations in balance; choice of motor strategies to disturbances in balance were noted (i.e., arm and leg counterbalancing vs. stepping strategy)	Maria was unable in all functional mobility activities. When placed and supported in upright (sitting) positions, Maria did not attempt to maintain her head or trunk erect over her base of support. There was no evidence of attempts to compensate for disturbance in balance with any compensatory strategies.
	Passive ROM tested by goniometry	Bilateral ankle dorsiflexion limited to 0°, otherwise without limitations throughout bilateral upper and lower extremities.
	Physiologic response: Monitoring of HR, respiratory rate, BP (continuous mechanical monitors at bedside)	Persistent hypertension and increased respiratory rate. Also, disproportional increase in physiologic response (HR and BP) to actual level of activity.
Consumption of age-appropriate diet by mouth	*Feeding and dysphagia:* Observation of spontaneous saliva swallow; assessment of perioral and oral sensation by response to tactile, thermal, and gustatory input; observation of intraoral control and swallow response when presented with small (1–3 mL) bolus of water and pureed fruits or vegetables	Jaw opened spontaneously and random tongue movements occurred when Maria was presented with pureed foods. Inadequate lip closure before swallow response noted. Exaggerated gag response and bite reflex when stimulus (spoon) introduced to middle third of tongue. Consumed 15 mL of pureed fruits and 5 mL of water with significantly delayed swallow and decreased laryngeal excursion, minimal coughing after swallow.

PEDI, Pediatric Evaluation of Disability Inventory; ROM, range of motion; HR, heart rate; BP, blood pressure.

applied over time, provide documentation of recovery. The PEDI served as a measure of functional performance in the case of Maria (Table 3–11).

On admission, normative standard scores were zero in all the functional skill domains (self-care, mobility, and social function) of the PEDI. Normative standard scores on the PEDI are based on a mean of 50 and a standard deviation of 10. All normative scores were less than 10, more than 4 standard deviations below the mean score for her age (Table 3–11, test 1, column 1). The use of normative standard scores did not provide any useful information for treatment planning. The authors of the PEDI suggest the use of the scaled scores when the child is functioning far below the expected age level because important clinical changes may not be noticeable from the repeated use of normative standard scores.[64] The scaled scores can be used to provide a baseline measure, highlight abilities, identify constraints for intervention, and provide objective measurements for the documentation of change over time irrespective of age or peer-level abilities.[64]

Constraining Factors

Detailed findings of the initial examination are shown in Table 3–10. It was evident that many constraining cognitive and physical limitations were present. Cognition, motivation, and the ability to interact with the environment were profoundly impaired. Maria was demonstrating relatively no interaction or interest in the environment. It was hypothesized, therefore, that Maria's level of cognition limited her ability to perform functional mobility in her environment.

Physical limitations were severe and numerous. These included no active movement of the right upper extremity and only minimal movement of the left arm and leg. Maria did not demonstrate any attempts to maintain postural control in upright positions (such as sitting) or attempt to respond to perturbations in balance. Impaired cognition and severe oral motor control problems were hypothesized to interfere with Maria's ability to consume age-appropriate diet textures (such as solids) and placed her at risk for aspiration.

Based on the examination results, an initial hypothesis to guide intervention was established: the inability to produce functional movement strategies for mobility within her environment was a result of Maria's impairments in attention, cognition, motor control, and postural responses. It was difficult to determine the extent to which each of these impairments influenced Maria's lack of initiation to interact or be mobile in her environment, but it was assumed that cognitive and attentional factors were severely limiting Maria's ability to engage in functional movement. The lack of movement in Maria's right upper extremity and only minimal movement of her right lower extremity (as well as a lack of variable movements in the right leg) were also hypothesized to be constraining factors. Maria's lack of any attempt to maintain the stability of her head or trunk over her base of support was also limiting her ability to produce successful functional movements

Results of Maria's PEDI Functional Skills Assessment at Admission (Test 1), Monthly Reassessment (Test 2), Discharge from Inpatient Care (Test 3), and Yearly Reassessment (Test 4)

TABLE 3–11

Domain	Test 1 (5.5 Wk After Injury)		Test 2 (9 Wk After Injury)		Test 3 (3.5 Mo After Injury)		Test 4 (20 Mo After Injury)	
	Norm Std* ± SE	Scaled Score ± SE	Norm Std ± SE	Scaled Score ± SE	Norm Std ± SE	Scaled Score ± SE	Norm Std ± SE	Scaled Score ± SE
Self-care	<10 ± —	0 ± —	<10 ± —	34.0 ± 2.0	<10 ± —	36.0 ± 1.9	23.2 ± 1.8	57.4 ± 1.6
Mobility	<10 ± —	0 ± —	<10 ± —	26.0 ± 2.8	<10 ± —	34.1 ± 2.0	21.8 ± 1.8	56.2 ± 1.6
Social	<10 ± —	0 ± —	<10 ± —	33.0 ± 2.1	<10 ± —	37.0 ± 1.9	21.8 ± 1.8	56.2 ± 1.6

Norm Std, normative standard score; SE, standard error; PEDI, Pediatric Evaluation of Disability Inventory.
*Normative standard scores are based on a mean of 50 with a standard deviation of 10.

in her environment. The impact of physical constraints such as ROM limitations, velocity-dependent muscle stiffness, and deconditioning were not expected to be completely evident until Maria performed "higher-level" functional activities (e.g., walking, running), but knowledge of typical sequelae led to the hypothesis that a contracture-prevention program would be needed.

A significant positive correlation between cognition and functional independence has been found in adults with TBI.[151] Additionally, it has been suggested that measures of cognitive impairment could be predictors of functional status in the adult population.[151] Motivation, and consequently the desire to move and interact with people, toys, and environmental obstacles, likely plays a similar role in the functional mobility of children. With anticipated improvements in Maria's cognition and attention we also expected increased and more meaningful attempts to interact and become mobile in the environment. Postural control factors would then become more salient. Further studies are indicated to determine the interrelationships of motivation, family support, and prior cognitive level with later functional mobility in children after TBI.

INTERVENTION

Treatments were designed to (1) reduce the influence of existing and expected impairments constraining function, and (2) facilitate the development of coordinated, timely, and efficient functional mobility through the provision of meaningful and functional practice. The plan of care was based on the guiding framework of the previously established functional goals in the context of the dynamic systems theory and the systems-based task-oriented approach. There were multiple considerations in treatment planning, which included the family's goals, desires, and educational needs; Maria's motivation and cognition; her age, previous functional status, and cognitive level; and the severity of her injury. Regardless of the underlying impairments, interventions were oriented toward the attainment of the previously established goals (e.g., related to functional mobility and the consumption of an age-appropriate diet) and facilitation of discharge home to her family. Age-appropriate play and strategic placement of enticing stimuli, such as familiar faces and toys, were used to provide Maria with the motivation to participate in the therapeutic activities.

Family Education

Throughout her rehabilitation stay, Maria's family became more frequently present and involved in her daily care activities. Family support, needs, and resources were assessed as soon as the family was available for collaboration. Interview of the family revealed goals that reflected the therapist's perceived importance of independence in functional mobility, communication, and the consumption of diet by mouth. Specifically, the family goals were for Maria to "talk and walk again." Maria's mother stated that she would be at home with her during the day and was willing to provide as much care as needed. Maria's family was incorporated into treatment sessions as much as possible to facilitate carryover of treatment and practice in daily care activities. When present, the family was instrumental in stimulation, motivation, and play activities. Additionally, the parents were encouraged to bring in some of Maria's favorite toys and videotapes from home; these were frequently used during treatment sessions.

The family was continually educated about their daughter's injury and anticipated progression of physical and cognitive recovery. The family was also informed of opportunities for the use of community resources and access to programs and education for persons with disabilities and was encouraged to become an advocate for Maria. Her family was empowered with information regarding rights for children with disabilities, specifically related to the Americans with Disabilities Act of 1990.[152] This is critical legislation related to civil rights for persons with disabilities. It was established for many reasons, but it was primarily designed to protect persons with disabilities and ensure that they have an equal opportunity to succeed and become active participants in society.[152] Title I of the Americans with Disabilities Act, which addresses equal-opportunity employment (in this case for persons associated with a child with a disability), was especially critical to Maria's father.[152] Maria's mother did not drive, so at discharge her father would be responsible for essentially all transportation to doctor and therapy appointments. With this responsibility her father recognized that he would miss many hours of work. He was educated regarding provisions afforded under the law and the possibility of requesting alternative work schedules during such instances.

Empowerment of the family by inclusion and active participation in the decision-making process and intervention was paramount throughout Maria's rehabilitation. The acknowledgment of family needs and the encouragement of active participation in the rehabilitation process has proved to be critical for many reasons. Strategies to maximize opportunities for involvement were implemented, but it was recognized by the rehabilitation team that family inclusion was limited due to a combination of factors (i.e., a need to return to work, transportation problems, stress). Fortunately, this did not result in any perceived conflicts between the family and the team members.

Physiologic Response

Active participation in functional activities, especially during early rehabilitation, was complicated by Maria's maladaptive physiologic response to activity and her limited endurance. Maria's exaggerated physiologic responses to movement included increased heart rate and blood pressure. A maladaptive blood pressure response (in the case of Maria, hypertension), a decreased heart rate, and an increased respiratory rate are signs of possible increased intracranial pressure.[69, 75] As a result, close monitoring of these parameters is necessary. Antihypertension medications and constant physiologic assessment were employed while Maria was at rest and during treatment sessions. The physician requested that all interventions be provided at bedside. The physician provided unacceptable physiologic parameters of heart rate less than 60 or greater than 160 and blood pressure less than 110/65 or greater than 150/100. With these guidelines to the progression of activity, therapy was often limited in order to safely adhere to the established parameters. Approximately 3 weeks after admission, her physiologic response to activity became more adaptive, thereby decreasing the need for constant monitoring. Maria continued, however, to require antihypertensive medications.

Reimbursement guidelines in the United States require at least 3 hours per day of intervention from the members of at least two disciplines in order to qualify for inpatient rehabilitation. Maria demonstrated severe limitations in her endurance during early stages of rehabilitation, which made it difficult to meet these standards. The obvious complexity of Maria's problems necessitated inpatient rehabilitation, however, so this level of care was provided. Initially, many physical therapy sessions involved cotreatment with occupational therapists or speech therapists and implementation of multiple short treatment sessions (≤30 minutes) to maximize the use of periods of attention and alertness. Throughout Maria's stay her endurance for therapy sessions and periods of alertness gradually increased. Initially Maria was able to tolerate only brief periods (less than 1 hour) of sitting in the wheelchair. Collaborative efforts by therapists and nurses progressively increased her wheelchair-sitting tolerance. Maria's improved physiologic response coincided with increased endurance for upright activities (e.g., supported sitting, supported kneeling) approximately 4 weeks after admission. This allowed greater age-appropriate perception of the environment and interaction with family members, peers, and therapists. Coordinated efforts such as these provided by the rehabilitation team produced maximal reinforcement of functional skills and an appropriate level of challenge to Maria's endurance limitations.

Preventive Measures and Range-of-Motion Activities

Knowledge of Maria's injury and the possible sequelae (e.g., bed rest with prolonged inactivity, increased muscle stiffness, as well as a femur fracture with external fixation) guided the decision to implement and instruct the family in daily ROM activities to prevent musculoskeletal complications. Clinical examination revealed a limited right ankle dorsiflexion ROM and an Ashworth score of 2. These findings prompted implementation of passive daily stretching, selectively provided to the right lower extremity. Although the dorsiflexion ROM was not constraining function at admission, once she was standing and walking, a plantar flexion contracture and increased velocity-dependent muscle stiffness would interfere with the normal gait pattern and needed to be prevented.[135, 137] Although the right femur had an external fixator device, there were no restrictions on performing passive ROM or weight-bearing activities (she was permitted "weight-bearing-as-tolerated" status after orthopedic surgeon consultation). Teaching family members to provide these simple measures to prevent contractures, especially during growth spurts, was expected to reduce the need for more aggressive and invasive procedures later. The external fixator remained on for an additional 5 weeks after admission to our hospital and was later removed without incident.

Functional Mobility

Initial examination revealed several constraints limiting motor performance. Interventions were oriented to reduce these limitations within the context of achieving the functional mobility goals of independence with bed mobility, assisted transfers, and assisted ambulation. In this case, active participation in functional activities, especially during early rehabilitation, was complicated by deficits in cognition (Rancho pediatric level III); attention and motivation; endurance; and maladaptive physiologic responses to activity. Maria was not making any attempts to interact with or be mobile in her environment. She was able to visually attend, however, for short periods of time. Meaningful activities at this time included the facilitation of visual attention to previously familiar faces and toys. For example, Maria was encouraged to maintain her head upright while supported in a sitting position and watching a favorite video.

Therapy tactics were needed to provide Maria with the opportunity to explore potential useful solutions to her movement problems. Initially, movements were spontaneous and random. In order to compensate for the constraints limiting functional movement, Maria was provided with graded active facilitation of transitional movements. An emphasis was placed on movement from one posture to another. All treatments were provided within age-appropriate conditions, incorporating play and motivation that were progressively modified according to her level of cognition. For example, rolling from a supine to a sidelying position was initially performed in the context of tracking familiar faces. When Maria was able to respond to simple commands, this same functional activity of rolling was followed by a transition to sitting and the placement of a toy in a bucket held by her mother (a higher-level cognitive skill, a two-step process). Graded movement exploration of anterior and posterior spaces in which to move her body was encouraged to stimulate appropriate postural stability and weight-shifting responses in upright positions. For instance, assisted forward leaning while seated on a child-size bench to play peek-a-boo with her siblings required anterior translation of her trunk relative to her base of support and the use of an appropriate postural response to prevent falling.

Opportunities such as these for the active practice of useful and meaningful functional activities that provided the sensation of successful and efficient movement were used to facilitate the development of adaptable motor skills. Adaptable motor skills are required for functional movement when task demands and environmental conditions change.[153]

Successful functional movement "patterns" or "synergies" are dependent on the input of sensory and perceptual information from tactile, somatic, proprioceptive, vestibular, and visual systems.[83, 153] The interplay of these multiple systems is essential for functional movement, especially with postural control activities. The use of unstable surfaces (i.e., her mother's lap or suspension equipment) as well as tactile and proprioceptive feedback (e.g., compression into selected weight-bearing surfaces) provided opportunities for multisensory input. For example, Maria enjoyed sitting on a suspended platform. This granted multisensory input from vestibular, proprioceptive, and tactile receptors in the context of a child-perceived "fun" activity. Additionally, the therapist was able to manipulate control parameters such as speed, stability, and the direction of platform movement to change the difficulty and the demands of the task.

The systems-based task-oriented approach emphasizes that children use a wide variety of movements to achieve mobility goals.[147] The repertoire of movements that share the same goal needs to be highly variable and adaptable to meet the demands of a constantly changing environment.[153] This theoretic framework was used to schedule practice under variable task conditions and environmental demands. Movements in and out of positions such as coming to a standing position were practiced using multiple movement strategies, rather than one single therapist-perceived "normal" or "appropriate" method. A wide variety of solutions, including backing off a chair, scooting to the edge of a chair and lowering herself down while facing forward, kneeling to stand, and a "bear" (quadruped with arms and legs extended) position for coming to a standing position, were all practiced to expose Maria to a variety of movement possibilities. Changes in the task condition and environment were also used to encourage learning and the transfer of present and emerging functional abilities to variable conditions, thereby making motor solutions more adaptable.[153] For instance, coming to a standing position from sitting was practiced from multiple surfaces such as an adult-sized chair, the floor, the grass, and her stroller.

The dynamic systems theory postulates periods of "phase shift" when movements become highly variable. Advocates of this theory emphasize that these periods may offer an opportunity to view how the child adapts and learns new tasks.[153] It has been our experience that during the acute rehabilitation period (usually the first 6 months after the onset of injury) when recovery is occurring at its most rapid rate, there are multiple periods when functional mobility skills become highly variable and transitions to higher level skills emerge. Although we recognize that it is difficult to claim that these periods are "phase shifts," we attempted to maximize our influence during these periods by practicing many different movement strategies to solve postural control problems and alleviate functional mobility limitations. We believed that we had a greater likelihood of "strengthening" the most efficient motor patterns during these periods of transition. Based on this belief, it was critical that Maria be exposed to opportunities to become more flexible in her selection and use of movement strategies.[153]

Feeding

At admission Maria was not able to consume age-appropriate diet textures. Many constraining factors limited Maria's feeding abilities including impaired cognition, motivation, and attention, and oral and pharyngeal motor control deficits. Maria was able to consume some pureed foods and thickened liquids by mouth, but her intake was not timely or sufficient for nutritional support. Pureed foods and thickened liquids were determined to be appropriate for Maria based on her examination findings (see Table 3–10). Because of their more cohesive texture, these foods provided greater "ease" of bolus formation during the oral phase. Pureed foods require little oral manipulation and no mastication so they were more energy efficient and simpler for Maria to consume. The increased viscosity of the thickened liquids provided additional oral transport time before the swallow. This "extra" time was valuable for Maria because it decreased the likelihood of penetration of food into an open airway before the initiation of the swallow (and subsequent airway closure).

Intervention strategies focused on the consumption of greater volumes of food and more solid textures. Treatment sessions focused on increasing the volume consumed and efficient consumption of more age-appropriate textures and thinner liquids. The progression of treatments was based on Maria's feeding efficiency and endurance.

Initially, Maria demonstrated a delayed swallow, coughing, and choking after the consumption of limited amounts of pureed foods. If a tracheostomy tube were present, suctioning could have been performed to determine if Maria had aspirated (e.g., suction of food colored with food dye through the tracheostomy tube). Because no tracheostomy tube was present, we were unable to determine if food, liquids, or saliva was penetrating the laryngeal vestibule. Bedside assessments have been found to be inadequate in the identification of silent aspiration.[140] VSF was therefore performed to determine the cause of the coughing. The VSF revealed an increased oral transit time, a delayed swallowing response, decreased laryngeal elevation and pharyngeal motility, and a residual in the valleculae after swallowing. Although Maria was at risk, penetration and aspiration were not noted, so oral feedings were continued within the limitations of her endurance. The family and team members were informed about the VSF findings and the signs of decreased endurance during feeding.

The family was continually informed and educated regarding Maria's feeding status. They were regularly instructed in feeding techniques, which included the provision of appropriate food textures and liquid consistencies, bolus size, timing of presentation, and response to signs of fatigue and aspiration. Maria was thought to be at greater risk for aspiration when fatigued, so safe parameters were provided to the family and team members. When available, family members (typically her mother) were encouraged to feed Maria. After competence in the use of the previously mentioned feeding guidelines was established, Maria's mother independently fed her and gradually progressed the quantity and texture of her daughter's diet with frequent therapist guidance. The family was encouraged to bring in some of Maria's favorite foods prepared in appropriate textures. It goes without saying that poor compliance with guidelines of feeding programs can be potentially dangerous. An early emphasis on family incorporation into the dysphagia program as described affords the therapist with improved adherence to guidelines and potentially greater facilitation of faster recovery.

REASSESSMENT

Progress toward the previously established functional goals was continually reassessed. This was done to examine the rate of progress and effectiveness of interventions, and to determine if services were being provided at the appropriate level of care. Ongoing questions were as follows: (1) Did Maria require intensive inpatient rehabilitation to continue to make cognitive and physical functional gains? (2) Could she be adequately cared for at home with the provision of outpatient therapy through a community-based rehabilitation program? Advocates of community-based rehabilitation programs say that the secure and familiar surrounds of home, in conjunction with support and guidance, can augment or replace intensive inpatient rehabilitation for some individuals.[150, 154] In the case of Maria, especially in the first 2 months after the injury, the complexity of her medical, cognitive, and physical limitations necessitated the more intensive level of inpatient rehabilitation care.

Results of reassessment findings at 2.1 months (monthly assessment), 3.5 months (discharge from inpatient rehabilitation), and 20 months after the onset of injury (yearly review) are reflected in Table 3–12. On each test occasion Maria was examined with previously described clinical procedures and the PEDI (functional skill scales) (see Table 3–11). Reassessment results were discussed with Maria's family and other team members to continually monitor progress toward and modify established goals.

Graphic representation of PEDI scaled scores on functional skills in each domain (self-care, mobility, and cognition) are presented in Figure 3–1. This graph clearly illustrates the gains made by Maria throughout her rehabilitation. Improvements were noted across testing periods with obvious intervals of dramatic progress, specifically, intertest period 1 to 2. Analysis of these results is described for each test occasion.

Test 2

At the time of her first reassessment, 9 weeks after the injury, Maria had participated in rehabilitation for 1 month (see Table 3–12, test 2). The PEDI functional skills assessment was administered at test 2. When the results of test 2 were compared with *normative standard scores* (comparison with age peers), there were no apparent changes in functional abilities in any domain (see Table 3–11), but when the results were considered in terms of s*caled scores* (change measured against her own previous performance), progress was revealed in every domain compared with test 1 (see Table 3–11). Maria made dramatic changes in self-care, mobility, and social skills in the period between test 1 and test 2. These improvements were related to the recovery of Maria's initiation of assistance with self-care activities, initiation of purposeful movement to change her physical location, and intentional social interactions with toys and people, as well as attempts to communicate.

Maria's cognition had improved to Rancho pediatric level II (responds to the environment), which corresponded with an improved score in the social domain of the PEDI (see Table 3–11, test 2). She attempted to use gestures and some single words such as *mama* and *no* for communication with the family and team members. Maria

Maria's Reassessment Results at 9 Weeks (Test 2), 3.5 Months (Test 3), and 20 Months (Test 4) After Injury

TABLE 3–12

Functional Goals	Measure	Reassessment Results		
		Test 2	*Test 3*	*Test 4*
Age-appropriate communication	Cognition	Rancho pediatric level II; responded to environment, selective attention for 3–4 min; easily distracted; initiated interaction with environment	Rancho pediatric level II; basic needs communication; followed 2-step commands; emotional lability	Rancho pediatric level II
Assisted with transfers Assisted ambulation in home Independence with bed mobility activities	Functional abilities	See text discussion of PEDI: functional skills assessment	See text discussion of PEDI: functional skills assessment	See text discussion of PEDI: functional skills assessment and caregiver assistance scales
	Motor control, muscle stiffness or spasticity, and somatosensory processing	Consistent purposeful movements of left upper and lower extremities, but severe ataxia of left arm limited functional activities; no movement of right arm; only slight activity of extensor muscles noted when upper extremity externally stabilized in weight bearing	Continued absence of right arm volitional movement, but spontaneous muscle activity noted in right arm extensor muscles with assisted weight bearing; ataxia continued to predominate in functional movements of left arm	Minimal volitional right elbow flexion noted; able to assist during dressing activities with right arm (e.g., push arm through coat sleeve); left arm dominated by ataxia
		Only minimal movements of right leg; unable to perform single-leg stance activities on either lower extremity	Poor control of hip, knee, and ankle extensor muscle groups (bilateral, right greater than left) during stance phase of gait; unable to even momentarily single-leg stand on either extremity	Able to single-leg stand momentarily (<5 sec) on left leg without upper extremity support (e.g., able to kick ball)
		Ashworth Score: 1+, right knee extensors and bilateral ankle plantar flexor muscle groups	Ashworth Score: 1, throughout bilateral lower extremity muscle groups; decrease in muscle stiffness especially noted in bilateral ankle plantar flexor muscle groups	Ashworth Score: 0, no stiffness noted in any upper or lower extremity muscle group
	Postural control	Responded appropriately to light touch and proprioceptive input; however, response was grossly diminished in the right extremities	Responded appropriately to light touch and proprioceptive input, but response remained grossly diminished in the right extremities	Responded appropriately to light touch and proprioceptive input; only slightly decreased in right extremities as compared to the left
	Musculoskeletal	ROM: no limitations with the exception of 0°–5° ankle dorsiflexion	ROM: no limitations with the exception of bilateral 0°–10° ankle dorsiflexion	ROM: no limitations noted

(continued)

(continued) **Maria's Reassessment Results at 9 Weeks (Test 2), 3.5 Months (Test 3), and 20 Months (Test 4) After Injury**

TABLE 3–12

Functional Goals	Measure	Reassessment Results		
		Test 2	*Test 3*	*Test 4*
Consumption of age-appropriate diet by mouth	Feeding	Consumed ¼–⅓ of diet by mouth; pureed foods with thickened liquids; attempted use of left arm for finger feeding; unsuccessful with utensils due to severe ataxia of left arm and no volitional movement of right arm	Consumed *all* nutrition by mouth; "mechanical soft diet" with thickened liquids; difficulty with mastication of meats; up to 1 hr required to complete meal; required nearly total assistance with self-feeding activities	Consumed regular diet with thin liquids; meals consumed within reasonable time (relative to siblings); completed less than half of self-feeding activities

PEDI, Pediatric Evaluation of Disability Inventory; ROM, range of motion.

demonstrated receptive abilities that were not present at admission, such as responding to her name and following very simple one-step commands in Spanish and English (i.e., "Touch the dolly"). Maria also initiated attempts to attain and play with toys. Previously, she did not show attempts at interaction with the environment (e.g., interest in toys or others or make any attempts at communication).

Maria demonstrated purposeful movements as described previously, primarily with her left arm. She also made attempts to assist with grooming, feeding, and dressing (i.e., she attempted to hold a brush with her left hand or pushed her leg through a pants leg). Maria's cognitive impairments and motor control limitations of bilateral upper extremities (e.g., severe ataxia of her left upper extremity and only minimal volitional movement of her right arm) limited her ability to completely perform these activities. Maria made purposeful attempts at movement in her environment, to change location or contact a family member or a toy. She also made brief attempts to maintain static postural control of her head and trunk during short sitting activities. Previously absent initiation of transitional

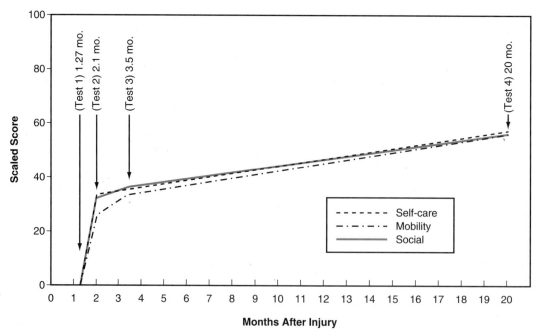

FIGURE 3–1. Maria's Pediatric Evaluation of Disability Inventory functional skills: scaled scores.

movements such as rolling from a supine to a sidelying position and coming from a supine to a sitting position were attempted at the time of test 2. Despite attempts at these activities, however, her efforts were typically unsuccessful, energy demanding, and lacking in variability and transferability to different task demands (e.g., using *only* a "sit-up" approach to attempt coming to a sitting position). When assisted, Maria was able to incorporate the use of her arms for stability when performing such transitional movements (assisted weight bearing through one or both arms). A lack of spontaneous functional use of her upper extremities continued to complicate Maria's lack of variability when performing such mobility skills.

Increased functional mobility skills were noted to coincide with improvements in cognition. It is difficult to speculate, however, about the extent of interdependence between functional mobility and cognition. It is possible that when attention and motivation are sufficient to produce the desire to move and interact in the environment, the child is provided with greater opportunities to practice functional mobility activities and use available motor control abilities. Conversely, when functional motor skills are sufficient to produce volitional movements and adequate postural control, the child is afforded with greater possibilities to interact with the environment and may demonstrate improvements in cognition, motivation, and attention.

At the time of test 2, Maria was dependent with feeding skills, but she was able to safely consume up to one-third of her pureed diet and thickened liquids by mouth. She was able to consume only a limited amount of her diet because of persistent endurance limitations and fatigue during feeding sessions. Maria was unable to consume solid foods effectively because of persistent oral motor control problems that limited her ability to form a cohesive bolus before the initiation of a swallow. She also continued to require thickened liquids because of a delayed swallow response and the previously mentioned oral motor control problems. Maria continued to require G-tube supplements for nutritional support.

Immediately *before* the first reassessment period, team members from each discipline noted that Maria was not recovering as rapidly as hoped for. At that time her functional status had not changed greatly since admission. These factors resulted in consideration of a revised discharge date. At that point it was believed that her family would be able to adequately care for her needs at home and facilitate cognitive and functional skill development with an outpatient program. Maria's parents were urged to practice caring for her and identify further training needs by taking her home overnight in preparation for discharge. In the following days, however, Maria became more alert and demonstrated increased interaction with the environment and signs of recovery (including decreased hypertension). Team members anticipated that Maria would continue to make dramatic improvements and would benefit from intensive and coordinated therapeutic intervention. As a result, early discharge was discarded in favor of continued inpatient rehabilitation. Anecdotally, in our experience this has been found to be a frequent occurrence after a visit home with family members. For *some* patients the stimulation of the well-known and typically comforting surroundings of home as well as intense interaction with family members has been found to be an opportunity for intervention to facilitate recovery. The practice of a home visit, for the day or overnight, is advocated by our rehabilitation team. Funding guidelines, however, often impose restrictions on this type of activity.

At test 2 it appeared that the previously established functional goals (independence with bed mobility, assisted transfers, assisted ambulation in the house) continued to be appropriate for Maria. When consulted, Maria's family continued to iterate similar goals as discussed shortly after admission. It was apparent, however, that Maria was recovering functional skills at a rate slower than expected. Therefore, the attainment of these goals would fall short of the established length of stay (6 to 8 weeks). It was believed that Maria would continue to make functional improvements, and she continued to require intensive and coordinated therapeutic intervention, so an additional 4 weeks of inpatient rehabilitation was projected. Maria's impairments of severe ataxia of the left arm and only minimal use of the right arm continued to be problematic for the performance of self-care and functional mobility activities. Interventions continued to focus on the reduction of impairments and the development of efficient functional mobility skills, as well as family education with an increased emphasis on readying Maria and the family for her discharge.

Test 3

Test occasion 3 was completed on discharge from inpatient rehabilitation, 3.5 months after the injury (see Table 3–12, test 3). Maria had participated in her rehabilitation program for 9 weeks. She demonstrated continued improvements in cognitive skills although her Rancho pediatric level had not changed (she remained at level II). Maria was able to communicate her basic needs with good accuracy and was able to express approximately 10 single-word responses (i.e., names of objects and people). She also demonstrated self-initiation of simple and familiar play activities such as "high five" and "patty-cake." Maria remained unable to perform problem-solving activities, play with her peers, or exercise age-appropriate judgments about safety (i.e., demonstrate caution around dangerous objects such as a hot stove). Maria also demonstrated frequent outbursts of emotional lability, crying, and hitting.

Improvements in PEDI scaled scores in the period between tests 2 and 3 were not as pronounced as previously seen (see Fig. 3–1). At test 3, relatively few changes in social, functional, and self-care functions were noted (of those that were measured by the PEDI). The only social domain changes were seen in cooperative play with peers and comprehension of directional commands (e.g., the ball is *under* the table). The only noted improvements in self-care abilities were related to the recovery of the ability to consume a soft diet and attempt some finger feeding of selected foods. Mobility improvements were associated with improved postural control while in an unsupported sitting position and, most significantly, an ability to ambulate with assistance (with right ankle-foot orthosis [AFO] and hand-held assistance). Short distance assisted ambulation and limited manual wheelchair propulsion with her left arm were Maria's primary forms of locomotion. Although these skills were limited, they did offer Maria opportunities to independently interact with her environment.

Improvements in functional abilities not captured by the PEDI were also noted. She was able to sit unsupported (without external support or the use of her arms) on various surfaces including a toilet, a child-sized chair, or the floor. She was able to raise and lower herself into a sitting position from a supine or a quadruped position, with some use of rotational movements at her trunk. Maria demonstrated greater variability of solutions to movement problems, but she still showed limited access to these solutions. For instance, she was able to come to a standing from a seated position, but she was unable consistently, safely, and independently to perform the same activity when it was immediately followed by ambulation. She was unable to quickly establish the needed postural stability to safely execute the described task (she demonstrated many near-falling episodes). Maria's relatively ineffective solutions for postural stability demonstrated a readiness to perform the task, but the lack of a stable solution to the movement problem. Therapy tactics provided her with the opportunity to explore potentially useful solutions to such movement problems.

At the time of discharge, Maria demonstrated severe limitations in self-feeding, grooming, and dressing abilities. These were in part related to severe impairments in motor control abilities of both upper extremities; the right arm demonstrated only minimal volitional movement and the left exhibited severe ataxia. Nevertheless, she was able to offer cooperation and attempt assistance with dressing and grooming activities. Maria attempted self-feeding of finger foods, but it was difficult and energy- and time-consuming, as well as frustrating for her. She attempted grooming activities such as brushing her hair and teeth, but efforts were unsuccessful.

At the time of discharge Maria consumed all her diet by mouth. She was able to eat a mechanical soft diet with thickened liquids. Maria continued to demonstrate oral motor control problems, although they were improved since test 2. Her inability to consistently form and maintain a cohesive bolus limited her ability to consume a regular diet. No signs of fatigue, coughing, or choking during feedings were noted, but feedings required up to 1 hour to complete. Excessive time requirements for meal consumption were due to distractibility, extraneous tongue movements, and prolonged mastication before swallowing. Maria did not require additional G-tube supplements after feedings.

At the time of discharge Maria had completed approximately 9 weeks of inpatient rehabilitation. The expected length of stay was previously established in collaboration with team members and later Maria's family; the initial projection was exceeded by only 1 week. Ultimately, however, the strongest determinant of the discharge date was the family's strong desire to bring their daughter home in time for the approaching holiday season.

Previously established long-term family and team goals included (1) age-appropriate communication skills, (2) independence with bed activities, (3) assisted transfers, and (4) assisted household ambulation. At the time of discharge, Maria had nearly met the previously established functional goals. It was believed that the goals and the hypotheses on which treatments were based were appropriate with the employment of skillful intervention. Factors interfering in the attainment of goals included the severity of neurologic injury, a maladaptive physiologic response to activity, and severe cognitive impairments. On discharge it was believed that Maria had maximized her gains during the more rapid phase of recovery. It is hoped that intervention maximized the development of adaptable, efficient, and successful movement solutions to motor problems.

Equipment Needs

The need for equipment was continually assessed as Maria progressed through her rehabilitation. On discharge, an upright wheelchair was ordered for community mobility, including use at school and for family outings. Maria's family was able to transport her in a stroller for community mobility, but a wheelchair was needed for school bus transportation. The wheelchair provided a safe and energy-efficient form of mobility so her family could take her out into the community including the use of bus transportation. A solid polypropylene AFO for the right extremity was also issued. During ambulation activities Maria demonstrated a frequent knee extension thrust that, over time, could damage the structures in her knee. Although gait deviations were present bilaterally, the thrust was more forceful and functionally limiting on the right (e.g., a greater reduction in forward progression of the tibia). The AFO was issued to reduce the likelihood of future orthopedic complications such as damage to the tendons and ligaments of the posterior knee.

On discharge, Maria was referred to a school-based therapy program in her community. Based on her age and family financial constraints, this form of outpatient therapeutic intervention was her only option. During the interval between discharge from our facility and the initiation of the school-based program, Maria's family was given a home program aimed at a reduction in her impairments and challenge of her current functional abilities. Maria's parents were instructed in many intervention tactics to improve her functional mobility; these were to be performed throughout the day. These activities included the practice of successful and adaptable motor activities such as safe and independent transition from sitting to a standing position and the immediate initiation of ambulation from *home*-specific surfaces such as *her* toilet and booster seat. Progressive independence of ambulation within her home was also encouraged, including the performance of activities while walking such as pushing open a door. Maria's parents did not have time to practice isolated "exercise" activities. As a result, a focus on the incorporation of continual reinforcement of emerging abilities into daily life activities was more appropriate for her family's hectic lifestyle.

Throughout the rehabilitation process Maria's family was educated regarding the previously described aspects of the injury, the anticipated progression of recovery, and the expected needs for continued medical and therapy follow-up care. The family was informed about the proper use of issued equipment (e.g., AFO, wheelchair), safe car transportation (e.g., car seat laws), and proper body mechanics during transfers. They were also informed about entry into school. As a result of her injury, Maria now qualified for a special education preschool. Finally, her family was educated about access to appropriate and needed community resources. Such resources may include the National Brain Injury Association (state and local chapters).

Test 4

Test 4 was performed 20 months after the injury, when Maria was 5 years and 5 months old. In addition to previously described reassessment procedures and PEDI functional skill scales (see Table 3–12, test 4), the PEDI caregiver assistance scales were also administered (Table 3–13). It was not until test 4 that Maria's raw scores on the functional skill scales were able to be transformed into meaningful normative standard scores (see Table 3–11, test 4), but she was performing at nearly 1½ standard deviations below the mean. Analysis of scaled scores showed dramatic progress since admission (see Fig. 3–1). At the time of reassessment, Maria received 1 hour of school-based occupational and speech therapies per week. She received physical therapy services only on a consultation basis. Her parents reported that ongoing physical therapy was discontinued because "she can do her program at home."

The period between tests 3 and 4 showed notable improvements in all domains of the functional skills scales on the PEDI (see Table 3–11 and Fig. 3–1). These improvements were representative of recovery in the areas of the ability to consume an age-appropriate diet, bowel and bladder control, transfers, locomotion, social interactions with others, and expressive communication. It was not until test 4 that mobility skills scaled scores "caught up" with the scores of social and self-care skills. This was likely due to improved independence with transfers and locomotion. According to the PEDI, remaining limitations were in the categories of grooming and dressing activities, independence with all transfers, speed of locomotion, functional communication, problem solving, and safety.

Maria had made significant cognitive improvements, although she remained at Rancho pediatric level II. Maria demonstrated greater comprehension and expressive communication skills. Her parents reported that she understood simple 2- to 3-step commands and time concepts. Maria was able to communicate in 2- or 3-word sentences as well as talk about abstract concepts such as her emotions. For example, Maria was able to say phrases in Spanish such as "I love you Mama (or Papa)" or "I'm mad at you." Play skills incorporated more interactions with her peers and siblings as well as symbolic and pretend play (i.e., "feeding her baby"). Of great significance to her parents was the fact that Maria demonstrated some safety awareness such as caution near the stove. She also attempted to assist with family chores such as cleaning.

Maria also made notable improvements in functional mobility skills including transfer skills and locomotion. Maria was able to independently transfer herself in and out of bed, on and off an adult-sized chair, and on and off the toilet, but she continued to require assistance for getting into and out of the bathtub. Maria was able to walk without support for limited community distances (approximately 2 or 3 blocks), but her speed was slow. At the time of reassessment she continued to use her right AFO for most ambulation activities. The AFO continued to provide assistance with controlled tibial progression and decrease the force of the knee extension thrust during stance. Figure 3–2 illustrates Maria walking up an incline without her AFO. She demonstrated decreased forward progression

Maria's Results of PEDI: Caregiver Assistance Scales 20 Months After Injury (Test 4)

TABLE 3–13	Domain	Normative Standard Score ± SE	Scaled Score	Modification Frequency
	Self-care	30.3 ± 3.0	54.6 ± 3.5	0
	Mobility	35.0 ± 2.9	60.1 ± 3.5	1 (hand-held assist, use of wall or railing)
	Social function	20.4 ± 3.6	42.8 ± 4.2	0

PEDI, Pediatric Evaluation of Disability Inventory; SE, standard error.
*Scaled scores range from zero to 100.

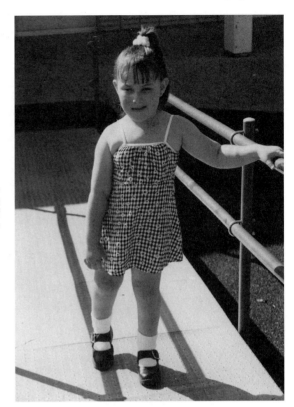

FIGURE 3–2. Maria ascending a ramp. She did not incorporate the use of her right extremity (holding side rails) or demonstrate a reciprocal arm swing. (Courtesy of Rancho Los Amigos Medical Center, Pediatric Brain Injury Service, Downey, Calif.)

of her right tibia at the transition between stance and swing. Her trunk and pelvis show excessive backward rotation that also decreases forward progression during walking.[155] (Refer to Perry[155] for further discussion of terminology and treatment in normal and abnormal walking and Sutherland and colleagues[156] for development of walking in children.) Maria showed adaptability of her ambulation efforts such as walking over even surfaces, accommodation to changes in terrain, and dealing with environmental obstacles (Fig. 3–3). The required adaptability for changes in the demands of a task and environmental constraints were performed with minimal difficulty, but she had problems with ambulation over very rough surfaces such as dense grass or gravel. Previously, Maria was unable to perform any stair locomotion. At test 4 she was able to walk up and down 4 to 5 steps with upper extremity assistance (e.g., a railing, a wall, or a parent's hand). Figure 3–4 illustrates Maria's stair locomotion skills. She consistently used the railing with her left upper extremity and demonstrated a marking time pattern, placing both feet on one step before advancing to the next level. Maria was able to alternate the lead limb when prompted. Community ambulation skills were limited by impaired endurance, a slow velocity, and an inability to independently ascend or descend curbs (for which she required upper extremity assistance).

Maria still demonstrated great difficulty with the performance of grooming, self-feeding, and dressing activities. Her parents reported that she required maximal assistance with all self-care activities with the exception of toileting. She was able to consume a regular diet with thin liquids in a reasonable amount of time (compared with her younger siblings). Severe ataxia of her left arm and a lack of functional control of her right arm continued to significantly limit self-feeding abilities, including the use of utensils or even effective lifting of a spouted cup to her mouth, so her parents performed nearly all the feeding activities. Figures 3–2 and 3–4 illustrate the lack of incorporation of the right upper extremity into functional mobility activities. She did attempt to perform simple grooming and dressing activities with assistance (e.g., cleaning her face and brushing her teeth), but she was unable to manage more complex tasks such as the placement of

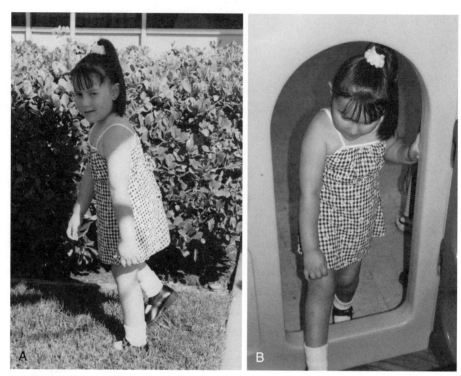

FIGURE 3–3. Maria negotiating environmental obstacles: grass *(A)* and the threshold of the door to a play house *(B).* (*A* and *B,* Courtesy of Rancho Los Amigos Medical Center, Pediatric Brain Injury Service, Downey, Calif.)

toothpaste, zippers, or buttons. Of great importance to Maria's parents was the recovery of bowel and bladder continence; she was completely "potty-trained." Although she continued to demonstrate significant self-care limitations, improvements in toileting accounted for improved PEDI scores on functional skills.

Information regarding the caregiver assistance scales was available only for test 4 (see Table 3–13), so we were unable to compare the "burden of care" or amount of assistance required to carry out functional activities to that on previous occasions. Maria's parents reported the necessity of modification to the environment when Maria climbed stairs, such as a hand-held assist, holding a railing, or holding onto a wall during stair climbing. Her family reported that she required maximal assistance in nearly all areas of self-care and for selected transfers, and moderate-to-maximal assistance with expressive communication, problem solving, safety, and play with peers.

RECOMMENDATIONS FOR CONTINUED CARE

We believe that the most rapid phase of recovery has occurred for Maria. Throughout Maria's lifetime we expect new concerns to arise as she grows and continues her recovery. As therapists for children who have experienced TBI we can guide and promote continued functional recovery, providing and discontinuing intervention as appropriate. The child's and the family's goals should continue to guide interventions.

Functional limitations in Maria's self-care abilities (feeding and grooming) may be the greatest source of excessive burden of care responsibilities for her family. At the last test period, 20 months after injury, Maria's parents provided essentially all her self-care with the exception of toileting. Maria's two younger siblings (27 months old and nearly 4 years old) required a high degree of constant care and supervision. The perceived severity of Maria's limitations and their impact on the family, therefore, may not be evident to her parents until her siblings are older and do not demand as much intensive care, assistance, and supervision. Likewise, Maria's cognitive limitations may become even

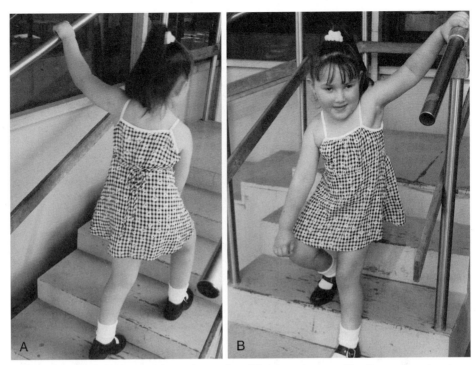

FIGURE 3–4. Maria ascending *(A)* and descending *(B)* stairs using a marking time pattern: however, she was able to alternate extremities when so instructed. (*A* and *B,* Courtesy of Rancho Los Amigos Medical Center, Pediatric Brain Injury Service, Downey, Calif.)

more evident when she is unable to cognitively play or engage in "higher-level" activities that interest her siblings.

Persistent severe motor control deficits of Maria's bilateral upper extremities (minimal volitional control of the right and severe ataxia of the left) continue to limit Maria's ability to perform functional movements with her arms (e.g., self-care and transitional mobility activities). Future interventions may be aimed at teaching Maria strategies to reduce the influence of her upper extremity ataxia by reducing the complexity of the desired movement through minimizing the number of moving segments and the rate at which they move.[81] For example, weight-bearing or stabilizing her proximal arm while performing feeding or grooming activities may enhance success with these activities and encourage more independent performance. Biofeedback and relaxation training have also been found to be effective treatments for ataxia in adults related to feeding abilities.[146]

Physical inactivity is a major public health concern. This concern is even greater for those individuals with severe disabilities.[157] The *Surgeon General's Report on Physical Activity and Health*[157] outlines the importance of regular activity for the prevention of heart disease, diabetes, hypertension, and depression, for weight control, and for the maintenance of healthy bones, joints, and muscles. As Maria grows older it will become increasingly important that regular exercise be a part of her daily regimen.

The potential for affective and behavioral problems in the future exists. This is anticipated to be of concern to the family, so they must be educated regarding the most effective solutions to manage these problems as they arise. At our facility, outpatient support groups are provided for families to learn to cope with such problems. There are support groups and many community resources that would be beneficial for Maria's parents. Additional reported strategies for coping may include planned time away and participation in activities away from the home (and the person they were caring for), as well as prayer or meditation.[149]

Periodic reassessments provide the opportunity to monitor cognitive and functional mobility status and gains, assess home program effectiveness, and provide equipment recommendations. Optimally, a multidisciplinary team with specialized knowledge of children with TBI should monitor the status of these children throughout the recovery process. School-based therapy programs often provide these services. At these reassessment periods parental education regarding expected future needs for medical care and therapy can be updated. We expect that as Maria grows older and her cognition improves, she will play a greater role in the establishment of her own goals. Education should shift its focus toward empowering Maria to make decisions and advocate for her needs.

REFERENCES

1. Ward JD: Pediatric issues in head trauma. New Horiz 3:539, 1995.
2. Finney JW, Christophersen ER, Friman PC, et al: Society of Pediatric Psychology Task Force Report: Pediatric psychology and injury control. J Pediatr Psychol 18:499, 1993.
3. Kraus JF, Fife D, Conroy C: Pediatric brain injuries: The nature, clinical course and early outcomes in a defined United States population. Pediatrics 79:501, 1987.
4. Interagency Head Injury Task Force Reports: National Institute of Neurological Disorders and Stroke, National Institutes of Health, Bethesda, MD, 1990.
5. Sosin DM, Sniezek JE, Thurman DJ: Incidence of mild and moderate brain injury in the United States, 1991. Brain Inj 10:47, 1996.
6. Kalsbeek WD, McLarin RL, Harris BSH, et al: The national head and spinal cord injury survey: Major findings. J Neurosurg 53:S19, 1980.
7. Raphaely RC, Swedlow DB, Downes JJ, et al: Management of severe pediatric head trauma. Pediatr Clin North Am 27:715, 1980.
8. Brink JD, Garrett AL, Hale WR, et al: Recovery of motor and intellectual functions in children sustaining severe head injuries. Dev Med Child Neurol 12:565, 1972.
9. Bruce DA, Schut L, Bruno L, et al: Outcome following severe head injuries in children. J Neurosurg 48:679, 1978.
10. Cartlidge NEF, Shaw DA: Head Injury. *In* Walton Sir JN (ed): Major Problems in Neurology, vol 10. WB Saunders, Philadelphia, 1981, p 34.
11. Mayer T, Walker ML, Johnson DG, et al: Causes of morbidity and mortality in severe pediatric trauma. JAMA 245:719, 1981.
12. Gilchrist E, Wilkinson M: Some factors determining prognosis in young people with severe head injuries. Arch Neurol 36:355, 1979.
13. Goldstein FC, Levin HS: Epidemiology of pediatric closed head injury: Incidence, clinical characteristics and risk factors. J Learn Disabil 20:518, 1987.
14. Bruce DA: Head injuries in the pediatric population. Curr Probl Pediatr 10:67, 1990.
15. Eiben CF, Anderson TP, Lockman L, et al: Functional outcome of closed head injury in children and young adults. Arch Phys Med Rehabil 65:168, 1984.
16. Humphreys RP: Outcome of severe head injury in children. Concepts Pediatr Neurosurg 3:191, 1983.
17. Wagstyll J, Sutcliffe AJ, Alpar EK, et al: Early prediction of outcome following head injury in children. J Pediatr Surg 22:127, 1987.
18. Jennett B: Head injuries in children. Dev Med Child Neurol 14:137, 1972.
19. Mamelak AN, Pitts LH, Damron S: Predicting survival from head trauma 24 hours after injury: A practical method with therapeutic implications. J Trauma 41:91, 1996.
20. Berney J, Froidevaux AC, Favier J: Paediatric head trauma: Influence of age and sex. II: Biomechanical and anatimo-clinical correlations. Childs Nerv Syst 10:517, 1994.
21. Carlsson C-A, von Essen C, L'fgren J: Factors affecting the clinical course of patients with severe head injuries. J Neurosurg 29:242, 1968.
22. Chestnut RM, Marshall LF, Klauber MR, et al: The role of secondary brain injury in determining outcome from severe head injury. J Trauma 34:216, 1993.
23. Jaffe KM, Massagli TL, Rivara JB, et al: Pediatric traumatic brain injury: Acute and rehabilitation costs. Arch Phys Med Rehabil 74:681, 1993.
24. Boswell WC, Boyd CR, Schaffner D, et al: Prevention of pediatric mortality from trauma: Are current measures adequate? South Med J 89:218, 1996.
25. Hazinski MF, Francescutti LH, Lapidus GD, et al: Pediatric injury prevention. Ann Emerg Med 22:456, 1993.
26. Kraus JF, McArthur DL: Epidemiologic aspects of brain injury. Neurol Clin 14:435, 1996.

27. Clifton GL, McCormick WF, Grossman RG: Neuropathology of early and late deaths after head injury. Neurosurgery 8:309, 1981.

28. Miller JD, Butterworth JF, Grudeman SK, et al: Further experience in the management of severe head injury. J Neurosurg 54:289, 1981.

29. Dobkin BH: Traumatic brain injury. *In* Neurologic Rehabilitation. Contemporary Neurology Series, vol 47. FA Davis, Philadelphia, 1996, p 257.

30. Gennarelli TA: Mechanisms of brain injury. J Emerg Med 11(suppl 1):5, 1993.

31. Berker E: Diagnosis, physiology, pathology and rehabilitation of traumatic brain injuries. Int J Neurosci 85:195, 1996.

32. Gennarelli TA, Thibault LE, Adams JH, et al: Diffuse axonal injury and traumatic coma in the primate. Ann Neurol 12:564, 1982.

33. Dimitrijevic MR: Restorative neurology of head injury. J Neurotrauma 6:25, 1989.

34. Levin HS: Head trauma. Curr Opin Neurol 6:841, 1993.

35. Povlishok JT, Christman CW: The pathobiology of traumatically induced axonal injury in animals and humans: A review of current thoughts. J Neurotrauma 12:155, 1995.

36. McIntosh TK: Novel pharmacologic therapies in the treatment of experimental traumatic brain injury: A review. J Neurotrauma 10:215, 1993.

37. Faden AI: Pharmacological treatment of central nervous system trauma. Pharmacol Toxicol 78:12, 1996.

38. Clifton GL: Systemic hypothermia in treatment of severe brain injury: A review and update. J Neurotrauma 12:923, 1995.

39. Bouma CJ, Muizelaur JP: Cerebral blood flow in severe clinical head injury. New Horiz 3:384, 1995.

40. Johnston MV: Neurotransmitters and vulnerability of the developing brain. Brain Dev 17:301, 1995.

41. Sharples PM, Stuart AG, Matthews DS, et al: Cerebral blood flow and metabolism in children with severe head injury. Part I: Relation to age, Glasgow Coma Score, outcome, intracranial pressure, and time after injury. J Neurol Neurosurg Psychiatry 58:145, 1995.

42. Dobkin BH: Plasticity in motor and cognitive networks. *In* Neurologic Rehabilitation. Contemporary Neurology Series, vol 47. FA Davis, Philadelphia, 1996, p 3.

43. Dobkin BH: Biologic mechanisms of recovery. *In* Neurologic Rehabilitation. Contemporary Neurology Series, vol 47. FA Davis, Philadelphia, 1996, p 46.

44. Sabatini U, Toni D, Pantano P, et al: Motor recovery after early brain damage. Stroke 25:154, 1994.

45. Merzenich M, Recanzone G, Jenkins W, et al: Cortical representational plasticity. *In* Rakic P, Singer W (eds): Neurobiology of Neocortex. John Wiley, New York, 1988, p 41.

46. Riolo-Quinn L: Motor learning considerations in treating brain injured patients. Neurol Rep 14:12, 1990.

47. Coster WJ, Haley S, Baryza MJ: Functional performance of young children after traumatic brain injury: A 6-month follow-up study. Am J Occup Ther 48:211, 1994.

48. Ewing-Cobbs L, Fletcher JM: Neuropsychological assessment of head injury in children. J Learning Disabilities 20:526, 1987.

49. Rivara JB, Jaffe KM, Fay GC, et al: Family functioning and injury severity as predictors of child functioning one year following traumatic brain injury. Arch Phys Med Rehabil 74:1047, 1993.

50. Jennett B, Snoek J, Bond MR, et al: Disability after severe head injury: Observations on the use of Glasgow Outcome Scale. J Neurol Neurosurg Psychiatry 44:285, 1981.

51. Aisinkinen I, Kaste M, Sarna S: Patients with traumatic brain injury referred to a rehabilitation and re-employment programme: Social and professional outcome for 508 Finnish patients 5 or more years after injury. Brain Inj 10:883, 1996.

52. Klonoff H, Low MD, Clark C: Head injuries in children: A prospective five year follow-up. J Neurol Neurosurg Psychiatry 40:1211, 1977.

53. Klonoff H, Clark C, Klonoff PS: Long-term outcome of head injuries: A 23 year follow up study of children with head injuries. J Neurol Neurosurg Psychiatry 56:410, 1993.

54. King ML, Lichtman GS, Steinberg JS: Heart-rate variability in chronic traumatic brain injury. Brain Inj 11:445, 1997.

55. Fay GC, Jaffe KM, Polissar NL, et al: Outcome of pediatric traumatic brain injury at three years: A cohort study. Arch Phys Med Rehabil 75:733, 1994.

56. Whitlock JA Jr, Hamilton BB: Functional outcome after rehabilitation for severe traumatic brain injury. Arch Phys Med Rehabil 76:1103, 1995.

57. Chaplin D, Deitz J, Jaffe KM: Motor performance in children after traumatic brain injury. Arch Phys Med Rehabil 74:161, 1993.

58. Telzrow CF: Management of academic and educational problems in head injury. J Learn Disabil 20:536, 1987.
59. Young B, Rapp RP, Norton JA, et al: Early prediction of outcome in head-injured patients. J Neurosurg 54:300, 1981.
60. Filley CM, Cranberg LD, Alexander MP, et al: Neurobehavioral outcome after closed head injury in childhood and adolescence. Arch Neurol 44:194, 1987.
61. Dombovy ML, Olek AC: Recovery and rehabilitation following traumatic brain injury. Brain Inj 11:305, 1996.
62. Wong PP, Dornan J, Keating AM, et al: Re-examining the concept of severity in traumatic brain injury. Brain Inj 8:509, 1994.
63. Jennett B, Bond M: Assessment of outcome after severe brain damage. A practical scale. Lancet 1:480, 1975.
64. Haley SM, Coster WJ, Ludlow LH, et al: Pediatric Evaluation of Disability Inventory (PEDI), 1st version. New England Medical Center Hospitals, Boston, 1992.
65. Data Management Service of the Uniform Data System for Medical Rehabilitation and the Center for Functional Assessment Research: Guide for the Use of the Uniform Data Set for Medical Rehabilitation Including the Functional Independence Measure (Version 3.1). State University Of New York at Buffalo, Buffalo, 1990; Uniform Data System for Medical Rehabilitation, Buffalo, 1986.
66. Data Management Service of the Uniform Data System for Medical Rehabilitation and the Center for Functional Assessment Research: Guide for the Use of the Functional Independence Measure for Children (WeeFIM™) of the Uniform Data Set for Medical Rehabilitation. State University of New York at Buffalo, Buffalo, 1989.
67. Teasdale G, Jennett B: Assessment of coma and impaired consciousness. Lancet 2:81, 1974.
68. Michaud LJ, Duhaime AC, Batshaw ML: Traumatic brain injury in children. Pediatr Clin North Am 40:553, 1993.
69. Brink JD, Imbus C, Woo-Sam J: Physical recovery after severe closed head trauma in children and adolescents. J Pediatr 97:721, 1980.
70. Massagli TL, Michaud LJ, Rivara FP: Association between severity indexes and outcome after severe traumatic brain injury in children. Arch Phys Med Rehabil 77:125, 1996.
71. Massagli TL, Michaud LJ, Rivara FP, et al: Predictors of survival and severity of disability after severe brain injury in children. Neurosurgery 31:254, 1992.
72. Mayer T, Walker ML, Shasha I, et al: Effect of multiple trauma on outcome of pediatric patients with neurologic injuries. Childs Brain 8:189, 1981.
73. Mayer T, Matlak ME, Johnson DG, Walker ML: The modified injury severity scale in pediatric multiple trauma patients. J Pediatr Surg 15:719, 1980.
74. Oddy M, Humphrey M: Social recovery during the year following severe head injury. J Neurol Neurosurg Psychiatr 43:798, 1980.
75. Hoffer M, Brink J, Marsh JS, et al: Head injuries. *In* Lovell WW, Winter RB (eds): Pediatric Orthopaedics, vol 2. JB Lippincott, Philadelphia, 1986, p 479.
76. Ommaya AK: Trauma to the nervous system. Ann R Coll Surg Engl 39:317, 1966.
77. Pediatric levels of consciousness. *In* Rehabilitation of the Head Injured Child and Adult: Selected Problems. Downey, Calif. Professional Staff Association of Rancho Los Amigos Hospital, Inc., 1982, p 5.
78. Malkmus D: Integrating cognitive strategies into the physical therapy setting. Phys Ther 63:1952, 1983.
79. Rappaport M, Dougherty AM, Kelting DL: Evaluation of coma and vegetative states. Arch Phys Med Rehabil 73:628, 1992.
80. Ansell BJ, Keenan JE: The Western Neuro Sensory Stimulation Profile: A tool for assessing slow-to-recover head-injured patients. Arch Phys Med Rehabil 70:104, 1989.
81. Bastian AJ: Mechanisms of ataxia. Phys Ther 77:672, 1997.
82. Iloeje SO: Measurement of muscle tone in children with cerebellar ataxia. East Afr Med J 71:256, 1994.
83. Westcott SL, Lowes LP, Richardson PK: Evaluation of postural stability in children: Current theories and assessment tools. Phys Ther 77:629, 1997.
84. Gill-Body KM, Popat RA, Parker SW, Krebs DE: Rehabilitation of balance in two patients with cerebellar dysfunction. Phys Ther 77:534, 1997.
85. Brandt T, Paulus W: Postural training in exceptional populations. *In* Woollacott MH, Shumway-Cook A (eds): Development of Posture and Gait Across the Life Span. University of South Carolina Press, Columbia, SC, 1989, p 299.
86. Jeka JJ: Light touch contact as a balance aid. Phys Ther 77:476, 1997.
87. Horak FB, Henry SM, Shumway-Cook A: Postural perturbations: New insights for treatment of balance disorders. Phys Ther 77:517, 1997.

88. Sobus KML, Alexander MA, Harche HT: Undetected musculoskeletal trauma in children with traumatic brain injury or spinal cord injury. Arch Phys Med Rehabil 74:902, 1993.

89. Blasier D, Letts RM: Pediatric update #7. The orthopedic manifestations of head injury in children. Orthop Rev 18:350, 1989.

90. Hoffer MM, Garrett A, Brink JD, et al: The orthopedic management of the brain-injured children. J Bone Joint Surg Am 53:567, 1971.

91. Meyler WJ, Bakker H, Kok JJ, et al: The effect of dantrolene sodium in relation to blood levels in spastic patients after prolonged administration. J Neurol Neurosurg Psychiatry 44:334, 1981.

92. Becker E, Bar-Or O, Mendelson L, et al: Pulmonary functions and responses to exercise of patients following craniocerebral injury. Scand J Rehabil Med 10:47, 1978.

93. Sullivan SJ, Richer E, Laurent F: The role of and possibilities for physical conditioning programmes in the rehabilitation of traumatically brain-injured persons. Brain Inj 4:407, 1990.

94. Rothstein JM, Echternach JL: Hypothesis-oriented algorithm for clinicians: A method for evaluation and treatment planning. Phys Ther 69:559, 1989.

95. Mackey L, Bernstein B, Chaoman P, et al: Early intervention in severe head injury: Long term benefits of a formalized program. Arch Phys Med Rehabil 73:635, 1992.

96. Walker WC, Kreutzer JS, Witol AD: Review of subject: Level of care options for the low-functioning brain injury survivor. Brain Inj 10:65, 1996.

97. Granger CV, Divan N, Fiedler RC: Functional assessment scales: A study of persons after brain injury. Am J Phys Med Rehabil 74:107, 1995.

98. Piper M, Darrah J: Motor Assessment of the Developing Infant. WB Saunders, Philadelphia, 1994.

99. Chandler L, Andrews M, Swanson M: Movement Assessment of Infants. Rolling Bay Press, Rolling Bay, Wash, 1980.

100. Russell D, Rosenbaum P, Gowland C, et al: Gross Motor Function Measure, 2nd ed. Gross Motor Measures Group, McMaster University, Hamilton, Ontario, Canada, 1993.

101. Bruininks R: Bruninks-Oseretsky Test of Motor Proficiency. American Guidance Service, Circle Pines, Minn, 1978.

102. Fewell R, Folio R: Peabody Developmental Motor Scales. Developmental Learning Materials Teaching Resources, Allen, Tex, 1983.

103. Hislop HJ, Montgomery J: Upright motor control. *In* Daniels' and Worthingham's Muscle Testing: Techniques of Manual Examination, 6th ed. WB Saunders, Philadelphia, 1995, p 320.

104. Gajdosik CG, Nelson SA, Gleason DK, et al: Reliability of isometric strength measurements of girls 3–5 years: A preliminary study. Pediatr Phys Ther 6:206, 1994.

105. Lunsford BR, Perry J: The standing heel-rise test for ankle plantar flexion criterion for normal. Phys Ther 75:694, 1996.

106. Backman E, Odenrick P, Henriksson KG, et al: Isometric muscle force and anthropometric values in normal children between 3.5 and 15 years. Scand J Rehabil Med 21:105, 1989.

107. Horvat M, Croce R, Roswal G: Intratester reliability of the Nicholas Manual Muscle Tester on individuals with intellectual disabilities by a tester having minimal experience. Arch Phys Med Rehabil 76:808, 1994.

108. Shumway-Cook A, Horak FB: Assessing the influence of sensory interaction on balance: Suggestion from the field. Phys Ther 66:1548, 1986.

109. Horak FB: Clinical measurement of postural control in adults. Phys Ther 67:1881, 1987.

110. Crowe TK, Deitz JC, Richardson PK, Atwater SW: Interrater reliability of the Pediatric Clinical Test of Sensory Interaction for Balance. Phys Occup Ther Pediatr 10(4):1, 1990.

111. Westcott SL, Crowe TK, Deitz JC, Richardson P: Test-retest reliability of the Pediatric Clinical Test of Sensory Interaction for Balance (P-CTSIB). Phys Occup Ther Pediatr 14(1):1, 1994.

112. Deitz JC, Richardson PK, Atwater SW, Crowe TK: Performance of normal children on the Pediatric Clinical Test of Sensory Interaction for Balance. Occup Ther J Res 11:336, 1991.

113. Richardson PK, Atwater SW, Crowe TK, Deitz JC: Performance of preschoolers on the Pediatric Clinical Test of Sensory Interaction for Balance. Am J Occup Ther 46:793, 1992.

114. Pelligrino TT, Buelow B, Krause M, et al: Test-retest reliability of the Pediatric Clinical Test of Sensory Interaction for Balance and the Functional Reach Test in children with standing balance dysfunction. Pediatr Phys Ther 7:197, 1995.

115. Stuberg WA, Fuchs RH, Miedaner JA: Reliability of goniometric measurements of children with cerebral palsy. Dev Med Child Neurol 30:657, 1988.

116. Gajdosik CG, Bohannon RW: Clinical measurement of range of motion: Review of goniometry emphasizing reliability and validity. Phys Ther 67:1867, 1987.

117. Bohannon RW, Smith MB: Interrater reliability of a modified Ashworth scale of muscle spasticity. Phys Ther 67:206, 1987.
118. Peel C: The cardiopulmonary system and movement dysfunction. Phys Ther 76:448, 1996.
119. Ciesla N: Chest physical therapy for patients in the intensive care unit. Phys Ther 76:609, 1996.
120. Hammon WE, Martin RJ: Chest physical therapy for acute atelectasis. Phys Ther 61:217, 1981.
121. Lazarus C, Logemann JA: Swallowing disorders in closed head trauma patients. Rehabilitation (Stuttg) 68:79, 1987.
122. Zablotny C: Evaluation and management of swallowing dysfunction. *In* Montgomery J (ed): Physical Therapy for Traumatic Brain Injury. Clinics in Physical Therapy. Churchill Livingstone, New York, 1995.
123. Baum B, Hall KM: Relationship between constructional praxis and dressing in the head-injured adult. Am J Occup Ther 35:438, 1981.
124. Neistadt ME: Perceptual retraining for adults with diffuse brain injury. Am J Occup Ther 48:877, 1994.
125. Guercio J, Chittum R, McMorrow M: Self-management in the treatment of ataxia: A case study in reducing ataxic tremor through relaxation and biofeedback. Brain Inj 11:353, 1997.
126. Campbell SK: The child's development of functional movement. *In* Campbell SK, Vander Linden DW, Palisano RJ (eds): Physical Therapy for Children. WB Saunders, Philadelphia, 1994, p 3.
127. Goldberger ME: Recovery of movements after CNS lesions in monkeys. *In* Stein DG, Rosen JJ, Butters N (eds): Plasticity and Recovery of Function in the CNS. Academic, New York, 1974, p 235.
128. Nelson JR: Neuro-otologic aspects of head injury. Adv Neurol 22:107, 1979.
129. Baker LL, McNeal DR, Benton LA, et al: Clinical uses of neuromuscular electrical stimulation. *In* Neuromuscular Electrical Stimulation: A Practical Guide, 3rd ed. Rehabilitation Engineering Program, Los Amigos Research and Education Institute, Downey, Calif., 1993, p 45.
130. Reed B: The physiology of neuromuscular electrical stimulation. Pediatr Phys Ther 9:96, 1997.
131. Carr JH, Shepherd RB (eds): Movement Sciences: Foundation for Physical Therapy in Rehabilitation. Aspen, Rockville, Md, 1987.
132. Fisher B, Woll S: Considerations in restoration of motor control. *In* Montgomery J (ed): Physical Therapy for Traumatic Brain Injury. Clinics in Physical Therapy. Churchill Livingstone, New York, 1995.
133. Mosely AM: The effect of casting combined with stretching on passive ankle dorsiflexion in adults with traumatic brain injuries. Phys Ther 77:240, 1997.
134. Hill J: The effects of casting on upper extremity motor disorders after brain injury. Am J Occup Ther 3:219, 1994.
135. Wilson DJ, Childers MK, Cooke DL, et al: Kinematic changes following botulinum toxin injection after traumatic brain injury. Brain Inj 11:157, 1997.
136. Dobkin BH: Problems of medical management. *In* Neurologic Rehabilitation. Contemporary Neurology Series, vol 47. FA Davis, Philadelphia, 1996, p 128.
137. Almeida GL, Campbell SK, Giroloami GL, et al: Multidimensional assessment of motor function in a child with cerebral palsy following intrathecal administration of baclofen. Phys Ther 77:751, 1997.
138. Vitale AE, Jankoski LW, Sullivan SJ: Reliability of a walk/run test to estimate aerobic capacity in a brain-injured population. Brain Inj 11:67, 1997.
139. Rossi C, Sullivan SJ: Reliability of motor fitness tests in children and adolescents with traumatic brain injury. Arch Phys Med Rehabil 77:1062, 1996.
140. Silverman EH, Elfant IL: Dysphagia: An evaluation and treatment program for the adult. Am J Occup Ther 33:382, 1979.
141. Serio CD, Kreutzer JS, Witol AD: Family needs after traumatic brain injury: A factor analytic study of the Family Needs Questionnaire. Brain Inj 11:1, 1997.
142. Rivara JB: Family functioning following pediatric head injury. Pediatr Ann 23:38, 1994.
143. Wade S, Drotar D, Taylor HG, Stancin T: Assessing the effects of traumatic brain injury on family functioning: Conceptual and methodological issues. J Pediatr Psychol 20:737, 1995.
144. Sokol DK, Ferguson CF, Pitcher GA, et al: Behavioral adjustment and parental stress associated with closed head injury in children. Brain Inj 10:439, 1996.
145. Waaland PK, Burns C, Cockrell J: Evaluation of the needs of high- and low-income families following paediatric traumatic brain injury. Brain Inj 7:135, 1993.

146. Osberg J, Brooke M, Baryza M, et al: Impact of childhood brain injury on work and family finances. Brain Inj 11:11, 1997.
147. Shumway-Cook A, Woollacott M: Motor Control: Theory and Practical Applications. Williams & Wilkins, Baltimore, 1995.
148. Woollacott MH, Shumway-Cook A, Williams HG: The development of posture and balance control in children. *In* Woollacott MH, Shumway-Cook A (eds): Development of Posture and Gait Across the Life Span. University of South Carolina Press, Columbia, SC, 1989, p 77.
149. Sanders AM, High WM, Hannay HJ, et al: Predictors of psychological health in caregivers of patients with closed head injury. Brain Inj 11:23, 1997.
150. Freeman EA: Community-based rehabilitation of the person with a severe brain injury. Brain Inj 11:143, 1997.
151. Kaplan CP, Corrigan JD: The relationship between cognition and functional independence in adults with traumatic brain injury. Arch Phys Med Rehabil 75:643, 1994.
152. Lowes LP, Effgen S: The Americans With Disabilities Act of 1990: Implications for pediatric physical therapists. Pediatr Phys Ther 8:111, 1996.
153. Case-Smith J: Analysis of current motor development theory and recently published infant motor assessments. Inf Young Children 9:29, 1996.
154. Kay E, Dunleavy K: Community-based rehabilitation: An international model. Pediatr Phys Ther 8:117, 1996.
155. Perry J: Gait Analysis: Normal and Pathological Function. Slack, Thorofare, NJ, 1992.
156. Sutherland DH, Olshen RA, Biden EN, et al: The development of mature walking. Clin Develop Med 104:33, 105:55, 1988.
157. Report of the Surgeon General: Physical Activity and Health, 1996. US Department of Health and Human Services, Centers for Disease Control and Prevention, Atlanta, 1996.

Children with Multiple Disabilities

K a r e n   Y u n d t   L u n n e n, MS, PT

There is increasing recognition that retarded individuals are more like us than they are different; that they need, just as we all do, love, joy, activity, a chance to grow and progress, and a chance, wherever possible, to become independent.[1]

Senator Hubert H. Humphrey

The focus of this chapter is the child with severe cognitive impairment, complex deficits in adaptive function, and multiple associated impairments and disabilities. This child challenges us in our decision making to carefully select from a long list of problems those for which creative intervention will make a difference. The chapter first sketches a picture of what this child with multiple disabilities might look like and then describes how, as physical therapists, we can participate effectively and meaningfully in comprehensive assessment and intervention. The chapter closes with a representative case study of a 5-year-old girl with multiple disabilities.

DEFINING THE PROBLEM

What distinguishes the focus population from those in other chapters of this text is the degree of cognitive impairment. Volumes have been written about mental retardation and about intelligence, and controversy persists over many of the prevalent theories. The discussion here is basic. A variety of behaviors are considered to be reflective of intelligence: "the ability to learn and profit from experience . . . the ability to reason . . . the ability to adapt to changing conditions . . . and the will to succeed."[2] Mental retardation refers to "substantial limitations in present functioning . . . characterized by significantly sub-average intellectual functioning, existing concurrently with related limitations in two or more of the following applicable adaptive skill areas: communication, self-care, home living, social skills, community use, self-direction, health and safety, functional academics, leisure, and work. Mental retardation manifests before the age of 18."[3] The key elements in the definition are *capabilities* (or competencies), *environments,* and *functioning* (Fig. 4–1).[3]

Classification of Mental Retardation

The definition and classification of mental retardation set forth by the American Association on Mental Retardation (AAMR) in a 1992 publication by Luckasson and colleagues[3] represents a dramatic paradigm shift away from a focus on deficits or disorders present within the individual. Instead of categories like *mild, moderate, severe*, and *profound* based on intelligence quotients (IQs), the new paradigm focuses on "the intensity and pattern of changing supports needed by an individual over a lifetime."[3] The focus shifts

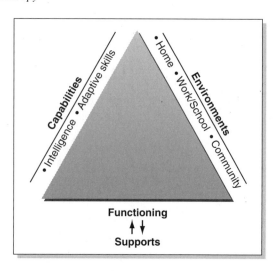

FIGURE 4–1. General structure of the definition of mental retardation. (From Luckasson R: Mental Retardation: Definition, Classification, and Systems of Support, American Association on Mental Retardation, Washington, DC, 1992, p 10.)

from the individual to the interaction of the individual within a complex, changing environment over time. The older labels are still used as descriptors of an individual or population, but the intent is not to remain focused on the individual.

The AAMR process for diagnosing the presence of mental retardation contains three steps and encompasses four dimensions:

1. *Step 1.* Diagnosis of mental retardation
   Dimension I: Intellectual functioning and adaptive skills
   a. IQ by standardized intelligence test of 70 to 75 or below
   b. Adaptive skill limitations by an appropriately normed and standardized instrument
   c. Age of onset below 18 years
2. *Step 2.* Classification and description (identifies strengths and weaknesses across the remaining three dimensions)
   Dimension II: Psychologic and emotional considerations
   Dimension III: Etiologic, physical, and health considerations
   Dimension IV: Environmental considerations
3. *Step 3.* Profile of needed supports across the four dimensions, according to the level of intensity required (intermittent, limited, extensive, or pervasive)

Focus Population

The intent of the AAMR classification to avoid pejorative categorization is recognized and valued. Physical therapists, however, are presented with particular challenges when dealing with the population with very low IQs. Subsequent discussion addresses those individuals with more severe levels of cognitive impairment based on the four dimensions described by the AAMR.

AAMR Dimension I: Intellectual Functioning and Adaptive Skills

The prevalence of mental retardation is about 2.5 to 3 percent of the general population, making the actual numbers 6.2 to 7.5 million people in the United States (based on 1990 census data).[4] One out of every 10 families is directly affected by mental retardation.[4] The focus population generally has an IQ of less than 35 (previously, 20 to 35 was termed "severe" mental retardation and zero to 19 was termed "profound" as measured by the Cattell or Stanford-Binet standardized tests).[5] Those with IQs this low represent only about 4 percent of the total population who are mentally retarded.[6]

On adaptive measures, those with severe mental retardation "require continuing and close supervision, but may perform self-help and simple work tasks under supervision."[5] Those with profound mental retardation "require continuing and close supervision for survival, but some may be able to perform simple self-help tasks."[5] Children at these levels of intellectual function reach an ultimate mental age of less than 6 years, and those who are more involved may never progress out of Piaget's sensorimotor period,[7] the first stage in the development of cognitive systems.[8] Thus, the caregiver or caregivers must play a pivotal role in decision making.

There are many theories and considerable controversy about the development of individuals who are retarded compared with those with normal intelligence.[9] Weisz and Zigler developed one of the more popular theories, the "similar sequence hypothesis,"[7] based on Piagetian concepts. The hypothesis holds that "during development retarded and nonretarded persons traverse the same stages in precisely the same order and differ only in the rate of development and in the ultimate ceiling they attain." Some theorists believe that the hypothesis is valid only for those persons with mild retardation, thus in essence proposing a different sequence of cognitive development for individuals who are severely or profoundly retarded and who may have brain damage or genetic impairment. Weisz and Zigler, however, drew evidence from three longitudinal and 28 cross-sectional studies of developmental phenomena described by Piaget and found that the evidence supported their hypothesis with respect to every subject group, with the "possible exception of individuals with pronounced electroencephalogram abnormalities."[7]

In decision making with this population, it is logical to assume that one can use appropriate developmental tests and anticipate that development will progress in a predictable manner. The similar sequence hypothesis does *not* dictate, however, that a child must master each stage in the developmental sequence before being allowed to progress to the next stage. A persistent focus on functional outcomes and the prevention of secondary impairments should guide this type of decision making.

AAMR Dimension II: Psychologic and Emotional Considerations

The interrelationship of cognitive impairment and mental illness is a controversial and complex area that presents unique problems for diagnosis and intervention.[10] "Without exception, studies on prevalence of psychopathology in mentally retarded persons have shown rates much higher than the general population."[11] The prevalence of the dual diagnosis of mental retardation and mental illness is difficult to determine because of a number of complicating factors, but studies indicate that 15 to 35 percent of all noninstitutionalized persons with mental retardation carry the dual diagnosis, with increasing frequency (as high as 50 percent) at the lower IQ levels.[10] Types of mental illness include schizophrenic disorders, organic brain disorders, adjustment disorders, personality disorders, and affective disorders.

Serious self-injurious behaviors are found in 20,000 to 25,000 individuals in the United States.[11] The specific cause is unknown, but a variety of factors are thought to contribute. These include "neuroanatomical, physiological, and chemical abnormalities; social and environmental deprivation; need for stimulation due to sensory deficits; and operant and respondent learning."[11] Mulick and Kedesdy would add to this list social reinforcement and the avoidance of recurrent aversive events.[12] Current theorists postulate the potential contribution of endogenous opioids, either that the individual has abnormally high levels causing an elevation of the pain threshold, or that self-injury results in the release of naturally occurring endogenous opioids that are highly reinforcing and addictive.[14] Self-injurious behaviors cause serious social and personal consequences for the individual, and the annual cost of care may exceed $100,000 per case.[13]

Less serious, but still an interfering factor in more meaningful exploration of the environment, are stereotypic (repetitive) behaviors found in approximately half of the individuals below the age of 13 who reside in institutions.[15] The most common behaviors are repetitive motor behaviors (e.g., rocking or head banging) and unusual object manipulations (e.g., spinning objects). Stereotypic behaviors are common in normal infants but are replaced by more flexible and complex behaviors in a normal developmental progression.[15] In children with disabilities, stereotypic behaviors are more likely to appear later, last longer, and be less sensitive to environmental influences.[16] Stereotyped mannerisms of children who are cognitively impaired vary with the environmental setting and the nature of ongoing activities, and the frequency of stereotyped behavior appears to be inversely related to the potential for alternative activity. This is true for infants as well as for older persons.[17]

Sensory-processing abnormalities, especially tactile defensiveness, have been implicated in the development and maintenance of stereotypic behaviors.[18–21] These behaviors have been demonstrated to be a consequence of increased arousal[22] as well as a modulator of arousal level.[19] Instruments like the Stereotyped Behavior Checklist,[23] a 54-item questionnaire, or the Sensory Profile developed by Dunn[24, 25] have value in quantifying and describing these behaviors.

AAMR Dimension III: Etiologic, Physical, and Health Considerations

Cause

The cause, notably absent in the earlier AAMR definition and classification of mental retardation,[5] is now a primary consideration. Several hundred conditions are known to cause mental retardation. Variability is found in the reports of cause among the population with severe or profound retardation. Stevenson and associates studied 2106 residents of institutions in South Carolina (approximately 75 percent had IQs less than 20) and found that genetic causes accounted for 19.6 percent (this included chromosome anomalies, single-gene defects, and multifactorial causes) and environmental causes accounted for 26.8 percent (this included trauma, infection, chemical exposures, and prematurity).[26] The cause was unknown in 53.6 percent of cases. In the population studied, 29.1 percent had low birth weights (less than 2500 g).

Intervention viewed as support for the individual is not dependent on the cause, but the cause is relevant for practice, research, and policy.[27] The cause can also help determine the prognosis and in that way influence decision making. Understanding the cause of cognitive impairment is a critical first step for the development of appropriate technology aimed at prevention. In 1971 (with modifications in 1976), the President's Committee on Mental Retardation called for reducing the incidence of mental retardation from biomedical causes by at least 50 percent by the year 2000.[28] Stevenson and coworkers set forth three components that are essential to meet that goal: "availability/development of technological capacity for prevention, the will of the reproducing population for prevention, and a system to advocate for the goal to monitor progress."[26]

Physical and Health Considerations

General. Neurobiologic factors are the primary cause of severe and profound retardation, and it is logical that medical problems would be concurrent. If one uses a functional definition of health, it is often hard to diagnose poor health in those who have multiple severe disabilities and difficult to judge whether a specific treatment will improve the quality of life for these individuals. Severe medical complications accompanying cognitive impairment are a major concern in planning residential environments and other services.[29]

With severe and profound levels of retardation, there are almost always diffuse brain abnormalities and neurologic insult. One study reported autopsies conducted on 1410 individuals with severe or profound retardation over a 14-year period and found that 97.5 percent had neurologic damage.[30] In the population studied by Stevenson and coworkers, 47.4 percent of the individuals had had two or more seizures unrelated to febrile illnesses.[26]

Conley states that almost 95 percent of individuals with IQ levels less than 30 and almost 78 percent of individuals with IQ levels between 30 and 55 have at least one major physical disability, the frequency and severity roughly proportional to the degree of IQ deficit.[31] Capute and associates examined children with cognitive impairment at a nonresidential treatment facility and found the major presenting signs to be overall slowness, motor disability, language disorder, and behavioral disturbances.[30] Many children also had defects in physical growth (stunting of skeletal development),[32] and 21.7 percent had structural birth defects.[5]

Mortality and Morbidity. In the study by Capute and associates, children who were profoundly mentally retarded had mortality rates 50 percent higher than those with severe mental retardation.[30] In a population studied by Cleland and coworkers, aspiration of food was found to be the direct cause of 3.5 percent of deaths of individuals with profound retardation (the seventh leading cause),[33] and aspiration pneumonia is a common medical complication. Rempel and colleagues found clinical signs of gastroesophageal reflux or aspiration in 72 percent of the children with multiple disabilities that they studied.[34]

Tecklin defines respiratory failure as a "condition in which impairment of gas exchange within the lungs poses an immediate threat to life."[35] He reviews the general, structural, and metabolic factors in the normal pediatric population that make the respiratory tract susceptible to respiratory failure in times of stress. The majority of factors that contribute to the susceptibility to respiratory failure are factors that are more significant in the focus population than in the typical pediatric population. These include poor development of abdominal muscles needed for coughing, a high incidence of respiratory tract infections, and compromised respiratory musculature.

Orthopedic Considerations. Orthopedic intervention with the child who has multiple disabilities must be "long range continuum care" rather than "episodic" because of the complexity of the problems and the necessity of considering a multitude of contributing factors.[36] Three phases of orthopedic treatment are prevention; control and support; and correction. Fraser and colleagues review these various treatment phases for spinal curvatures and upper and lower extremity deformities.[36]

The question arises whether the potential benefits of orthopedic surgery are worth the risks. Hoffer and Bullock estimate that the length of hospital stay for those with severe mental retardation is two to four times longer than usual, and the rehabilitation period is complicated by the patient's inability to comprehend what has occurred or to cooperate maximally.[37] Financial considerations are a significant factor in the decision-making process relative to surgical intervention for this population because of current trends toward shortened hospital stays and managed care plans that generalize the care needed based on diagnostic categories. Pettitt listed what she believed to be the legitimate reasons for considering surgery for individuals with severe mental retardation: (1) alleviation of pain, (2) improvement of posture for wheelchair mobilization, and (3) increased ease of nursing care.[38] Lindsey and Drennan would add to that list the achievement or maintenance of ambulation.[39]

Samilson provides a comprehensive review of the incidence, cause, and management of problems in the spine among the mentally retarded.[40] He found that the incidence of scoliosis in patients with cerebral palsy (CP) who were ambulatory was 7 percent and among those who required total bed care, 39 percent. Of 232 patients with scoliosis, 193 had spastic quadriplegia, 68 percent had fixed pelvic obliquity, and 81 percent had deformity of one or both hips that ranged from soft tissue contracture to dislocation.

Under what conditions surgery is indicated for scoliosis is often a difficult decision. Rinsky believes that the most common indications for spinal fusion in neurogenic curves of patients who are retarded include the following:[41]

- Pelvic obliquity interfering with sitting tolerance or causing ischial breakdown
- Collapsing curves requiring the use of the upper extremity to maintain sitting balance
- Pain (usually rib impingement against the iliac crest)
- Progressive curves when the use of a brace is not feasible
- Interference with the ability of others to care for the patient

Even with these problems, Rinsky does not believe that the child who is profoundly retarded with multiple disabilities would realize enough benefit from the surgery to warrant the risks involved.

Askin and colleagues used subjective and objective measures pre- and postoperatively to assess outcomes in 20 patients with significant spinal deformity and truncal imbalance who had surgery to realign and stabilize their spines.[42] The level of physical independence (ability to sit, ambulate, and perform activities of daily living) was examined preoperatively and again 6 and 12 months after surgery. Parents and other caregivers were also questioned about the patient's experience of pain, the effect on caregiving functions, and cosmesis. Only 4 of the 20 patients in the population studied had severe mental retardation, but the outcomes were comparable. The authors conclude that "at best, surgery stabilizes function." A significant decrease in independent physical capabilities was seen until at least 6 months postoperatively, and function was not improved after 12 months. Patients, parents, and other caregivers all commented positively about improved cosmesis. The authors recommend that if surgery is performed, it should be done early, before the deformity is severe.

Dental Care. Prophylactic care and management of dental problems is seldom mentioned in the literature but is a critical component of comprehensive medical care and one fraught with difficulties. Few dentists specialize in pediatrics, and even fewer are comfortable with the complex problems of children who are mentally retarded. Sedation or total anesthesia is often necessary to perform even routine work, and reimbursement is minimal or nonexistent. Third-party payers like Medicaid reimburse approximately one-eighth to one-third of the fee charged in the average dental office, so many dentists refuse to accept Medicaid patients.[43] A lack of incentives and countless roadblocks impede the provision of adequate dental care to individuals who are mentally retarded.

Medication. The use of medication to moderate or alter behavior, to control seizure activity, and to manage a wide variety of concurrent medical problems is often a necessity in this population, but considerable controversy exists. Psychotropic drugs, used to treat behavioral problems, include stimulants (used primarily to treat hyperactivity), neuroleptics (major tranquilizers, antipsychotics), antianxiety agents (minor tranquilizers), antidepressants, hypnotics, and sedatives.[44] Common reasons for using antipsychotic medications (which act through general sedation) include hyperactivity, combativeness, hostility, and negativism.[45] The numerous side effects that occur with this category of medications are sometimes referred to as *neuroleptic syndrome*. The syndrome can include "suppression of spontaneous movements and complex behavior . . . [and the reduction of] initiative and interest in the environment, [and] displays of emotion or affect, . . . slowness in response to external stimuli and drowsiness."[45] Baldessarini further describes a variety of neurologic syndromes that can occur with the use of antipsychotic drugs, including strong subjective feelings of distress or discomfort, parkinson-like symptoms, and tardive dyskinesia.[45] The possibility that a child may be overmedicated is an essential consideration for all professionals involved with this population.[46]

Aman summarizes current trends in psychopharmacology in mental retardation.[47] He notes the decreased use of neuroleptic medications because of the serious side effects but also the possibility of new antipsychotic drugs being developed. The increasing use of beta-adrenergic blocking agents is of concern to Aman because of the lack of research about efficacy. Many of the new medications that mimic neurochemicals have interesting potential application with the focus population. Major research activity is directed at isolating diagnostic groups among mentally retarded individuals that are analogous to groups with known psychiatric conditions among the nonretarded population and treating them with diagnostic-specific agents. Aman believes, however, that as the severity of functional disability increases, the relevance of traditional classification schemes becomes increasingly suspect.

Medications used to control seizure activity (anticonvulsants or antiepileptics) are another common type of drug therapy used with this population. In a study by Richardson and colleagues, almost half of the individuals with an IQ of less than 50 had experienced one or more seizures by the age of 22, most occurring during the first year of life.[48] Drugs used to treat epilepsy generally work by inhibiting the firing of certain cerebral neurons, usually by increasing the inhibitory effects of endogenous compounds or by altering the movement of ions across the neuronal membrane.[49] Antiepileptic drugs are powerful central nervous system (CNS) depressants whose side effects can include sedation, ataxia, vitamin K deficiency, paresthesias, anorexia, nausea, ataxia, tremors, nystagmus, insomnia, dizziness, headaches, anemia, skin conditions, and movement disorders.[49]

A problem that is common, but frequently neglected, is nutrient-drug interactions. As an example, disorders of vitamin D, calcium, and bone metabolism result with long-term use of phenytoin or phenobarbital, or both, especially when taken by a person unable to ambulate.[50] In a population in which the adequacy of nutrition is a significant consideration, knowledge about this kind of side effect is important.

Language. Language problems in those with cognitive impairment are four times as common as in the general population, and the frequency and severity are generally inversely proportional to IQ.[30] Difficulties with language may be caused by the cognitive deficits or by associated neurophysiologic problems. Piaget believed that the cognitive structures necessary for the development of meaningful expressive language are not present until an individual is functioning at the sixth stage of the sensorimotor period,[51] and many individuals with profound retardation function below this level. Piaget based this belief on the premise that no mental images are formed during the first five stages of the sensorimotor period.[51] Research by Kahn,[52] who compared the language abilities of persons with profound mental retardation with their sensorimotor level of function (as tested with the Uzgiris-Hunt Ordinal Scales of Psychological Development[53]), supported Piaget's hypothesis.

The authors of the Mobility Opportunities Via Education (MOVE) curriculum[54] implemented a program for children with multiple disabilities to teach them symbolic representation. They progressed the students through a series of prompts to the point where they could point to a picture of a cup (starting with an actual cup with their favorite drink in it). They found that students who had any sort of mobility skills (crawling, rolling, or squirming) were able to succeed in the program and make meaningful choices, but those who lacked any sort of mobility were unable to make meaningful choices.

Growth. One of the common complications for children in the focus population is short stature and failure to thrive, often associated with feeding problems. Campbell and Wilhelm recommend routinely including growth measures (head and limb circumference, weight, length, and weight for length) in the assessment of children with CP.[55] They compared two groups of infants younger than 25 months, 21 with CP and 36 without CP, and found significant differences between groups on all assessed growth measures.

A positive correlation exists among short stature, the degree of mental retardation, and motor dysfunction.[56] The causes of growth failure in this population are still not fully understood, but brain damage, a lack of physical activity, and poor nutrition have been implicated.[34, 57] Physical activity and weight bearing are known to directly affect bone mass and development.[58] Bone mineral density measurements of children with CP who were nonambulatory were one-third to one-half less than those of age-matched peers without disabilities.[58]

Decreased caloric intake and poor nutrition may result in part from the overall dependency that limits children's ability to request food, express food preferences, search independently for food, or self-feed. Reilly and Skuse conducted a home-based observational study of a sample similar to the focus population and found that feeding times were relatively brief, children were positioned poorly (often not in available customized seating), and food was of relatively low caloric density (commercially prepared baby food).[56] In a study by Gisel and Patrick, children with CP took 15 times longer than children who were neurologically intact to eat a mouthful of food.[59] They comment that some children with severe feeding problems eat so inefficiently that they would need to eat constantly during waking hours to meet their growth and energy requirements.

Rempel and colleagues[34] and Shapiro and associates[60] examined the impact of gastrostomies on the growth of children with multiple disabilities. They found that by ensuring caloric intake for these children by means of feedings through the gastrostomy tube, they could effect significant gains in weight and gains in weight-for-length ratios, but only minimal gains in length. Conclusive studies have not been done on the impact of the nutritional status on cognitive and psychomotor development or on morbidity and mortality rates, leaving the debate open on whether gastrostomies are indicated for some children in the focus population. Certainly weight gain alone is not sufficient justification to warrant the associated risks, especially when increased weight can negatively affect independent function and caregiving.

Pollitt, in an article summarizing the developmental impact of nutrition, states that "in the United States there is not a single, definitive work that has adequately tested the developmental impact of supplementation in early life" with the exception of prevention of iron-deficiency anemia.[61] In the latter it is clear that infants and children who have iron-deficiency anemia perform worse on developmental and cognitive testing and that iron-repletion therapy supplementation dramatically improves performance. Orthopedic surgeons Lee and Lyne report a high incidence of vitamin D abnormalities (42 percent) among children with repeated skeletal fractures and a corresponding decrease in fractures with supplementation.[62] Adequate nutrition is a critical factor in preventing skin breakdown in individuals with little or no independent mobility.[63]

Altering the diet or using nutritional supplements to affect the actual intellectual functioning or behaviors of children who are mentally retarded is an area of continuing controversy. Critics maintain that results have been exaggerated and treatments turned into a profitable market directed at families clutching at any offering of hope. Proponents speak about the relatively harmless side effects of a basic approach they believe has been proved effective. Harrell and associates maintain that nutritional supplements can improve both the IQ scores and the functioning of some children who are severely mentally retarded.[64] They conducted an experiment with 16 children (initial IQ levels ranging from 17 to 70) who were given nutritional supplements or placebos over an 8-month period. Those children receiving supplements had statistically significant increases in their IQ scores when compared with those on placebos. The researchers had particular success with children who had Down syndrome. Hitchings reported several case studies in which the basic diet was changed to one high in protein and low in carbohydrates and supplemented with megadoses of vitamins and minerals.[65] His clinical impression was that this treatment is beneficial for children with autism, schizophrenia, brain damage, and the learning disabilities that may arise as a result of these disorders.

In health care guidelines for individuals with Down syndrome, which were prepared for the Down Syndrome Medical Interest Group, Cohen categorizes nutritional supplementation as an "alternative therapy."[66] Cohen states that "nutritional supplements including vitamins, minerals, amino acids, enzymes and hormones in various combinations represent one form of therapy. There have been a number of well-controlled scientific studies that have failed to show any benefit from megadoses of vitamins. Supplemental zinc and/or selenium may have an effect on immune function or susceptibility to infection, but studies thus far have been inconclusive."[66]

AAMR Dimension IV: Environmental Considerations

The so-called normalization movement of the 1970s was a concerted attempt to end the segregation of individuals who were cognitively impaired in large state institutions and had its roots in political, social, and legal activities. In the period from 1970 to 1995, populations at state institutions for persons with developmental disabilities were reduced by two-thirds.[67] New educational and residential environments were created in which children with cognitive impairment received services and physical therapists found employment on multidisciplinary teams. Federal funding for facilities that provided medical or rehabilitation services, or both, according to strict standards resulted in a significant growth in this area, including the development of Intermediate Care Facilities for the Mentally Retarded or ICF/MR Group Homes. The Home and Community Based Services or Waiver program of 1981 supported less regulated alternatives or community-based facilities. The results of a study by Conroy, however, raise the question of whether individuals' quality of life improved sufficiently to justify the costs associated.[68] Strauss and Kastner conducted a study comparing the mortality rates of people with mental retardation in institutions with those in the community and found that for the population studied, mortality rates were 72 percent higher for persons living in the community.[69]

The most significant federal laws in the United States in the past few decades are the Education for All Handicapped Children Act of 1975 (Public Law 94-142),[70] which guaranteed special education in the least restrictive environment and included physical therapy as a related service; the Education of the Handicapped Act Amendments of 1986 (Public Law 99-457),[71] which established services in natural environments for preschoolers, infants and toddlers; the Individuals with Disabilities Education Act of 1990 (Public Law 102-119),[72] which extended the provisions of Education for All Handicapped Children Act; and the reauthorization of the Individuals with Disabilities Education Act in 1997 (Public Law 105-17).[73] A pediatric practice survey done in 1990 indicated that schools are the most common employment setting for physical therapists who are members of the Section on Pediatrics of the American Physical Therapy Association (46 percent of the respondents).[74] Standards and guidelines of the U.S. Public Laws dictate the professional services provided and the nature of the assessment, planning, interdisciplinary communication, and intervention that occurs in educational environments.

In decision making, the importance of understanding the environment in which a child interacts and the role of the physical therapist in that environment cannot be underestimated. A critical paradigm shift in pediatric physical therapy in the past 20 years is the use of a service delivery model that has moved away from center-based, child-centered intervention toward naturalistic, family-centered intervention.[75] The shift to family-centered service delivery is particularly important with the focus population. Whereas cultural familial factors are the leading cause of mild retardation, the majority of parents of children who are severely or profoundly retarded have characteristics similar to those of the general population in terms of education and social status.[76] These parents are faced with tremendous emotional strains, the need to make critical decisions (sometimes beginning prenatally), and the responsibility for a person who will, for all of that person's life, require supervision and have special needs. Before the normalization movement of the 1970s, parents had basically two alternatives: to send their children away to large state or private institutions (often a choice encouraged by professionals because of a hopeless outlook) or to keep them at home with virtually no support and no services. Fortunately, many alternatives now bridge the large gap between home care and institutionalization.

Minnes[77] and Sparling and coworkers[78] summarized research related to the stress associated with having a family member who has developmental problems. Stress in families varies depending on the stressor event, the family's internal and external resources, the perceptions of parents concerning the meaning associated with the child with special needs, parents' coping strategies, and the effects of stress accumulate over time.[79] In general, parents of children who are mentally retarded experience greater stress than parents of children who are normally intelligent with physical disabilities, and families of children who are moderately or severely retarded report significantly greater limits on family opportunities and more concern regarding life-span care and terminal illness than parents of children who are mildly retarded.[77] A strong correlation exists between the dependency and management needs of children and parental stress.[80] Barabas and associates used a concept termed "care-loads" in an attempt to quantify the time required to assist children who have chronic neurologic disability with basic activities of daily living.[81] These authors emphasize the critical need for respite services for families caring for these children at home.

Wikler and colleagues found that the parents of a child who is disabled, rather than progressing through the usual mourning process within a given time frame, often experience a state of "chronic sorrow," defined as the long-term internalization of a depressive mood.[82] The majority of parents depicted a pattern of periodic adaptation with emotional distress and upheaval recurring at significant transitional stages in the child's development. These transitional stages can be milestones from any number of domains: when their child is 12 to 13 months of age (the usual time for independent ambulation), or 9 years of age (when other children are registering for Little League baseball), or any of the major transitional periods (e.g., enrolling in kindergarten). In a related research study, social workers were found to overestimate the stress experienced by parents in the early period and underestimate the impact of later experiences.[82] Research lends support to the importance of services that recognize the ongoing needs of parents and families, particularly at transition periods in the development of a child with disabilities.

OVERVIEW

The focus of this chapter is a child who has limited intelligence and, concurrently, limited ability to learn and profit from experience, to reason, or to adapt to changing conditions. Motivation is difficult to ascertain. Little or no means of interactive communication is typical. The child almost certainly has diffuse neurologic damage, small stature, and at least one major physical disability. The child is likely to have associated sensory deficits, psychopathologic problems, and a seizure disorder and is most likely receiving medication on a routine basis, with potentially significant side effects. Health may be compromised by the many adverse sequelae of relative inactivity, poor levels of physical fitness, compromised nutritional status, and chronic respiratory problems. The child will require lifelong care and support of an intensive nature.

The child's parents are likely of normal intelligence, with characteristics of the normal population, but they experience considerable stress and chronic sorrow. Constant demands are made on their time, their physical and emotional health, and their financial well-being. The whole family experiences limitations in the kinds of activities in which they can participate. A long list of agencies and professionals are involved with the child's care. Many times the parents' interactions with these professionals provoke, rather than reduce, stress.[77] In their interactions with professionals over many years, it is likely that the parents have been confronted with reactions along a continuum ranging from resignation and apathy to overzealous, exhausting devotion to intensive intervention.

It is critical that physical therapists use a balanced approach in assessment and in planning their contribution to intervention. They must appreciate the role that they are expected to play, which will vary depending on the setting, what has transpired before, and any requirements mandated by residential or educational programs. If there are other physical therapy providers involved, whether specialists (e.g., at a seating clinic), on-site providers of care, or consultants, effective communication is important.

The physical therapist must make a unique contribution, not duplicating the work of others, but functioning as a contributing member of the team. Resources should be a constant consideration, including those of time, personnel, expense, and the emotional and mental resources of the family or other caregivers. There must be sensitivity to the fact that transitional periods and issues related to custodial care are some of the most stressful aspects of parents' experience. It will be important to involve parents in all aspects of intervention, assisting them to define and shape the goals for their child and guiding them to think ahead to the long-term outlook in order to prevent secondary impairments, while remaining aware of the stress created by these issues and by the demands of the intervention itself. The therapist should bring positive energy to the child, family, and professional team, but within a realistic context that is empathetic. Education, about the child's condition, available resources, intervention plans, and prognosis, should be provided, as necessary, at a level appropriate for those receiving instruction.

FRAMEWORK FOR SERVICE DELIVERY

The inclusion in 1975 of physical therapy as a related service in the educational environment as part of Public Law 94-142[70] undeniably changed the assumptions about the delivery of physical therapy to children. Pediatric therapists were, and continue to be, challenged to define both individually and collectively the models of service delivery that allow them to optimally meet the needs of the child and the family and to contribute to the team process and communication. Before Public Law 94-142 the majority of pediatric physical therapy occurred in clinical settings by referral of physicians with relatively few constraints from third-party payers on the frequency or duration of treatment. In today's terminology this is considered *isolated, direct* therapy: *isolated* in that it occurs outside the environments in which the child functions and *direct* in that the therapist develops, implements (or delegates to a physical therapist assistant), and maintains responsibility for the outcomes of the intervention plan.

A place still exists for this model of service delivery, but under the guidelines that drive the delivery of services in educational environments it is no longer acceptable for physical therapists to work in isolation. More common now is *integrated* service (taking place in the environments where the child lives, plays, or goes to school) and *indirect* (responsibility may be delegated to parents, school personnel, or others who have regular contact with the child). Monitoring and consultative modes of delivery are examples of indirect service. Figure 4–2 summarizes various models of service delivery, and a number of sources provide further description.[83–86] A critical aspect of decision making with the pediatric population is determining what type of intervention will be most effective when delivered under a specific model of service provision.

Various models for team interaction are possible, although the transdisciplinary model has several advantages with this population. The transdisciplinary approach is based on "the common need for integration of philosophy, personnel, and services."[87] In this model, parents are active participants on the team; comprehensive assessments are conducted as a team; a service plan is developed by all members of the team, based on the priorities, needs, and resources of the family; a primary service provider is assigned to implement the plan with the family; and there is a commitment among team members to plan, work, and learn across disciplinary boundaries.[88] The complexity and long-term nature of problems, the tremendous impact of caretaking on parents, and the necessity of coming to a consensus on priorities for intervention when interfacing professionally with children who have multiple disabilities and their families makes the conceptual framework behind the transdisciplinary model a good fit. A similar framework for team interaction is the collaborative model described by Rainforth and coworkers.[89]

Several factors have contributed to the gradual shift in the past 20 years from isolated, direct service delivery to integrated, indirect models of care. These include the U.S. Public Laws mentioned previously, changes in the mechanisms of third-party payment, and shifting assumptions about the theoretic foundations for pediatric physical therapy. Regardless of the cause, a clear focus is now directed to the goals and needs of the child and the child's caretakers expressed in functional terms. As stated in Chapter 1, "Clearly stated goals lead naturally to effective tactics for achievement of objectives."

The Hypothesis-Oriented Algorithm for Clinicians (HOAC) proposed by Rothstein and Echternach[90, 91] and described in Chapter 1 provides a framework for decision making with the focus population. Establishing functional goals, based on the problems and concerns stated by the patient or caregivers, or both, forms the basis for the subsequent assessment; intervention strategies and tactics; reassessment; analysis; and reflection. Almost without exception, the adult caregivers will be the ones in this instance to state problems, rather than the patient. A variety of caregivers may be involved in giving feedback, including parents, educators, other professionals, respite workers, and staff from a residential facility. Problems are likely to be complex and require a transdisciplinary approach, perhaps on many levels. Caregivers may initially be better able to express problems, which they can then be helped to reshape into goals.

A common example is a mother's complaint: "My back hurts all the time from lifting Johnny." Possible goals and interventions might include a nutritional plan to get

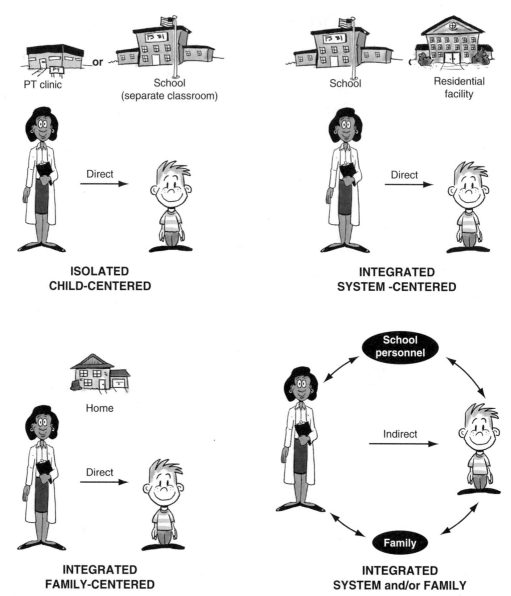

FIGURE 4–2. Various models of service delivery.

Johnny's weight under control; a trial with a lift or other adaptive equipment; medical assessment for the caregiver and a physical therapy plan for instruction in back care and proper lifting; a goal for Johnny that he will assist at least 50 percent in a pivot transfer; a behavior modification program to structure the training for assisted transfers; training for the staff and family who will carry out the program as part of Johnny's daily routine; redesign of living space to adjust the height or arrangement of furniture; and possibly respite care for Johnny or short-term placement in a residential facility.

A tool like the Canadian Occupational Performance Measure[92] is helpful to guide the process of shaping problem statements into goals. The Canadian Occupational Performance Measure describes an individual's performance as a balance among three areas: self-care, productivity, and leisure. The client or caregiver is not only involved in problem definition but is asked to weight the importance of the problem. Five goals are selected and prioritized by the caregiver. A baseline score on each goal provides objectivity for subsequent reassessment and follow-up.

PHYSICAL THERAPY ASSESSMENT

One of the outcomes of legislation on behalf of children who are disabled is the mandate in educational environments that "a variety of assessment tools and strategies [be used] to gather relevant functional and developmental information," and that any standardized tests used "have been validated for the specific purpose for which they are used."[73] In part, the intent of this legislation is to ensure more comprehensive and valid assessment of the population that is multiply handicapped or severely or profoundly retarded, for whom "previous testing, if it was done at all, was accomplished with a hodgepodge of modified instruments originally designed for a less severely involved group."[93] Resources are available that provide an annotated listing of a variety of assessment tools appropriate for children with disabilities,[94, 95] and American Physical Therapy Association measurement standards provide a guide to assessing the quality of tests and measures.[96]

The multiple disabilities of the focus population challenge the professional team to plan an assessment process that is meaningful (based on functional outcomes important to the child or caregivers, or both), coordinated (efficient and effective use of various team members), and comprehensive. It must incorporate measures that are valid, reliable, and sensitive to change over time, so that reassessment is a meaningful indication of the efficacy of intervention.

Play-based assessment is a relatively new category of assessment designed to use a team approach to observing a child in a structured play situation. Play can be defined as "a spontaneous activity that involves interactions with objects in a pleasurable manner."[97] It is such an all-encompassing activity for children that it is possible to observe all domains (cognitive, language, motor, social, and emotional). A major advantage of play-based assessment is that the child is observed performing spontaneous behaviors that can provide insight into developmental organization across domains, personal preferences, learning styles, and function that are not easily observed in other assessments.

Corresponding to Piaget's stages, the earliest form of play is sensorimotor play and consists of infants assimilating objects into their existing sensorimotor action schemes.[98] A norm-referenced measure that evaluates the sensorimotor stages described by Piaget is the Uzgiris-Hunt Scales of Infant Psychological Development.[54] The last scale, schemes for relating to objects, can be helpful in capturing levels and styles of play in children. Many of the play scales do not encompass the lower developmental ages, or if they do, the items in the lower ranges are very similar to items on standardized developmental tests. For that reason, some of these scales may have limited use with the severely involved child with multiple disabilities. Play-based assessments vary widely in the amount of structured interaction required and the specificity of the scoring and coding. Most start with an opportunity for the child to interact spontaneously with an object and then progress to various levels of facilitation of play by the parent or examiners, or both. Other children may be involved as well.

The Transdisciplinary Play-Based Assessment (TPBA) by Linder has items for developmental ages from 6 to 72 months.[99] Linder's model involves using a transdisciplinary team approach with one member of the team generally serving as play facilitator. Four domains are assessed: cognitive; social-emotional; communication and language; and sensorimotor. An assessment session is composed of six phases of play: (1) unstructured facilitated, (2) structured facilitated, (3) child-child interaction, (4) parent-child interaction, (5) motor play, and (6) snack. Sessions are videotaped and observations recorded on observational worksheets for each domain. The physical therapist is usually responsible for scoring the sensorimotor domain.

The child from the focus population is likely to have limited capacity to cooperate or to follow directions, a short attention span, poor imitation skills, questionable motivation or sense of task completion, behavioral problems, decreased or absent curiosity and will to achieve, and an inability to give verbal feedback. Flexibility in assessment must be maintained in order to recognize and appropriately adapt to these constraints.

It is important that the documentation of the assessment be meaningful to the intended readers (including the family and the teachers) and related to functional performance within relevant environments. Linehan and colleagues reported on educators' expectations for students with severe disabilities based on the type of assessment report they read.[100] They found that teachers who read *ecologic reports* (documentation of a student's observed competencies in the daily environment) had higher expectations for the student's performance than teachers who read *developmental reports* (documentation with mental and developmental ages based on standardized tests).

Background Information

It is essential to obtain a general knowledge base by reviewing available records and talking with family members, teachers, and other important individuals who interact with the child. What is the structure of the basic family unit and what attitudes are displayed by various members? Multiple problems often make the child eligible for a variety of services and programs. What agencies are involved? In what programs is the child participating? For what services and financial support systems is the child eligible?

What medical care has the child received, and who provided it? Ideally, a primary care physician has assumed a leadership role and summarized or coordinated health care from a variety of providers, although more often the medical history must be put together from multiple sources, like the pieces of a puzzle. Is there a history of seizures, and if so, what type? Are the seizures controlled with medication, or is the child on any other type of medication? Have side effects from these medications been observed? Is there evidence of recurrent problems as one reviews the medical history? For example, recurrent pneumonia is a red flag to carefully assess oral motor function and feeding behaviors. Has there been surgical intervention for physical deformities or other problems? Have hearing and vision been evaluated, and with what result? What equipment is available for the child's use, and how is it being used?

It would seem, at times, that the specialty skill one needs most in pediatrics is the ability to establish sufficient rapport to gain the cooperation of the child in performing activities and allowing handling or positioning. Encouraging imitation is one of the "tricks" sometimes used to gain cooperation from children. It is fairly well-documented, however, that individuals with severe retardation lack spontaneous imitative behavior, although they can be trained to copy the behavior of others.[101] This limited imitation ability may be directly attributable to diminished intelligence, to sensory deficits, or to some experiential concomitant of retardation such as institutionalization;[102] it also may be the result of perceptual inconsistency and the subsequent difficulty of distinguishing self from the outside world.[103]

Because expressive and receptive communication skills are often absent or delayed, and behavioral problems are common among children with multiple disabilities, it is important to obtain information about the child's abilities in these areas before testing. Are there characteristic behaviors, reinforcement schedules, or communication aids developed for the child that should be used to facilitate cooperation? Many nonverbal children have been instructed in alternative modes of communication. Nonspeech communication modes used with those who are cognitively impaired include mime, manual sign language, Blissymbolics, or a variety of communication boards.[52] Basic familiarity with these systems is strongly recommended for anyone working with this population.[93, 104] The reliability and validity of the assessment may depend on how effectively behaviors are managed and communication established.

Assessment Structured by the Five-Dimensional Disability Model

In this section the Five-Dimensional Disability Model set forth by the National Center for Medical Rehabilitation Research[105] is used to direct attention to characteristic problem areas that must be considered when conducting a definitive assessment of children with multiple disabilities. For organizational purposes, various aspects of the assessment are discussed separately, but these functions often cannot be isolated in practice.

Disability Dimension I: Pathophysiology

It is important that physical therapists review and understand the implications of the existing pathophysiology (underlying processes at cellular and tissue levels, which are usually assessed by medical personnel or through laboratory tests) and the interplay among systems. It is unlikely that a therapist would actually conduct assessment in this area, but the therapist may recognize symptoms during the initial screening or subsequent intervention that would indicate a need for referral to the appropriate medical professional. When well-described syndromes are present, pathophysiology provides a clue to the child's potential.

Disability Dimension II: Impairment

Certain organ and system disorders potentially impair functioning at the person level. Children in the focus population have multiple impairments, only some of which contribute to functional limitations (for either the child or the caregivers). The focus in decision making must be on function. Therapists must also integrate knowledge of the underlying pathophysiology and existing impairments to determine potential areas of secondary impairment and associated risk factors. Research about secondary impairments is just moving from the "hunch" of experienced clinicians to a more scientific base. It may be possible with additional research to predict the occurrence of secondary impairments based on various constellations of primary impairments.[106]

Reflex Development

Extensive brain damage may be manifested in the persistence of early tonic reflexes that interfere with normal development and predispose to asymmetries in muscle tone, sometimes leading to serious deformity.[40, 107] Recognition of a child's inability to suppress the effect of tonic reflexes on motor behavior can be useful in making appropriate recommendations about positioning and handling, pharmacologic intervention, and the use of adaptive equipment. Many standardized and normed assessments for the pediatric population now include at least some reflex items at various developmental ages. Capute and colleagues developed an instrument, the Primitive Reflex Profile, that attempts to give consistency and objectivity to the assessment process.[108, 109] Fetters, however, encourages therapists to consider the possibility that the persistence of primitive reflexes may be an adaptive response; that is, the reflex is still useful to the infant or child and enhances the child's function.[110]

Postural Stability

Postural reactions (as distinguished from reflexes) are based on the interplay of multiple input modalities and require cortical integrity for effective motor output. Functionally, they serve the purposes indicated by their descriptive subgroups: righting, protection, and equilibrium. Their presence enables a child to gain movement or postural stability against the force of gravity and is critical to the development of higher-level skills.

Postural stability as defined by Westcott and coworkers is the "ability to maintain or control the center of mass in relation to the base of support to prevent falls or complete desired tasks."[111] Postural stability is often diminished in children with multiple disabilities. It is a complex function and difficult to assess even in children who are developing in a typical manner. *Balancing* is the process used to maintain postural stability and can be either static or dynamic. General systems theory of motor control proposes that three primary systems are involved in the process of balancing: (1) sensory, (2) motor, and (3) biomechanical. Westcott and associates review currently available pediatric tools for the assessment of postural stability and include the measurement of all three systems.[111] They conclude that relatively few tests have acceptable reliability and validity documentation. In addition, the majority of the tests require a level of functional performance and behavioral cooperation not possible for the focus population.

Muscle Tone

Muscle tone must be carefully assessed and judgments made about whether abnormal tone is interfering with functional abilities or contributing to the development of secondary impairments, or both. Because primitive reflexes can greatly influence tone and movement,[112] assessment should be based on observation and handling of the child in a variety of positions and postures. Hypotonia is a common characteristic of children with mental retardation when CP and other defined neuromusculoskeletal problems are excluded. Objective measurement of muscle tone is difficult, but assessments like the Movement Assessment of Infants[113] and the modified Ashworth Scale[114] have attempted to quantify aspects of muscle tone.

Muscle Strength and Function

It is very difficult to test muscle strength objectively in the focus population because of the child's inability to follow instructions or adapt to a changing stimulus. Connolly has included a chapter on assessing muscle strength in the pediatric population in the most recent edition of Daniels and Worthingham's classic text on manual muscle testing, which is useful as a guide.[115] In general, one must extrapolate muscle capabilities from observation of the child's general motor activity, functional movement, and posture. Information gained from observation would be about muscle groups, not individual muscles, and would be quantified using a gross scale such as *muscle activity present, trace muscle activity,* or *no muscle activity observed*, rather than the normal five-point scale.

Joint Range of Motion and Muscle Length

The physical therapist must determine if the child has adequate joint mobility for functional performance and must anticipate and prevent secondary impairments. In some circumstances, regression on standardized assessments like the Gross Motor Function Measure (GMFM)[116, 117] may be an adequate measure of the joint's range of motion or muscle length. In other circumstances, mobility should be assessed with baseline goniometric measurements of the range of key joints (e.g., knee extension) as well as the length of key muscle groups (e.g., hamstrings and hip flexors). Both interrater and test-retest reliability of goniometric measurement of a joint's range of motion can be problematic with a child who has multiple disabilities. The results of two studies on the reliability of goniometric measurements performed by different therapists indicate that 10 to 15 degrees of variability over time does not signify meaningful change in a child with CP.[118, 119] Functionally, however, the loss of even 5 degrees of knee extension can be critical.

Hip dislocation or subluxation is one of the secondary impairments that warrants particular attention, particularly in those individuals who are nonambulatory or have abnormal muscle tone, or both.[120] Efforts directed toward prevention should start early and continue.[121] Samilson found the incidence of hip subluxation or dislocation among individuals who were severely involved, neurologically immature, or developmentally retarded to be about 28 percent.[40] The mean age when hip problems were discovered was 7 years; 62 percent of those with hip problems were patients with quadriplegia who required total care. Postures that predisposed to dislocation were hip flexion, adduction, and medial rotation; scoliosis; and pelvic obliquity with rotation and inclination. Analysis of torsional and rotational alignment of the pelvis and lower extremities using reliable measures may be an important contribution.[122]

Lindsey and Drennan conducted a study of persons who were cognitively impaired and residing in institutions, excluding those with CP or other recognizable neuromuscular disorders.[39] Hypotonia, ligamentous laxity, and delayed motor milestones were characteristic of this population. From a total of 1600 residents, they found 48 (24 with Down syndrome) who had either isolated major foot problems or a combination of foot and knee disorders. In this study, Lindsey and Drennan found that knee problems were uniformly associated with foot problems. The most common problem was genu valgum associated with various degrees of joint laxity and sometimes chronic patellar dislocation, but normally no interference with function. The most common functional knee deformity was flexion contracture that can be attributed to the prolonged use of a wheelchair or the stance adaptation of a crouch gait.

Posture

Sherrill defines posture as "good body alignment and proper body mechanics" and stresses that posture assessment should be based on dynamic postures (e.g., walking, sitting, stair climbing, and lifting and carrying objects) rather than a single static stance.[123] A pictorial description of positions that predispose to posture problems is provided by Kendall and Kendall[124] and is helpful in evaluating individuals from the focus population who may be "locked in" to positions as a result of abnormal tone and primitive reflex posturing. Kyphotic deformities in children who are mentally retarded may be secondary to an absence of the normal lumbar lordosis (because of tight hamstrings) or to an increased lumbar lordosis (with hip flexion contractures).[40] Excessive lumbar lordosis, like kyphosis and scoliosis, may be functional or structural. Tight hip flexors, weak hip extensors, and weak abdominals are commonly associated problems.

Sensory Processes and Integration

Sensory information bombards the individual in everyday experiences. Abnormalities in sensory perception can be the result of dysfunction at the level of the receptor; the afferent pathways that carry the sensory information to higher centers; or the interpretation or integration of the information by higher centers to shape perception, cognitive processes, and motor acts. It is an intricate and complex subsystem that we know relatively little about. The diffuse nature of the brain damage in the focus population suggests that there would be dysfunction in the transfer or processing of sensory information at one or more of the levels described.

A lack of accurate sensory feedback makes it difficult to refine motor acts. The reverse may also be true. Poorly coordinated movement may distort sensory feedback. In Piagetian theory, concrete action precedes and makes possible the use of the intellect, and sensorimotor experiences are the foundations of mental development.[125] Stated another way, intelligence may be viewed as a progressive transformation of motor patterns into thought patterns. Certainly the child who lacks the motor control to act on the environment or to move purposefully experiences sensory deprivation at some level. What is the effect of sensory deprivation or abnormal sensory input on cognitive and motor development? What kind of compensatory mechanisms and responses develop? Is the underlying level of arousal affected? Mental state? Self-awareness? Motivation?

Sensory integration is one aspect of sensory processing. Ayres developed sensory integration theory to describe the observed relationships among behavior, sensorimotor function, and academic performance.[126] She states that sensory integration is "the neurological process that organizes sensation from one's own body and from the environment and makes it possible to use the body effectively within the environment."[126] Sensory integrative dysfunction has been implicated in stereotypic and self-injurious behaviors, altered arousal states, and abnormal or delayed motor development. The population that was the focus of most of Ayres' study was composed of those who demonstrated learning disabilities, clumsiness, or other evidence of difficulty organizing responses to sensory information. She did not extend her theory to those with obvious causes of brain dysfunction such as "mental retardation, peripheral sensory loss [and] neurological damage or abnormalities."[127] Although many children who are mentally retarded display behaviors similar to those of children with sensory integrative dysfunction, it is an extrapolation of Ayres' theory to apply the same principles to the focus population, in which neurologic damage is almost universal.

Clinically, we know that sensory problems are common in the focus population and intricately entwined with other systems and behaviors. How do we assess the sensory status in a child with multiple disabilities? Fisher and colleagues' publication *Sensory Integration: Theory and Practice*[127] is the most comprehensive reference since Ayres' classic text published in 1976.[126] Another resource for physical therapists and occupational therapists that condenses information on the applicable theories of Ayres is Montgomery's article on the assessment and treatment of the child with mental retardation.[128] Although general principles are discussed, the emphasis is on specific assessment and treatment strategies for visual, auditory, tactile, olfactory-gustatory, proprioceptive-kinesthetic, and vestibular functions.

A common strategy for obtaining information about a child's sensory-processing abilities is to have the parent or other caregiver complete a history. The Sensory Profile is a fairly new instrument that has 125 behaviors reflecting a child's response to sensory events in daily life.[24, 25] It is an attempt to not only evaluate the impact of sensory processing on functional performance, but also to consider how children regulate or modulate sensation. The standardized evaluation tool developed by Ayres, the Sensory Integration and Praxis Tests,[129] has too many cognitive components to be applicable to the focus population. It is possible to use Ayres' Southern California Test of Postrotary Nystagmus,[130] but with caution about interpretation of the results.

Respiratory Status

Respiratory problems are common in the child with multiple disabilities and can interfere with phonation, feeding, and general good health. A single cause of respiratory problems is uncommon. The problems frequently result from a combination of (1) improper positioning, which can cause deformities of the rib cage, pooling of secretions in dependent areas of the lung, and poor chest excursion; (2) abnormal breathing patterns; (3) weakness, incoordination, or spasticity of the respiratory muscles, resulting in an ineffective, weak cough and poor chest expansion; (4) incoordination of oral motor and respiratory movements and absent or depressed protective reflexes resulting in chronic aspiration; (5) increased saliva production and ineffective means of clearing the saliva so that it tends to collect in the throat; (6) an increased incidence of allergies causing respiratory symptoms; and (7) a lack of exercise and overall poor cardiovascular and respiratory fitness.[131–133] In a study of the dynamic and static lung volumes of school-aged children with CP, Bjure and Berg found that the children's total lung capacity averaged 85 percent of the predicted normal values.[134]

Tecklin summarizes the characteristics of the pediatric respiratory system and describes the components of an assessment of children with respiratory disorders.[35] The therapist should observe the general coloration of the skin (looking especially for cyanosis or general pallor), the use of accessory muscles for breathing, the size and shape of the thorax, and the development of thoracic musculature. The respiratory rate provides an important baseline. The normal rate per minute for a full-term neonate is 30 to 40, decreasing to 25 to 30 for a 2-year-old and 12 to 15 for a normal adult.[133] In addition to the rate, the therapist should observe the regularity of breathing, the ratio of inspiration to expiration, the synchronous motion of the thorax and abdomen, and the movement of the chest wall.[35] Auscultation, or listening to lung sounds with a stethoscope, requires experience to distinguish abnormal (adventitious) lung sounds like wheezes and crackles from transmitted sounds originating in the upper airways. The ability to breathe through the nose is important, as the obligatory mouth breather has problems coordinating respiration and feeding, and a tendency to aspirate food. As mentioned earlier, aspiration and aspiration pneumonia are significant causes of death among those with multiple disabilities.

Disability Dimension III: Functional Limitations

Motor Development

Literature reports vary about the extent of motor deficit in persons who are mentally retarded. In general, research indicates delays in sensorimotor development among those who are mentally retarded—the extent of the delay roughly paralleling the extent of intellectual impairment.[135] Many of the published assessments of those who are severely and profoundly retarded include a motor performance checklist, which is essentially a yes-or-no format for indicating accomplishment of the basic motor milestones. What the physical therapist can and must contribute to the completion of that checklist is a description of motor behaviors and deductive reasoning as to the causes of delays. The physical therapist's role is an analysis of the contribution to deficient sensorimotor performance being made by behavior, motivation, cognition, perception, strength, muscle tone, posture, contractures, joint limitation, sensory processing, and reflexes. An assessment like the GMFM, which has been shown to be sensitive to subtle improvements or regression in developmental skills, can be useful with this population as a baseline for measuring change.[116, 117]

Motor development is commonly separated into gross motor, fine motor, and oral motor areas. These three areas are discussed separately in the section to follow, although the interplay among the various areas must be appreciated.

Gross Motor. The child should be observed in the supine, prone, and sitting positions and should be given the opportunity to make transitions between these positions. The GMFM is useful because it looks at the maintenance of positions as well as the attainment of positions (transitions).[116] Even if motor skills are rudimentary, it is important to observe the child's abilities in the upright position (supported standing). The child can often demonstrate improved head and trunk control as well as improved performance of fine motor skills when upright. The child's ability to accept even partial weight can enable him or her to assist with a standing transfer. Avoiding a total lift from location to location can make a significant difference for parents or caretakers, especially as the child grows.

Ambulation is a complex task dependent on the intricate interaction of biomechanical, neuromuscular, kinesiologic, cognitive, and perceptual components. An excellent overview of more recent research related to the development of gait is provided by Stout in the chapter Gait: Development and Analysis in Campbell and coworkers' *Physical Therapy for Children*.[136] The current thinking, that locomotion is controlled by a central pattern generator, located either in the brainstem or spinal cord, has interesting implications for the focus population. It is believed that the central pattern generator organizes the activation and firing sequence of muscles during walking and that the "neural foundations for locomotion are present at a very early stage in prenatal development."[136] The active period of myelination that occurs during the first year of life contributes to the neural organization required for independent ambulation. Thelen and colleagues, however, suggest that sufficient extensor strength is the critical variable for independent locomotion, not pattern-generating or postural control capabilities.[137]

It is difficult to predict the ambulatory potential of children who are cognitively impaired. Illingworth predicts that children with mental retardation but without CP may walk if they have an IQ less than 20 and will walk if they have an IQ above 20.[138] Of those with an IQ less than 40 who do learn to walk, the onset is delayed in approximately one-third.[30] Based on their study of 152 children with profound mental retardation, Shapiro and associates concluded that the major determinant for learning to walk was not cognition but a lack of damage to the motor areas of the brain.[139] In their study, 92 percent of children who had no neurologic impairment walked (median age of 20 months), but only 11 percent of children who had both mental retardation and CP learned to walk (at a median age of 63.5 months).[139] Molnar and Gordon, in a prospective study of 233 children with CP, found a positive correlation between the ability to ambulate by 8 years of age and the ability to sit at 2 years of age, suppression of obligatory primitive reflex activity by 24 months, and intelligence.[140] The findings of Watt and colleagues, with a smaller prospective study of children with CP who had been cared for in a neonatal intensive care unit, were similar, although there was an even stronger correlation between the ability to sit at 2 years of age and ambulation by 8 years of age.[141]

If one looks at the population of individuals with mental retardation but no identified neuromuscular problems, some characteristic gait patterns are evident. Lindsey and Drennan refer to the "Chaplinesque" gait of those who are mentally retarded.[39] The hips are in moderate lateral rotation, the knees are in flexion and valgus, the tibias are in lateral rotation, and the feet are placed with the medial longitudinal arch as the presenting aspect of the foot accompanied by marked heel valgus and forefoot pronation.

Many children with cognitive impairment walk in a crouched posture, which can lead to fixed flexion deformities of the hips and knees. One reason for the development of this type of gait pattern is the delay in motor maturation and balance.[39] Some children initially stand with a normal posture of full extension at the hips and knees but develop a crouched posture as they approach adolescence. An interesting postulate for this, proposed by Lindsey and Drennan, is that children have a "predetermined functional height."[39] Once they reach that functional height, they compensate for continued skeletal growth by assuming a crouched posture, which enables them to maintain their head position at a constant distance from the floor. It would seem to be an attempt to maintain consistency in specific types of sensory feedback. It is also common to see children with cognitive impairment walk with a wide base of support and arms held in a high guard posture. Both the crouched posture and the high guard and wide-based stance may represent a child's attempt to lower the center of mass and enlarge the base of support to improve stability and prevent falls.

Toe walking is a typical isolated finding in populations that are severely and profoundly retarded. Three reasons for toe walking are postulated: (1) hypertonicity in the gastrocnemius-soleus muscle group increased by assumption of the upright posture, (2) behavioral aberrancy (i.e., "It feels good" for whatever reason), or (3) in the absence of CP or spasticity, a problem of sensory dysfunction. Montgomery and Gauger theorize that the latter group of children are generally hypotonic and hyperflexible and demonstrate vestibular dysfunction exacerbated by tactile defensiveness.[142] Weight bearing on the toes triggers a persistent influence of the positive support reaction (seen normally in infancy) and gives them additional extensor tone to resist the force of gravity. This type of toe walking must be differentiated from that seen in individuals with CP who may have structural change in the triceps surae muscle or tendon or excessive contraction of the triceps surae.[143] Whereas surgical release and bracing or inhibitive or serial casting may be indicated in the child with contracture or excessive contraction, it would not benefit the child with primarily sensory dysfunction.

Several other aspects of gait should receive attention as part of an observational assessment of gait. Is there an overflow of muscle tone when the child is upright (evidenced possibly by tight elbow flexion with retraction of the scapulae and subsequent interference with the normal use of the arms for balance)? Is there reciprocal, coordinated movement of the arms with the legs? Where is the focal point of the eyes? Children with poor equilibrium may keep their eyes on the floor as they walk, rather than looking straight ahead.[144] Is the head maintained in midline? Tilting of the head to one side or the other may indicate sensory dysfunction, poor integration of primitive reflexes, asymmetric muscle tone, or visual problems. Are the hips relatively stable? Is there a good heel-to-toe pattern? The common foot problems often result in flat feet and a concomitant inability to establish a good heel-to-toe gait. What type of shoes are usually worn? Is there a difference in the gait with and without shoes? If a child has orthotics or casts, the child should be carefully checked to ensure an appropriate fit, and the child should be observed ambulating with and without them.

Although the physical therapist's assessment of gait will emphasize the problematic physical components, it is often true that cognitive and affective factors are the most important determinants of the functional use of walking. Some aspects of intelligence not measured by tests are the awareness of a goal, the will to succeed, and the motivation to safely perform a skill as a means to an end. It is often difficult to make a motor task like ambulation meaningful to a child who is severely or profoundly retarded and therefore reinforce its execution sufficiently that it will occur spontaneously.

Fine Motor. Assessment of fine motor skills is typically the focus of the occupational therapist rather than the physical therapist, but it is important to get at least a sense of the effective use of fine motor skills for functional tasks like reach, grasp, manipulation, self-feeding, and the use of assistive technology devices. It is also helpful to examine the effects of positioning, or use of orthotics, on the quality of fine motor skills.

Oral Motor. An occupational therapist, a physical therapist, or a speech and language pathologist may be the person on the team who takes the lead in the area of oral motor function, depending on the environment and the experience and comfort level of individual professionals. The development of normal oral motor patterns for feeding, respiration, phonation, speech, and language is a complex process influenced by reflexes, muscle tone, positioning, sensory processing, and behavior. It is one of the most important areas in the evaluation of the focus population because problems are so common.

Behaviors like drooling or messy eating, over which the child has no control, may be aversive to caretakers and may affect social interaction, possibly resulting in isolation. Feeding, which should be a pleasurable experience for the child and a time of positive interaction, becomes instead a tension-filled experience. The lack of speech as a result of oral motor dysfunction can prevent meaningful communication and affect the type of interaction in which the child is engaged.

A number of resources are available for both the assessment and the management of oral motor ability, feeding, and swallowing.[145–148] Detailed information on oral motor assessment cannot be included in this chapter, but the following guidelines may be useful as a basis for organizing the approach to this important area of development:[146, 149]

1. *General.* An assessment should begin by observation of the child and caregiver in a typical feeding situation and attending to positioning; the use of special equipment (e.g., chairs, spoons, cups, plates); the type, texture, and temperature of food; the sequence of presenting food; and the quality of social interaction that occurs. A useful feeding scale is part of a comprehensive assessment of caregiver-child interaction developed as part of the Nursing Child Assessment Satellite Training.[150] Especially if a nutritionist is not part of the evaluative team, information should be obtained about the child's basic diet. This is particularly important if the child's weight or height is below the 5th percentile or weight is inappropriate for height. The Parent Eating and Nutrition Assessment for Children with Special Health Needs (PEACH) is an easily administered one-page survey that reportedly has a predictive value of 88.6 percent for nutritional problems.[151] Dietary supplements may be helpful, warranting the involvement of the primary care physician or referral to a nutritionist, or both.
2. *Oral reflexes*
3. *Muscle tone and sensitivity of oral motor structures (cheeks, lips, and tongue)*
4. *Feeding behaviors.* Knowledge of the normal developmental sequence is essential to determine the difference between normal, delayed, and abnormal patterns. Mindful that aspiration is a possibility, the physical therapist should observe the coordination of breathing and swallowing. Referral for a barium swallow study may be indicated. Except in unusual circumstances, the child's head should be in midline, stabilized if necessary, and the child's upper body inclined at least 45 degrees from horizontal.
   a. *Sucking.* There should be smooth, rapid initiation and a rhythmic pattern
   b. *Spoon feeding.* The mouth should be quiet when the food is presented, with mouth opening graded, lip closure around the spoon, food cleaned from the spoon with the upper lip, effective mobility of the tongue and jaw, and a persistent stable position of the head.
   c. *Cup drinking.* There should be graded jaw excursion, sufficient stabilization of the jaw to allow normal placement of the cup, and adequate lip closure.
   d. *Biting and chewing.* There should be a mature rotary motion of the jaw (as opposed to up and down "munching"), adequate lateral tongue movement to keep the food between the teeth, and good lip closure.
5. *Self-feeding.* Observations should include both finger feeding and feeding with

utensils. Considerations include the use of adaptive equipment, any necessary prompts, either verbal or physical, and the types of food that can be managed.

Assistive Technology

The inclusion of assistive technology services as part of the legislative mandates included in the Individuals with Disability Education Act (Public Law 102-119)[72] and the Technology-Related Assistance for Individuals with Disabilities Act (Public Law 100-407)[152] gave credence to the importance of comprehensive, focused multidisciplinary assistive technology services for children with disabilities. As defined in the 1997 Amendments to Individuals with Disabilities Education Act (Public Law 105-17),[73] the term *assistive technology device* refers to "any item, piece of equipment, or product system, whether acquired commercially off the shelf, modified, or customized, that is used to increase, maintain, or improve functional capabilities of a child with a disability." This would include adaptive equipment, postural support systems, wheeled mobility, augmentative and alternative communication, environmental control units and automated learning devices (switches).[153] Physical therapists have been involved with assistive technology, at least peripherally, for a long time. The public law formalizes the process for implementing assistive technology services: the evaluation, recommendation, purchase, and selection of assistive devices. Assessment of the child's function with the various pieces of equipment designated for the child's use, as well as a projection of potential benefit from other types of adaptive equipment, is critical.

Behavior

The behavior manifested at any particular time has its origins in an intricate matrix of physiologic and environmental systems. Hutt and Gibby devoted several chapters in their book *The Mentally Retarded Child: Development, Training, and Education* to discussion of social, emotional, and psychologic development, comparing children who have normal intelligence with those who have mental impairments and factors in their environment that influence personality and may contribute to maladaptive behavior.[154] Behavior is the substrate of a child's response system and must therefore be assessed and taken into consideration when determining potential and establishing a treatment program. Deviant behavior can be more of a deterrent to the success of a treatment program than deficient intelligence.

Disability Dimension IV: Disabilities

Disabilities result when functional limitations persist and children are unable to fulfill life roles or gain independence in activities of daily living as a result. Most measures of adaptive behavior include the more or less standard list of self-help skills like dressing, grooming, and feeding. The Vineland Adaptive Behavior Scales[155] and the Pediatric Evaluation of Disability Inventory (PEDI)[156] are two that are often used. Based on interviews with parents of children who resemble those in the focus population, the authors of the MOVE curriculum[54] developed the list of basic minimal activities necessary for a functioning adult in the home and community shown in the box:

IN THE HOME	IN THE COMMUNITY
Eating with family or peers	Shopping
Bathing or showering	Going to appointments
Getting in and out of bed	Eating in restaurants
Dressing and grooming	Attending social activities both indoors and outdoors
Toileting	Using public rest rooms
Communicating	Riding on public transportation or in regular cars
Participating in leisure activities	

These basic daily living skills must be kept in mind as long-term goals for functional behavior. The more of these skills that are attained, the less stress the caregivers experience and the less likely it is that alternative living arrangements will need to be considered. Both the PEDI and the Vineland Adaptive Behavior Scales address the majority of the home-based functions listed as important by parents but address very few of the community-based functions.

Disability Dimension V: Societal Limitations

This dimension of dysfunction results when societal barriers prevent an individual from functioning at the highest level at which that individual is capable. "Problems such as these often fall outside the usual purview of rehabilitation specialists and must be addressed through problem identification and action at the community and societal level."[157] Advocacy efforts are necessary to continue to influence public policies and attitudes related to full inclusion in society of individuals with multiple disabilities.

PHYSICAL THERAPY INTERVENTION

Decision making with the focus population is complicated by the complexity of both the problems and the matrix within which the child functions and receives services. Identifying the problem or problems is not difficult. There are likely to be long lists. Applying knowledge about the underlying pathophysiology to understand the interplay among various problems, the potential for developing secondary impairments, the problems that are amenable to intervention, and the design of appropriate plans of care is challenging. These considerations must be meshed with the demands and opportunities in the environments within which the child functions; other services and programs the child participates in; the goals and needs of the caregivers; and the available resources. Resources include financial (both public and private), personnel, time, and the emotional reserve of the family or other caregivers.

Regardless of the intervention planned, the temporal element for all aspects of the model is stretched for the focus population. The attainment of goals (even stated in incremental steps) is likely to take months, not days or weeks, and reassessment may be relatively infrequent, depending on the level of intervention and the model of service delivery. The maintenance of function or musculoskeletal status is often a difficult goal to achieve, yet one that is not "good enough," in most cases, for third-party reimbursement of professional intervention. In the population with multiple disabilities reported on in the MOVE curriculum,[54] 99 percent of the children regressed on the developmental scale after they reached the age of 7 or 8 years. As the children increased in size, "gravity became an enemy to already weak muscles, positioning became more difficult, and deformities developed."[54]

The discussion of physical therapy for children with multiple disabilities that follows is divided into two areas that affect decision making: (1) theoretic approaches to treatment as they relate to the focus population, and (2) selected intervention strategies that have particular value with children who have severe cognitive impairment.

Theoretic Approaches to Treatment

In the first half of the century the predominant view of motor development was based on neural-maturationist theory.[8] The theory is based on the assumption that development proceeds in a predetermined pattern based on hierarchic maturation of the neural control structures. Environmental factors were thought to support but not alter the evolution of motor development. Neurophysiologic approaches used by physical therapists in treating the pediatric patient that were developed based on neural-maturationist theory include the neurodevelopmental, sensorimotor, and sensory integrative techniques of Bobath and Bobath,[158] Semans,[159] Rood and Stockmeyer,[160, 161] and Ayres.[126]

These approaches to treatment are based on the following assumptions, as summarized by Ostrosky: (1) "the brain controls movement, not muscles"; (2) "a patient's movement patterns can be altered by applying specific patterns of sensory stimulation, especially through proprioceptive afferent pathways"; (3) "the CNS is hierarchically organized," and therefore, "abnormal movement patterns and tone disorders are assumed to result from a lack of inhibitory control by the higher centers"; (4) "recovery from brain damage follows a predictable sequence that parallels the development of normal motor behavior from infancy"; and (5) "all motor phenomena associated with brain damage have a neurophysiological basis."[162] As stated by Montgomery, the neurophysiologic approaches seem particularly appropriate for the child with mental retardation because they emphasize functions that are relatively automatic for the individual (i.e., based on normal reflex and sensorimotor development) and therefore demand learning at a subcortical level.[128]

Neuro-Developmental Treatment

The aim of Neuro-Developmental Treatment (NDT), developed by Karl and Berta Bobath is to normalize postural tone and improve the quality and control of movement, following the normal developmental sequence as closely as possible.[158, 159] This is accomplished by using reflex-inhibiting patterns with manual control at key points to normalize postural tone. With tone normalized, active automatic reactions are facilitated to develop elements of the normal postural reflex mechanism. The handling techniques used in NDT are designed to elicit active, automatic movements from the child, and therefore do not require that the child cooperate at a cognitive level. As the Bobaths stated, "It is this aspect of the approach which has made this [NDT] treatment so eminently adaptable to the needs of the mentally subnormal and uncooperative child."[158]

Sensorimotor Theory

Stockmeyer has described an interpretation of Rood's approach to the treatment of neuromuscular dysfunction.[160, 161] It is an approach that "seeks to activate the movement and postural responses of the patient in the same automatic manner as they occur in the normal, without need for conscious attention to the response itself."[161] Reliance on automatic reactions makes Rood's approach, like Bobath and Bobath's, applicable to the child with severe or profound retardation.

Several premises form the basis for Rood's approach to treatment.[161, 162] First, motor and sensory functions are inseparable. Stimuli, carefully chosen to activate, facilitate, or inhibit motor responses, are an important part of the treatment program. The effect of various stimuli on not only somatic but also autonomic and psychic function is an ongoing consideration. Second, there are two major sequences in motor development that are distinctly different and yet inextricably interrelated: skeletal functions and vital functions. Third, skeletal function can be separated into four sequential levels of control: mobility (shortening and lengthening of the agonist with its antagonists), stability (cocontraction of agonists and antagonists), mobility superimposed on stability in a weight-bearing position (proximal part moving on fixed distal part), and mobility superimposed on stability in a non–weight-bearing position (free distal part moving on a proximal part that is dynamically holding). Fourth, children normally traverse a specific skeletal function sequence (also termed *ontogenetic motor patterns*). This sequence is the guideline Rood proposed for the assessment and treatment of neuromuscular dysfunction.

Sensory Integrative Techniques

Ayres developed a comprehensive theoretic basis for sensory integrative therapy and a rationale for its use with children who had brain damage.[126] She informally defined sensory integration as the ability to organize sensory information for functional use in producing an adaptive response and believed that this ability is the essence of perception. A motor act is a typical response to a perception, and the sensory feedback gained from the motor act enables the child to evaluate the accuracy of the perception and the effectiveness of the response (Fig. 4–3). Ayres believed that a strong relationship exists among cognitive function, motor development, and reflex integration, but that the child first experiences the environment through information conveyed by afferent pathways. An inability to accurately receive or organize sensory input causes dysfunction in the whole process of learning by means of sensorimotor experience. Sensory integrative therapy is directed not toward the mastery of specific tasks or skills but toward improving the brain's capacity to perceive, to remember, and to plan motor activity.

Several studies have investigated the effectiveness of sensory integrative therapy with individuals who are severely and profoundly retarded. Children with IQs less than 50 were the subjects of Montgomery and Richter's study, which compared the effectiveness of three different motor programs on neuromotor development.[144] On a test battery that assessed gross, fine, and perceptual motor skills and reflex integration, the children receiving sensory integrative therapy showed the greatest gains. The investigators concluded that neuromotor development may be enhanced more effectively by activities that facilitate improved postural responses than by practice of specific motor skills. A pilot study by Norton indicated improved motor skills in preschoolers who were profoundly retarded after they participated in a program of sensory stimulation.[163] A study by Clark and associates found that a sensory integration program elicited increases in eye contact and vocalization and promoted postural adaptation in adults who were profoundly retarded.[164]

Controlled vestibular stimulation is one of the most popular types of sensory stimulation. In a review article, Ottenbacher relates that "controlled vestibular stimulation has had positive effects on arousal level, visual exploratory behavior, motor development and reflex integration."[165] Ottenbacher and colleagues used a group of 38 children who were severely or profoundly retarded, nonambulatory, and developmentally delayed to compare the results of sensorimotor therapy alone or sensorimotor therapy combined with controlled vestibular stimulation.[166] They found that the group receiving the combined therapies "made significantly greater gains on measures of reflex integration and gross and fine motor development." Magrun and colleagues found that vestibular stimulation prior to a monitored free play situation increased the spontaneous use of verbal language in children who were trainably mentally retarded.[167]

Bright and associates assumed sensory deprivation was at least a partial cause of

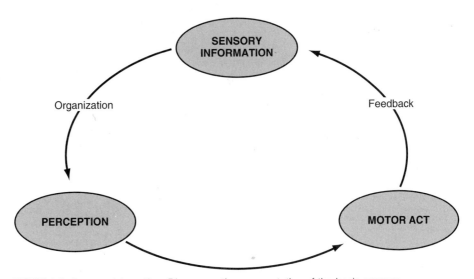

FIGURE 4–3. Sensory integration. Diagrammatic representation of the basic process.

the self-injurious behavior of an adult who was profoundly retarded, and they were successful in reducing the frequency of the behavior using sensory integrative techniques.[168] Evans was able to reduce the hyperactive behavior of three adolescents who were profoundly mentally retarded by increasing the visual and auditory stimulation in their environment.[169]

Controversy persists about the scientific basis for sensory integration theory and the effectiveness of treatment. Arendt and coworkers reviewed eight studies that described the application of sensory integration procedures with individuals who were mentally retarded and concluded that "there exists no convincing empirical or theoretical support for the continued use of sensory integration theory with that population [mentally retarded] outside of a research context."[170] Ottenbacher provides a valuable overview of the existing research in sensory integration and some of the issues that make conclusive findings difficult.[171] He clarifies that many studies that proclaim to use sensory integration techniques are really using sensory stimulation. A sensory integration approach requires the individual to make an adaptive response.

Theoretic Approaches

Dramatic and rapidly expanding research in how the nervous system functions has caused physical therapists to question some of the more traditional approaches to the treatment of neurologic problems in the pediatric population. A variety of new theories have emerged.

Motor control theory assumes that "every movement is a response to a motor problem presented to the CNS," and it looks to a more circular, distributed neural control system.[162] Carr and Shepherd, two of the major clinical proponents of this model, encourage therapists to select meaningful, functional goals that are task specific and difficult but obtainable, and to clearly communicate these goals to the patient.[172] Therapist-guided active movements are minimized, a problem-solving approach is established so that carryover is maximized, and the patient is encouraged to practice both overtly and mentally.

Motor control theory places great emphasis on the importance of cognitive processes, both conscious and subconscious, such as reasoning, memory, and judgment to optimize performance. "Variables might include arousal, motivation, anticipatory strategies, and the selective use of feedback, practice, and memory."[173] The literature does not specifically address the impact of severe cognitive deficit on the application of motor control principles, but the problems are apparent because the approach relies on the cognitive involvement of the client.

Dynamic systems theory, as proposed by Thelen and colleagues, links the internal development and maturation of the organism with factors in the external environment.[137] "Development of a particular motor pattern depends on a combination of mechanical, neurologic, cognitive, and perceptual factors in addition to environmental contributions specific to both the task and the context of the infant's action."[8] Intertwining systems make the experience of movement, especially self-directed movement, important to cognitive and perceptual development. Conversely, the inability, or lack of opportunity, to perform motor skills in a meaningful context can limit other areas of development.

As described by Shumway-Cook and Woollacott, task-specific movement is performed within the context of intent and motivation so that cognitive aspects of motor control must also be assessed.[174] Tactics recommended for intervention include the use of a structured environment and augmented feedback.

Horn and associates state that "combining the strengths of multiple techniques and procedures should be the first priority for investigators if the efficacy of early motor intervention is to improve."[175] These authors propose a hybrid approach to early motor intervention in the educational setting that they have termed *neurobehavioral motor intervention*. The approach combines behavioral programming (*how* to teach with an emphasis on functional activities) with an NDT approach (*what* to teach by means of focus on underlying components of movement). They believe that goals of therapy should not be motor milestones (e.g., raising the head from a prone position) but the functional outcome of the motor behavior (e.g., looking at a mobile hung over the crib). They also believe that a child must be able to generalize a learned behavior (with variation in both the stimulus and the response) for the intervention to be considered efficacious. Research on the efficacy of various treatment approaches and assessment of clinical outcomes should include measures for generalization.

Only minimal indirect reference is made in the literature to the application of any of these more recent theoretic approaches to the child who has severe mental impairment and multiple disabilities. Aspects of each of the theories has potential relevance with the focus population, but the hybrid approach of Horn and colleagues,[175] combining the strengths of multiple approaches, seems to have the greatest applicability.

Where Does Intervention Begin?

Neural-maturationist theory guided therapists to adhere closely to a normal developmental sequence in treatment. Atwater's presentation at the II Step Conference on Contemporary Management of Motor Control Problems summarized the ongoing debate about the importance of following the normal developmental sequence in treatment.[176] Particularly with the focus population, in which progress is measured in minute increments, there may not be time to progress through a normal developmental sequence. The authors of the MOVE curriculum[54] developed strategies with the underlying premise that children with multiple disabilities do not have time to work from "bottom up" (learning motor skills in a sequence taken from normal motor development) and propose instead going from "top down," focusing on the skills with the greatest functional importance to the child.

Guiding the decision making must be the functional outcomes that are most significant for the child or caregivers, or both, and the motor skills necessary to achieve them, not necessarily the next motor milestone. Think about the example given earlier of the mother who complained of back pain from lifting her son Johnny. The need is for her son to accept at least some of his weight during a standing pivot transfer so that she does not have to lift him. With this goal in mind, it certainly is not practical for therapy to start with teaching Johnny to crawl and then progressing to kneeling to half-kneeling to standing. Using the National Center for Medical Rehabilitation framework,[105] the therapist must ask, "What are the disabilities and impairments that limit function (i.e., his ability to accept weight in standing)?" Contractures, pain, apprehension, tactile defensiveness might all be factors further complicating his underlying problems with motor control and postural stability. Or is it the context? Is Johnny brought forward in his chair first with his feet planted firmly? Would a gait belt help? Would a handle that he could use for support make a difference? Are his shoes appropriate for the floor surface?

Intervention Particularly Relevant for the Focus Population

Behavior Management

Intervention programs are more likely to be successful with the focus population if attention is given to structured implementation within a behavioral context. One would expect to find not only an increase in the number of new behaviors learned and the rate at which they are learned, but also improvement in the child's ability to generalize these new behaviors in different environmental contexts.[177] Target behaviors should be clearly defined, with multiple opportunities for repetition. Identifying an appropriate reinforcer is often difficult with the focus population and requires coordinated efforts with all those involved in the child's care. The effectiveness of a particular reinforcer may last for a relatively short time period, so change or novelty is important.

Early work by Skinner on behavior modification techniques remains applicable to this population.[178] A target behavior is selected, and the specific responses that are desired are selected and defined. Correctly completed responses are immediately reinforced. By continued specific reinforcement and by successive and more generalized reinforcement procedures, the learning sequence is established, leading to the accomplishment of the target behavior. In establishing a behavior modification program, one must (1) specify target behaviors in an objective and measurable manner, often breaking down a desired behavior into many small increments; (2) determine the method of measuring changes; (3) choose appropriate reinforcers; (4) specify the conditions (contingencies) under which the desired behavior will be rewarded; (5) establish a plan that provides for consistent reinforcement and frequent "success"; (6) monitor the effectiveness of the contingencies; and (7) modify as indicated. Resources for the application of behavior modification with the focus population include *Behavior Modification with the Severely and Profoundly Retarded: Research and Application,*[179] *Behaviour Modification for People with Mental Handicaps* (2nd edition),[180] and an article by Hill entitled "Contributions of Behavior Modification to Cerebral Palsy Habilitation."[181] Clinical researchers have used behavior modification to reduce stereotypic behaviors[182] and to shape a variety of gross motor behaviors, including a reduction of the time in reverse tailor ("W") sitting,[183] the development of standing and walking,[184–190] raising an arm to pull a ring,[191] and the reduction of drooling.[192]

Behavior management strategies may also be important in the elimination or reduction of destructive behaviors, which are a serious problem in this population. The conclusions of the 1988 National Institutes of Health Consensus Conference on Destructive Behaviors in Persons with Developmental Disabilities included the following recommendations: "Most successful approaches to treatment are likely to involve multiple elements of therapy (behavioral and psychopharmacologic), environmental change, and education. Treatment methods may require techniques for enhancing desired behaviors; for producing changes in the social, physical, and educational environments; and for reducing or eliminating destructive behaviors."[12] Consistent implementation of the strategies developed is critical to the success of any program and, therefore, team involvement in assessment, planning and implementation across environments is essential.

The MOVE curriculum[54] incorporates some of the basic components of the neurobehavioral approach proposed by Horn and associates,[175] the intervention tactics proposed by Shumway-Cook and Woollacott,[174] and principles of behavioral management. The curriculum is structured around systematic instruction in functional mobility with frequent practice and incremental fading of required supports. "Our students with severe physical handicaps have repeatedly proven to us that they cannot acquire motoric skills without systematic instruction."[54] MOVE involves a six-step process: (1) testing, (2) setting goals, (3) task analysis, (4) measuring prompts, (5) reducing prompts, and (6) teaching skills. The goals in step 2 are always functional in nature (determined according to the needs and desires of the child or caregivers). Functional tasks are analyzed and broken down into components, which are targeted for instruction. Steps 4 and 5 involve systematic identification of the "physical, instructional prompts" used to assist a child in performing a task and the equally systematic reduction in the prompts until a maximal level of independent function is attained. A detailed scoring system promotes consistency in communication and the use of objective measures for assessing the effectiveness of intervention.

Biofeedback using automated learning devices is based on the principles of behavior modification—a concrete action immediately reinforced by a consequence with positive meaning—and can be very effectively applied with a population that is severely disabled.[153, 193, 194] In automated learning devices, a switch (either purchased or homemade) is interfaced between the power source (usually batteries) of the selected reinforcer so that the switch must be activated before the reinforcer will "perform." Switches can be of several types: a mechanical switch that requires a basic manipulation like light pressure or grasp to complete a circuit; a mercury switch that is activated by its position relative to gravity and can be placed on an individual in such a way as to be activated by a specific position of that body part in space; or a pressure-sensitive device. The reinforcer activated by the switch can be any battery-operated (or, with an adapter, electrically powered) device: for example, a toy, a small fan, a vibrating pillow, a light, or a tape recorder. Researchers have used automated learning devices to train patients in a wide range of behaviors, including head and trunk position,[194-200] range of motion,[201, 202] finger praxis,[203] and prehension.[204]

Prevention of Secondary Impairments

Many secondary impairments are predictable, and prevention measures should be incorporated into the intervention plan, including education for parents and other caregivers so that they have a rationale for certain intervention strategies and the knowledge to seek medical attention when needed.[106] It may be impossible to prevent all secondary impairments. The goal is to limit impairment and preserve function.

A variety of alternative positions and the appropriate use of assistive technology or adaptive equipment, or both, including postural support mechanisms, form the cornerstone of most prevention programs. An underlying assumption is that maintaining correct musculoskeletal alignment in a variety of body postures prevents deformity, although the definitive research is lacking. Carlson and Ramsey summarize the research on the benefits of external postural support mechanisms, which include improved pulmonary function; decreased myoelectric activity of the lumbar extensors; possibly enhanced upper extremity function, oral motor function, vocalizations, and social interaction; and improved pressure distribution and spinal alignment.[153]

Aspiration pneumonia associated with gastroesophageal reflux and dysphagia, as well as other respiratory problems, can be reduced or prevented by frequent changes in position and the use of postural support mechanisms.[205] Inverted positioning is of value in promoting the drainage of secretions into the segmental bronchi, where they can be more easily cleared by coughing.[133] Traditional postural drainage, however, with specific positioning to drain various lung segments, accompanied by percussion and vibration to those areas, is not indicated for upper airway congestion. Theoretically, the effect of postural drainage is to remove secretions, such as are produced in a lobar pneumonia, from the alveoli of specific lung segments. Its use for less serious upper airway congestion is not harmful, but neither is it likely to be particularly beneficial. In the classroom, beanbag chairs, wedges, large therapy balls, or ordinary pillows can be effectively used for comfortable, safe inverted positioning of children who would benefit from postural drainage positioning. It is important in establishing a postural drainage program (usually without percussion and vibration techniques unless supervision is adequate) that (1) it be done as a team effort between educational personnel and the physical therapist, (2) those responsible for implementing the program be instructed in the specific positions to be used as well as basic precautions, and (3) established time frames be adhered to. Another intervention of potential benefit for the prevention of respiratory problems is manual stretching and mobilization of the rib cage for patients with reduced thoracic compliance.[133]

Pierson and associates report on the use of botulinum toxin A injections into targeted muscles thought to be contributing to abnormal limb position based on objective and functional evaluation.[206] The results were positive: an increase of one point on the Ashworth scale, an increased range of motion, a decrease in the time required for ambulation, an increased tolerance of external supports (braces), decreased pain, and increased function.

Treatment of Oral Motor Problems

After a careful assessment of oral motor problems, remediation of the problem areas can be accomplished by following the guidelines provided by Morris and Klein[146] or others.[145, 147, 148] Consistency is particularly important in an oral motor program. Rarely can a therapist be available for all, or even most, of a child's feeding sessions, so that provisions for carryover to other mealtime situations are essential. It may be that the therapist will choose not to instruct others in specialized techniques like jaw control, but, if possible, there should be consistency in the position the child is in, the utensils used, and the type, texture, and temperature of foods offered.

It is important for therapists to support families or other primary caregivers in what can initially be a frustrating experience. Somehow, eating seems to be such a basic function that we just expect children to eat well. In the presence of a sloppy, slow eater who may have poor nutrition and choke frequently, this unmet expectation may lead to serious feelings of personal inadequacy or nonacceptance of the child on the part of a parent. Patience is essential. Feeding is such a habitual process that any change at first seems to worsen rather than improve the situation, and it takes time, sometimes as much as an hour and a half, to complete a meal when a new program is initiated. Mealtime should be a relaxed time, a sometimes rare opportunity for one-to-one interaction. In a book entitled *Mealtimes for Severely and Profoundly Handicapped Persons: New Concepts and Attitudes,* more than 50 professionals, as well as parents, volunteers, and persons with disabilities, describe and interpret the value of mealtimes.[207] Creative situations and mealtime atmospheres are described that can be the strata for positive interaction, development, and education.

Activities of Daily Living

Individuals who are severely and profoundly retarded are unable to be independently functioning members of society, but many will be capable of independence in at least some of the activities of daily living, and their independence should be encouraged by all possible means. They will be proud of their accomplishments, and their family or primary caretakers will be relieved of some of the many time-consuming aspects of basic care. The appropriate use of adaptive assistive technology and behavior modification can be very helpful in developing skills for daily living. Langley emphasizes the importance of a child's developing a sense of contingency awareness and a sense that the child can effect some control over the environment.[208] Examples of very basic control that should be incorporated, if possible, include some form of independent mobility, self-feeding, and augmentative communication systems to allow the child to make simple choices.

Assistive Technology

Especially for the child who has multiple disabilities and is nonambulatory, the proper use of assistive technology or adaptive equipment, or both, can be one of the most important aspects of a therapeutic program. Presperin states that "seating and positioning can have a direct correlation with the prevention of pressure sores, orthopedic deformities, and muscle contractures as well as with qualitative improvement of respiration, digestion, heart rate, and functional skills."[209] As summarized by Miedaner, other functions noted to have improved include speech intelligibility and vocalization, head control, self-feeding and drinking, and performance on psychologic testing.[210] Danquah noted a decrease in maladaptive behaviors among children with severe intellectual impairment who were nonverbal when given an opportunity to use Danquah Communication System Boards.[211] Selection of the appropriate equipment allows children with disabilities to interact more easily with their peers[212] and allows the educational staff to physically manage the student while teaching appropriate functional movement patterns.[54]

The process of selecting appropriate equipment requires consideration of its availability, cost, source of funding, portability, stability, ease of adjustment, ease of modifications, construction materials, and aesthetics.[213] Other considerations include the available space in the environment or environments in which the child functions, the ability of caregivers to lift or maneuver large equipment, the availability of a ramp, the type of transportation vehicle (e.g., interior room, height, two or four doors, storage space) and the lifestyle of the family or typical activities in the educational or residential environment. One piece of equipment can seldom do all the things caregivers would like it to do, but it is important to look at the big picture so that multiple needs can be considered and meshed, when possible.

Skills in correctly identifying equipment needs, locating resources for financial support, and obtaining the right piece of equipment (whether it is purchased or made) are some of the most important clinical decisions made by a pediatric physical therapist. The range of choices, the complexity of options, the expense entailed, and the availability of sophisticated technology such as simulators and computerized pressure mapping systems, is shifting much of the selection, ordering, and fitting to specialty clinics.

Positioning in adaptive equipment is often static, and care must be taken to provide opportunities for various positions, for mobility if possible, for free exploration of the environment, and for a frequent change of position. A child should have available a variety of positioning alternatives that are comfortable, that enable the child to perform functional tasks and interact maximally with the environment, and that provide the support necessary for the activity intended but still stimulate independent mastery of the necessary postural stabilization. Equipment must be correctly fitted and checked frequently for needed adjustments, and caregivers must demonstrate proficiency in the correct and safe use of the equipment.

The following areas should be assessed:

1. *Floor positions.* Several alternatives should be available for positioning on the floor.
   a. *Prone.* The child may benefit from a properly sized bolster or wedge. Size selection and positioning on the equipment depends on the developmental readiness of the child for head control, forearm support, or extended arm support.
   b. *Side-lying.* Commercially made side-lyers are available, but the appropriate use of bolsters and pillows may be sufficient.
   c. *Sitting.* There should be a seating arrangement that enables the child to participate in group activities with his or her peers at floor or table level.
2. *Seating.* Miedaner summarizes the results of 16 studies that demonstrate functional improvement from the use of appropriate adaptive seating.[210] Several different seating arrangements may be necessary for a child who has multiple disabilities. For instance, a child with athetosis may need a chair that provides maximal support (head, trunk, and legs) for eating or for fine motor activities. At other times during the day, a chair with less support allows the child opportunities to develop improved motor control. An excellent resource for postural support mechanisms is Carlson and Ramsey's chapter on assistive technology in *Physical Therapy for Children* by Campbell and associates.[153] Attention should be given to optimal seating for the following activities.
   a. *Feeding.* A chair that supports the head in midline and helps to minimize the effects of hypertonicity and abnormal movement patterns can be critical in promoting safe, effective feeding behaviors.
   b. *Fine motor skills.* For the child who is hypertonic, a well-fitted postural control chair may enable significant improvement in functional use of the arms and hands.
   c. *Interactive play.* Sufficient support allows the child's focus to be on interaction rather than on maintaining postural stability.
   d. *Transportation.* Federally approved adaptive seating that meets rigorous safety testing is a legal necessity. Only this type of approved seating should be used, and all directions as to its safe use should be adhered to, including not placing the child in front of airbags. When needed, tie-downs should be ordered for safe transport on school buses or vans.
3. *Mobility.* Previous discussions have illustrated the importance of self-directed motor activity.
4. *Supported weight bearing.* For a child who is nonambulatory, a standing program, starting at a chronologic age of 14 to 16 months, is an important component of intervention to maintain bone mass density (prevent calcium loss), to promote normal development of the acetabulum (prevent hip

dislocation), and to prevent soft tissue contractures.[214] Little definitive research is available to guide the therapist in the development of a standing program, but preliminary work by Stuberg indicates that to maintain bone mass a consistent program of supported standing of 60 minutes' duration three to four times per week is the minimum.[214] Options for supported weight bearing include a prone or supine board, with multiple adjustments available for standing or kneeling with optimal alignment; a standing box, which provides more behavioral than physical control; or a standing frame, which promotes a fully upright stance with foot, knee, and pelvic support. Additional considerations include ensuring adequate alignment and support of the distal extremity (custom orthotics)[215] and encouraging active participation of the child when possible. Therapists must also be aware of the load applied during weight bearing and maximize the load, as tolerated, or make adjustments in the frequency and duration of standing. This means adjusting commonly used prone or supine standers to a near-vertical position and minimizing support at the torso within the child's tolerance.

5. *General.* Finally, the physical therapist or occupational therapist must assess procedures for toileting, bathing, and dressing and identify the presence of architectural barriers preventing access to opportunities for recreation, education, and medical or dental care.

Electrical Stimulation

The use of neuromuscular electrical stimulation (NMES) is a fairly new intervention with the pediatric population that has shown promising results. The most common technique is to use surface electrodes and a portable battery-operated device to apply electrical current transcutaneously to superficial innervated muscle. Electrodes can also be surgically implanted into muscle tissue, a technique that allows stimulation of deeper muscle tissue.[216] "NMES has been used as an assist in muscle reeducation, strengthening, maintaining or increasing range of motion, decreasing spasticity or to serve as a functional orthosis."[217] Different outcomes are accomplished by altering basic parameters, including the waveform, stimulus frequency, stimulus intensity, ratio of on/off times, and ramp time. Two protocols are in increasingly common use. One is therapeutic electrical stimulation, developed in Canada in 1988.[218, 219] It uses low-intensity stimulation over long periods (8 to 12 hours) to promote growth in muscle tissue that is weak and atrophied. The presumed effect is to increase blood flow during a time of trophic hormone secretion (sleep). The intensity is below that required to produce muscle contraction and is comfortable enough to be tolerated by most children without interfering with sleep. In the second protocol, the therapist stimulates a particular muscle (by means of a remote control activator) as the child performs a functional activity at the time that the muscle would normally be acting.[220–224] NMES therefore supplements the volitional activation of the muscle and enhances sensory feedback. Critical to the success of NMES is selecting the correct muscles to stimulate at the correct time. Further research is needed to better define and validate the effectiveness of NMES as an intervention tool. The Fall 1997 special issue of Pediatric Physical Therapy, "An Overview of Electrical Stimulation for the Pediatric Population,"[225] is an excellent resource for information on NMES.

Cognitive impairment was not viewed as a contraindication for the use of therapeutic electrical stimulation,[218] but no specific mention is made in the literature of using NMES with children who have multiple disabilities. The likelihood that the child will not be able to comprehend the purpose of the NMES, provide adequate feedback about techniques or procedures, or work cognitively in an applied treatment session is a constraint to consider. The higher intensity would seem less desirable with the focus population because of the inability of the child to provide adequate feedback about techniques or procedures. Precaution is recommended (especially with application in the head and neck area) when using NMES with children who have a history of seizures, because some systemic absorption of the electric current occurs.[217]

The following case study illustrates the application of the principles for developing and evaluating a physical therapy plan of care for a child with multiple disabilities.

CASE STUDY

Nicole is a 59-month-old girl with multiple disabilities who lives in a small rural community. She was initially referred for developmental services by the follow-up clinic of the tertiary care hospital that managed her care during the neonatal period. Nicole received home-based services through an early-intervention program administered by the Developmental Evaluation Center, a state-funded regional program of transdisciplinary services for pre-school children who are at risk for, or identified with, developmental problems. A physical therapist was part of the transdisciplinary team that designed the intervention program for Nicole, and the physical therapist saw her with the early-intervention specialist in an indirect, integrated model of service delivery. Home visits were made monthly for the first year and then every 3 months. The physical therapist coordinated assessment and intervention with other members of the team (including the parents), adjusting the program as indicated, assisting with the acquisition of adaptive equipment, and generally being available for education, consultation, or problem solving.

At 3 years of age, Nicole made the transition from early-intervention to preschool services and participated for about 13 months in a center-based program. There she received direct physical therapy twice a week from either a physical therapist or a physical therapist assistant. Unfortunately, Nicole was withdrawn from the center because of frequent illness and a prolonged stay in pediatric intensive care with a respiratory virus. Another child with multiple disabilities from Nicole's class, who was hospitalized at the same time, subsequently died. Nicole's mother has just recently agreed to try center-based intervention again but is understandably uneasy about the risks. Nicole is referred for physical therapy assessment as part of the planning for her transition to services for school-aged children. The referral is to the Developmental Evaluation Center; the physical therapist making the assessment will assist other members of the transdisciplinary team to develop an intervention plan but will not be the one to provide any subsequent direct service.

The HOAC,[90, 91] described in Chapter 1, will be the basis for the approach used in decision making regarding Nicole's care.

INITIAL DATA COLLECTION

The first step in the model is data collection, obtained by reviewing the medical and educational records and interviewing significant caregivers. It is desirable to also interview the child, although this is not possible with Nicole.

Medical History

Nicole was born prematurely at 35 weeks of gestation. Her mother's pregnancy was complicated by premature labor, beginning at about 22 weeks of gestation, which was treated with medication and frequent hospitalizations for the duration of the pregnancy. Nicole was delivered at the small (65-bed) local hospital by emergency cesarean section due to abruptio placentae. Nicole required vigorous and prolonged resuscitation after delivery, after which she was transferred by helicopter to the neonatal intensive care unit of the closest tertiary care hospital, about 90 minutes from her home. There she was treated for respiratory distress and neonatal seizures and was discharged at about 3 weeks of age. No specific cause for her multiple disabilities is known, other than the presumed effects prenatally of a complicated pregnancy and perinatal hypoxia.

Ongoing medical problems for Nicole have included respiratory problems due to infections and difficulty gaining weight. Her current weight of only 21 pounds places her well below the 10th percentile for her age. Her seizure disorder has, at times, been difficult to control. The pediatric neurologist who followed her as a neonate continues to work with her pediatrician to manage her seizures. He referred her to a large specialty clinic at a medical teaching hospital about 120 miles away and continues to consult with those physicians about her care. Nicole is currently taking divalproex (Depakote), carbamazepine (Tegretol), and clonazepam for seizures.

Vision and hearing have been assessed to the degree possible and found to be within normal limits. Records indicate no history of surgeries or fractures. She has been seen at a state-funded orthopedic clinic about once a year since the age of 24 months. Screening for musculoskeletal problems and the review and approval required to obtain state funding for adaptive equipment for Nicole are accomplished at this clinic. A recent dental screening at the center resulted in a referral to a dentist in the closest city, about 90 miles away.

It would be difficult for her mother to seek employment outside the home. The myriad of professionals and specialists involved in service delivery for Nicole is staggering (Table 4–1).

Scheduling Nicole's appointments, transporting her to and from various professionals, and waiting in medical offices is the equivalent of a full-time job. This is not to mention the mental and emotional burden of coping with chronic problems and acute, sometimes life-threatening illnesses; interacting with professionals; interpreting recommendations; resolving conflicting advice; being an advocate; and carrying out home programs. Respite care has been a much appreciated opportunity for the mother to have a few hours a week for herself. A physical therapist met with the respite care worker to review basic handling and positioning techniques.

Medicaid covers the majority of Nicole's medical expenses. The family does not

Professionals and Specialists Involved in Nicole's Care, Their Distance from Her Home, and the Contribution They Make to Her Care

TABLE 4–1

Professional	Agency	Approximate Distance (miles)	Role
Local pediatrician	Private	25	Case coordination–medical management of routine problems
Developmental pediatrician	Specialty referral center	90	Assessment for diagnostic purposes
Orthopedist	State-sponsored clinic at county health department	5	Assessment and approval of adaptive equipment requests for state funding
Geneticist	Access through DEC	5	Assessment for diagnosis
Genetics counselor	Access through DEC	25	Consultation
Ophthalmologist	Private	30	Assessment
Neurologist	Private	90	Seizure management
Pediatric neurologist	Private	120	Specialized consultation–seizures
Audiologist	Speech and Hearing Center	25	Assessment—periodic
Early-intervention specialist	DEC	Home-based	Weekly intervention (until age 3)
Educational specialist	DEC	Home-based and/or center-based	Assessment, program planning, consultation
Occupational therapist	DEC	Home-based and/or center-based	Assessment, program planning, consultation
Orthotist	Private	90	Fabrication and fit of ankle-foot orthoses
Physical therapist 1	DEC	Home-based and/or center-based	Assessment, program planning, consultation
Physical therapist 2 (not specialized in pediatrics)	Local hospital	5	Treatment
Physical therapist 3	Tertiary hospital	90	Treatment when hospitalized
Physical therapist 4	Seating clinic	90	Adaptive equipment
Psychologist	DEC	Home-based and/or center-based	Assessment, program planning, consultation
Speech and language pathologist 1	DEC	Home-based and/or center-based	Assessment, program planning, consultation
Speech and language pathologist 2	Developmental day care	Center-based	Treatment
Teacher 1	Developmental day care	Center-based	Education
Teacher 2	Certified preschool	Center-based	Education

DEC, Developmental Evaluation Center.

have the financial resources for services that are not covered. Adaptive equipment that she currently uses was funded by another state program (Childrens' Special Health Services) with income guidelines similar to those for Medicaid.

Parent Interview

Several members of the transdisciplinary team were present for the interview to avoid repetitive questioning, but not the whole team for fear that the size of the group would be intimidating and inhibit conversation.

The mother says that Nicole is generally a happy child who enjoys social interaction and the attention of those around her. Nicole has a sister who is 4 years older. The mother is divorced from Nicole's biologic father, and he has not maintained contact. Nicole's stepfather is generally supportive and affectionate, but he is involved only marginally in the provision of care for Nicole or in decision making in relation to her needs.

Nicole is totally dependent in all aspects of daily living and requires round-the-clock care, often sleeping poorly at night. The mother's concerns have primarily focused on Nicole's health, because she is ill quite frequently and has required numerous hospitalizations, including the recent admission to the pediatric intensive care unit. In the past, seizures were sometimes of such severity that they were life threatening and required emergency medical management.

Nicole's mother speaks proudly of Nicole's interactive abilities (e.g., response to peekaboo) and minimizes problems. It is apparent that Nicole's small size and developmental level has, essentially, enabled the family to enjoy a kind of prolonged infancy state with her that is not particularly problematic at present—in fact, it is enjoyable. The medical concerns are where "reality" hits.

The mother mentions that Nicole's head is "to the top" of her car seat, and because she has outgrown her ankle-foot orthoses (AFOs), they have not been using her prone stander and are sure it needs to be adjusted. When questioned about bathing, the mother says she is still able to bathe Nicole in the kitchen sink on a towel, but that she loves the water, and the space is becoming confining.

In response to a comment by one of the examiners that it must be very difficult to keep up with all the appointments for Nicole, the mother noted that a system for managing appointments and facilitating communication with the various professionals, which she developed under the guidance of a case manager from the Developmental Evaluation Center, has made a very positive difference. A worry is that Nicole will be exposed to illness in the waiting rooms. The mother appreciates medical offices that allow her to take Nicole immediately to a clean examining room or other private area.

Teacher Interview

Nicole seems to have adapted well to the new environment at the center and loves to be around the other children and "part of the action." The teacher and classroom personnel are interested in finding ways to include Nicole in various activities in the classroom (arts and crafts, music, lunch and snack, and outdoor play). They are using her posture control chair for feeding her but would like adaptive seating that would allow her to be more at a level with the other children. They think she would enjoy using a swing outside. They have tried some "switch" toys with Nicole, which she is able to use, but they comment that she seems to lose interest in the stimulus fairly quickly. In general, she seems much more interested in human interaction than in toys and other objects.

Developmental Testing

Results of standardized and developmental testing done 1 year earlier indicate an approximate age-equivalent of 5 to 6 months. The Vineland Adaptive Behavior Scale[94] was used to assess adaptive behavior as part of the required documentation for placement decisions. Her mother was interviewed for the assessment with the following result:

Scale	Age Equivalent
Communication	0–11 mo
Socialization	0–9 mo
Daily living skills	0–10 mo
Motor skills	0–2 mo
Adaptive behavior composite	0–8 mo

In the documentation of those assessments, Nicole is noted to have good head control in all positions, but a tendency for a head tilt to the left and a functional C curve in her spine to the left when sitting upright. She was able to raise her head from supine and prone positions. She had difficulty using her arms for support in the prone position (e.g., forearm propping). She was able to right her head in response to lateral tilting, but trunk righting was more difficult. She had no protective extension response with her arms. She required minimal lower trunk or pelvic support to maintain ring sitting. She enjoyed supported standing. She tended to move in total patterns of extension or flexion and was strongly influenced by the asymmetric tonic neck reflex and the symmetric tonic neck reflex.

PROBLEM STATEMENTS AND RELATED QUESTIONS

The next step in the HOAC model, before assessment, is stating problems. Although it may seem an unusual sequence, the intent is to maintain a clear focus on the problems as presented by the patient or caregivers. From the review of Nicole's medical history, test results, and the parent and teacher interview, the following list of problems (in italic) was generated. In roman type are related questions or thoughts that will shape the decision making.

1. *She has a seizure disorder that is complex and only partially controlled with high doses of anticonvulsant medications.* What kind of side effects is Nicole experiencing from the medications? Are there times during the day when she is more alert? Is it possible that she is having petit mal seizures or subliminal seizure activity?

2. *She has adaptive equipment and assistive technology needs.*
   a. *There is a need for adaptive equipment and positioning alternatives in the classroom that enable her to participate more directly with her peers.* How does Nicole sit in a classroom chair of appropriate size? Adapting a chair like this and working on the required motor skills would be more functional than adding another piece of equipment. Would the corner chair that she uses at home work at the table in the classroom? Nicole's mother might be willing to loan it to the school and see if it worked. If so, funding sources for a school chair could be investigated.
   b. *AFOs no longer fit; as a result, Nicole is not weight bearing because she goes into severe pronation.*
   c. *A prone stander, purchased for Nicole to use at home, needs adjustment.* Might the prone stander work as an option to get Nicole at the table with the other children at school?
   d. *There is a lack of play opportunities for Nicole out of doors.* Is there a swing set that would accommodate an adaptive swing?
   e. *Bathing (done in the sink) is becoming more difficult as Nicole grows.* Does the family have a bathtub? Is it large enough to accommodate a bath chair? Will the mother, who is very petite, be able to safely lift Nicole in and out of the bathtub?
   f. *The car seat is almost too small.*
   g. *There is no means of independent mobility.*

3. *She has poor sleep patterns.* Is this a behavioral issue? Do any of the medications she is taking affect sleep? Is so, would adjustments in the schedule of administering medications make a difference? Is nighttime positioning safe and comfortable?
4. *She weighs only 21 pounds.* How do other anthropometric measures compare? Are there feeding problems? Is she getting adequate calories? Have supplements been tried? Is she getting recommended daily nutritional requirements, especially considering medications and inactivity? Has a nutritional assessment taken place? Were recommendations made that are not being carried out?
5. *She is at risk for musculoskeletal problems, including calcium resorption, hip dislocation or subluxation, soft tissue contractures, and spinal deformity.* All of these areas need to be assessed. Does her chair provide good spinal alignment? Will she tolerate prone positioning so that she is getting hip extension? What alternatives exist for supported weight bearing? Will it be possible to adjust the prone stander at home and could one be obtained for use at school? Should long leg braces (or shell splints for nighttime use) be considered as a positional assist? Or would these contribute to sleep problems? Is the mother able to be consistent with a home program of positioning and exercise? What alternatives are there for routine implementation of prevention strategies?
6. *The family focuses on the here and now, especially medical needs. They are not thinking about the future and what they need to be doing now to prevent problems as Nicole grows.* How much responsibility for long-term needs can the family assume on top of everything else they are coping with? With guidance would the stepfather take a more active role? This transitional period is likely to be particularly stressful. What attempts have been made to educate the family to the potential problems over the long term? What was the response? Can they handle adaptations in their routine at home and the responsibility of additional activities, and so forth? Would it be advisable to initiate programs at the center with other personnel and gradually educate the family and get their consent on aspects of the program from which they can realize direct benefit?

GOALS FOR INTERVENTION

The next step in the HOAC model is to establish goals based on the problem statements that are measurable, are functional, and include a temporal element. Questions and concerns related to overall management should be addressed by various team members but may need to be initiated by the physical therapist. Adaptive equipment needs seem to be a priority, and subsequent intervention is linked closely to the selection and acquisition of that equipment. Further clarification needs to occur about the best use of resources for consistent intervention. Any additional information needed may be gained by requesting additional records or contacting the appropriate professional or professionals.

For expediency, the primary care physician should be consulted and the necessary steps taken to initiate referrals to an orthotist and to the seating clinic where Nicole's chair was prescribed and fitted initially. The orthotist would make custom-molded bilateral AFOs and provide input to the team on the potential benefit of long-leg braces or shell splints for nighttime use. Specialized physical therapists and occupational therapists at the seating clinic would provide input on a car seat, bath chair, and swing, and on positioning in the classroom that would promote Nicole's interaction with her peers.

Goals for Nicole might resemble the following:

1. Nicole will be able to purposefully ambulate forward (supported in an appropriately adapted and adjusted wheeled walker with trunk support) at least 10 feet in less than 5 minutes within 3 months.
2. Nicole will be able to be physically present with her peers in the classroom

during at least two activities each day within 2 months after obtaining adaptive equipment.

3. Nicole will have well-fitted custom-molded bilateral AFOs within 2 months.
4. Nicole will be in a supported standing position with good alignment of her lower extremities for at least 60 minutes a day 3 to 4 days per week within 2 months (as described by Stuberg[214]).
5. Nicole's mother will comment positively about reduced stress in her daily routine and satisfaction with the benefit to Nicole of a new bath seat, car seat, and adaptive seating within 2 months after obtaining these pieces of adaptive equipment.
6. Nicole will have at least five identified positioning alternatives and will experience frequent changes of position (at least every hour) in both the home and the school environment.
7. Nicole will have no worsening of the contractures at her hips or knees as assessed by repeat goniometric measurements of hip and knee extension (plus or minus 10 degrees).

ASSESSMENT

Assessment is focused on gaining the information necessary to address the problems and achieve the goals. After discussion, members of the transdisciplinary team decide that the psychologist will administer the Stanford-Binet (a standardized measure of intelligence) and the PEDI[156] (a measure of adaptive behavior) as a means of classifying her level of mental retardation and making placement decisions. Subsequent discussion will identify strengths and weaknesses across the four dimensions according to the model for classification and description of mental retardation recommended by Luckasson and coworkers.[3] The team decides to jointly administer Linder's TPBA.[99] The case manager and physical therapist decide to use the Canadian Occupational Performance Measure[92] to involve the mother in setting goals and to stimulate discussion about her personal needs, as well as to provide a framework for prioritizing those needs and keeping reassessment focused at that level.

The physical therapist and occupational therapist decide to jointly address issues related to oral motor function and feeding, consulting with the nutritionist as needed about Nicole's energy needs, the adequacy of her diet, and the potential for drug-nutrient interactions.[226] To supplement the snack observation, which is one phase of TPBA,[99] they plan to schedule times to observe feeding sessions at home and at the center. An appreciation of the resources and constraints in both environments will be the foundation for meaningful, realistic intervention strategies. Because repeated respiratory problems and failure to grow and gain weight are problems noted in her medical history, particular attention will be given to clinical indications that she may be aspirating food or saliva and to the adequacy of her diet. Consultation with her physician and referral for a barium swallow study may be necessary.

The physical therapist decides to use the GMFM as a baseline motor assessment because it is comprehensive and sensitive to change even in the more severely involved population.[116, 117] Although postural stability is a significant problem, no tests with documented reliability and validity information are available that are applicable to children who also have very limited cognitive ability.[111] Assessment utilizing the MOVE curriculum[54] will be incorporated because of the goal for Nicole to have some type of independent mobility. Based on the problem list, further assessment would look at the current status of her respiratory function as well as skeletal and soft tissue structures that would be at risk, considering Nicole's typical postures and lack of weight bearing. An assessment of Nicole's adaptive equipment is also important.

The results of the physical therapy assessment and elements of the transdisciplinary testing are summarized as they relate to the problem list and goals as follows:

Play-Based Assessment. Eight different professionals were present for the "arena" assessment using the TPBA.[99] The physical therapist scored Linder's Observation Guidelines for Sensorimotor Development. Aspects of the guidelines appropriate for Nicole included the following:

1. *General appearance of movement.* Her movement is jerky and poorly coordinated with minimal isolated movement for functional purposes.
2. *Muscle tone, strength, and endurance.* Muscle tone fluctuates, with Nicole apparently making at least some intentional use of tonic reflexes to alter the tone for function.[110] Strength is difficult to assess. Endurance for sustaining functional postures is poor (e.g., midline head control).
3. *Reactivity to sensory input (touch, movement, auditory, and visual).* Nicole seems to enjoy tactile input of all kinds. She laughed with light touch ("tickle"), although it seemed to increase her overall tone. As related by her mother, she especially enjoys water play. Movement, too, was generally enjoyable. She loved being pushed in a wheeled cart or rocked over a large ball. Swinging in the hammock seemed a little stressful for her, but this may have been because of the semireclined position (which she dislikes) rather than the actual movement. Similarly, a trial in a borrowed swing seemed to bring a mixture of pleasure and apprehension (Fig. 4–4). Nicole is sensitive to unexpected, loud auditory stimuli like a telephone ringing or noise in the classroom, typically responding with an initial startle, apprehension, and increased muscle tone. Social interactions are accompanied by relatively good eye contact, but she gives very poor visual regard to objects or toys. Nicole has little interest in toys or objects and little motivation to reach, grasp, or manipulate them.
4. *Stationary positions used for play (prone, supine, sitting, supported standing).* In the prone position, Nicole has good head control, but her weight is shifted forward onto her chest, and she accepts only minimal weight on her arms, so she fatigues quickly (Fig. 4–5). She continues to be influenced by the

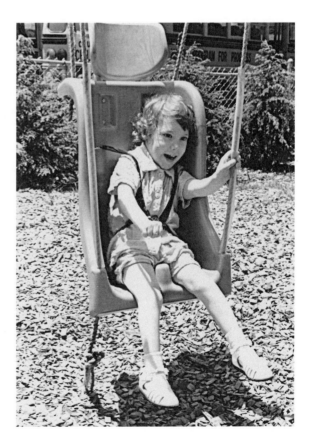

FIGURE 4–4. Nicole was tried in a swing already in place on the playground. She seemed to enjoy it, but the increased tone in her arms and legs indicates some apprehension and postural insecurity. Recommended for her use is a swing with an attached footplate with straps and a strap system for her trunk that includes a strap between her legs. Foam side supports will be tried to improve postural stability. She liked holding onto the upright of the swing assembly. It may be helpful to craft a lap tray with vertical handholds. Actual ordering of the swing will be coordinated by the school-based therapist in consultation with a specialist from a regional seating clinic.

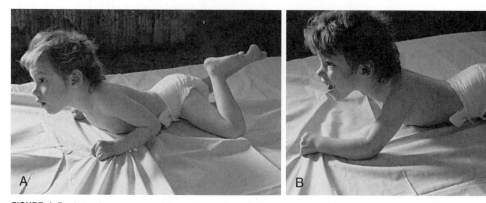

FIGURE 4–5. *A,* In the prone position, Nicole has good head control, but her weight is shifted forward, adding to the effort required. With her elbows behind her shoulders and her weight on her fisted hands, her arms contribute little to maintaining the position. *B,* With arms placed forward, she has more natural posturing throughout and weight is more appropriately shifted back toward her abdomen.

symmetric tonic neck reflex, so that changing the position of her head causes disconcerting alterations in tone (Fig. 4–6). She pivots in the prone position and occasionally "flips" over onto her back (without trunk rotation) but has very little controlled movement.

In the supine position, she actively thrusts her arms and legs, gaining some random mobility from the activity. She can lift her head briefly (Fig. 4–7). In a seated position, either in her chair or supported on the mat, Nicole is able to maintain a midline head and trunk position but seems to tire quickly and drift or sink into a position of lateral flexion to the left with accommodating head tilt, with no apparent anticipation of imminent falling. She actively straightens herself in response to her mother's verbal request. She does not like to be tilted back in her chair, preferring an almost totally upright posture, and strains forward with resulting head and trunk flexion if her seat back is angled. An attempt to use lateral head supports was met with obvious dismay

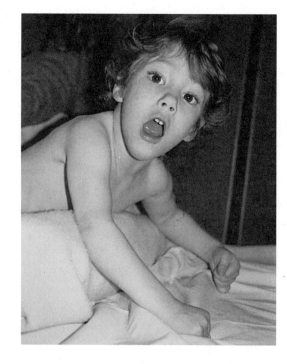

FIGURE 4–6. Prone over a wedge, Nicole is taking some weight on her hands, but still not on her elbows. Influence of the asymmetric tonic neck reflex results in flexion of the left arm as she turns her head to the photographer and in an inability to accept weight. Also noted again is overflow of abnormal muscle tone to her mouth.

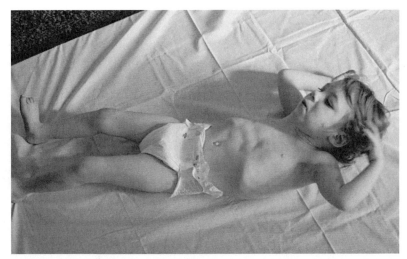

FIGURE 4–7. In the supine position, Nicole raises her head from the supporting surface with considerable effort and accompanying overflow of muscle tone to her mouth and flexion in her arms. The lateral rib cage is flared and the anterior-posterior diameter of her chest is decreased.

on Nicole's part. Nicole has relatively good head control and requires minimal support to maintain a ring-sitting position (Fig. 4–8).

More important functionally (than ring sitting) is how Nicole sits in a classroom chair of appropriate size. If this is a possibility, with minimal adaptation, it would avoid having to bring another piece of equipment into the classroom (Fig. 4–9). The authors of the MOVE curriculum[54] refer to two types of seating: *leisure* seating and *functional* seating. Leisure seating would be comparable to the positions most of us seek for entertainment, where the participant is passive. An example would be a recliner for watching television. For Nicole, her custom-adapted chair meets that need (when reclined). Functional seating involves support so that the individual is leaning forward, the way most of us do for active participation in our environment. This forward posture also places the diaphragm in a better position for breath support for vocalization or coughing.

FIGURE 4–8. In ring (tailor) sitting, Nicole briefly maintains the position if placed but has poor postural control and is unable to make the necessary adjustments to maintain an upright posture. She demonstrates acceptance of weight on her arms for propping but cannot use the support functionally to right herself.

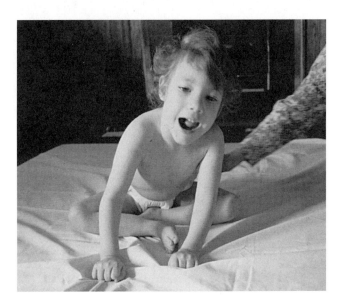

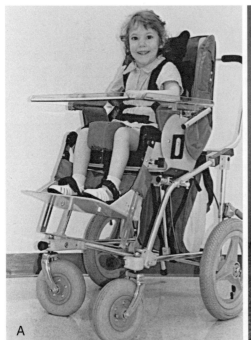

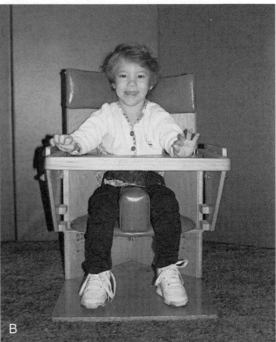

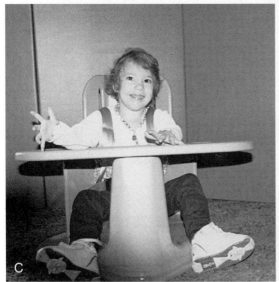

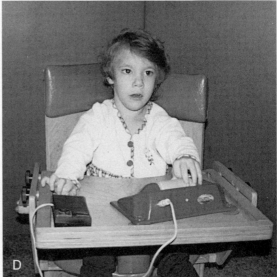

FIGURE 4–9. *A,* In custom-adapted seating, Nicole is well positioned for feeding and focused work on fine motor or cognitive skill development. She does not have to expend effort on maintaining her posture. The bulk and size of the chair and her fixed posture are constraints. Frequent "time out" is important. *B,* Nicole is well positioned in a corner chair with tray. Ankle-foot orthoses are in place and help with stabilizing her feet and legs. The position of her arms and left hand evidence the total extension she uses to maintain an upright head and trunk. *C,* Another type of corner chair allows her to be at floor height with the other children, but her legs are awkwardly positioned. She is not able to use her legs and feet for stability as effectively as in the corner chair shown in *B. D,* Positioned in her corner chair, Nicole activates a roller switch to play music. She is giving characteristically poor visual regard to the task and using her whole arm rather than isolated elbow, wrist, and finger movement to accomplish the task.

Nicole is unable to independently adjust her own position, either on a mat or in her adaptive-seating arrangement. She lacks any means of independent mobility. She really seems to enjoy supported standing, and although she uses total extension to maintain weight bearing, she has surprisingly good head and trunk control. She seems to understand her mother's request to "walk," but it is difficult for Nicole to maintain the extension required for weight bearing on one leg while flexing the other in preparation for a step. She is better at maintaining weight on her left leg and stepping with her right than vice versa. Some mottling of her legs occurs when she is upright, indicative of circulatory compromise.

5. *Communication.* Nicole lacks verbal expressive communication but is quite effective in communicating basic emotions through facial expression and a variety of vocalizations. The subtle, yet meaningful communication that occurs between the mother and the daughter in play situations is dramatic and was not duplicated in her interaction with others.

6. *Snack.* The snack that is included as part of Linder's TPBA was an opportunity to observe a relatively brief feeding session and was a basis for preliminary planning by the physical therapist, the occupational therapist, and the nutritionist for additional assessment in this area. Nicole is fed in her posture control chair at home and at the center and apparently becomes fussy if not fed on a regular routine of every 4 hours. She is fed strained or "junior" prepared infant foods or table foods blended to an appropriate consistency. During the observed feeding session, Nicole initially ate readily but seemed to satiate quickly and actively turned her head away from the spoon or pushed the food from her mouth. She actively opened her mouth in anticipation of receiving food, but there was little lip closure around the spoon and limited manipulation of the food once in her mouth. Periodic difficulty coordinating swallowing and breathing was noted, which would be anticipated to be worse if she were congested. In an attempt to maintain midline head position, both the mother and the center staff tended to support her head in a manner that placed her neck in extension, possibly compromising function of the glottis and allowing aspiration of food, although there was no overt choking.

Pediatric Evaluation of Disability Inventory.[155] Part I of the PEDI is a test of functional skills, with 197 discrete items. Nicole was rated on each item as either "unable, or limited in capability, to perform item in most situations," or "capable of performing item in most situations." Part II consists of 20 complex functional activities. The rating (zero to 5) is based on the amount of caregiver assistance required and any modifications used ("no modifications, non-specialized child-oriented modifications, rehabilitation equipment, or extensive modifications"). Both parts are further categorized into self-care, mobility, and social function domains. Because the PEDI was standardized on a normative sample, one can calculate both standard (normed) and scaled (criterion referenced) performance scores. The inclusion of the modification scale is particularly helpful in assessing a child with multiple disabilities.

Nicole's standard score establishes an objective measure of adaptive function for placement considerations. The criterion-referenced score provides a baseline measure of functional performance for subsequent comparison. Scores on individual items can be reviewed for a descriptive summary of her functional abilities and used as a basis for programming.

Nicole requires complete assistance with all aspects of dressing, feeding, grooming, toileting, and bathing. She is unable to initiate or actively participate in recreational pursuits. Her score on the PEDI was predictably low.

Canadian Occupational Performance Measure.[92] The Canadian Occupational Performance Measure provided a structured opportunity to discuss with the mother the need to incorporate measures to prevent secondary impairments that could reasonably be anticipated. For example, the mother, initially resistant to the idea of "braces," was amenable to their use once she understood the importance of weight bearing and the need for the AFOs to provide correct alignment during supported standing. She identified five prioritized goals, with the primary goal being to have some means of independent mobility for Nicole. She seemed overwhelmed at the prospect of adding any more activities to her basic routine with Nicole at home.

Gross Motor Function Measure.[116] The GMFM complements the results of other developmental assessments in the gross motor area and provides a sensitive measure as a basis for comparison over time.[117] Results on the GMFM, combined with traditional measures of musculoskeletal status (e.g., goniometry), should alert team members to any deterioration of Nicole's status.

Nicole's performance was as follows:

Dimension A (lying and rolling)	=	30 percent
Dimension B (sitting)	=	17 percent
Dimension C (crawling and kneeling)	=	2 percent
Dimension D (standing)	=	2 percent
Dimension E (walking, running, and so forth)	=	0 percent

Dimensions A, B, and D were determined to be goal areas, and the goal dimensions average score was 16 percent. Her overall average score was 10 percent. The results provide a baseline for subsequent assessment.

Mobility Opportunities Via Education.[54] Independent mobility as a prioritized goal indicates using the MOVE curriculum, and the Top-Down Motor Milestone Test is scored with this in mind. The test assesses a variety of functional motor behaviors and breaks them down into incremental steps that allow even a child with Nicole's limited motor ability to demonstrate success and progress over time. It provides a framework for establishing an intervention program of fading prompts and reinforcement of desired motor skills.

The summary of Nicole's test results on this portion of the MOVE assessment indicate that for static sitting and standing she is functioning at level II and for other mobility skills at level III. Completion of skills at level II ensures that the student will be able to "walk at least 10 feet with help from another person in maintaining balance and shifting weight. Lifting will be minimal due to help from the participant. A wheelchair will be required for distances of more than 10 feet."[54] At level III, completion of skills "improves bone health and functioning of internal organs and decreases the likelihood of joint deformities and pain."[54]

Musculoskeletal. Soft tissue contractures result in decreased hip and knee extension and ankle dorsiflexion. Limitations at the knee are the combined result of shortening of the hamstring muscles (straight leg raise to 40 degrees bilaterally) and involvement of the knee joint (lacking 5 degrees of full extension with hips neutral). For supported standing with AFOs, full knee extension, hip extension to neutral, and 5 degrees dorsiflexion would be desirable. Goniometric measurements taken of ankle dorsiflexion, knee extension, and hip extension and compared with measurements taken by the physical therapist at the last annual evaluation indicate a loss of 5 degrees in knee extension and 10 degrees in hip extension. Considering the interrater reliability problems in goniometry with children who have CP,[118, 119] this may or may not be significant but certainly warrants continued observation and preventive attention. No clinical evidence suggests structural problems with the hips or spine. With weight bearing, her feet collapse into severe pronation with heel valgus bilaterally, the right greater than the left (Fig. 4–10*A*). AFOs improve her alignment and stability (Fig. 4–10*B*). With AFOs in place, standing in a prone stander is accomplished with good alignment and comfort (Fig. 4–11).

Respiratory. Nicole has lateral rib flaring with relatively little movement of the rib cage during respiration. Her respiratory rate is 54 with approximately a 1:1 ratio of inspiration to expiration. She has a weak cough. She is able to breathe through her nose but prefers mouth breathing. Auscultation identifies upper airway "noise" but no adventitious breath sounds.

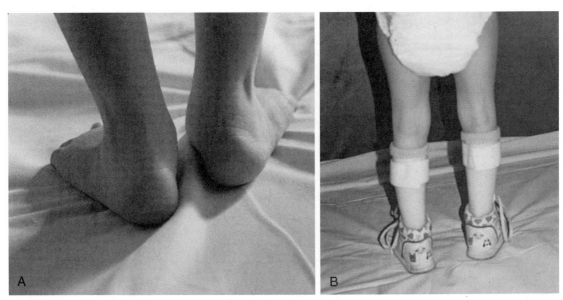

FIGURE 4–10. *A,* In supported standing, Nicole's feet (especially the right foot) collapse into severe pronation with heel valgus. *B,* Ankle-foot orthoses provide appropriate alignment for supported standing and also improve her stability in sitting.

FIGURE 4–11. Nicole is well supported in a prone stander wearing her ankle-foot orthoses. She is giving good visual regard to people. Her head is somewhat excessively extended. To gain the benefits of weight bearing, the goal would be to have her stand at least 60 minutes per day, 3 to 4 days per week, and to gradually increase the angle so that she is progressively more upright.

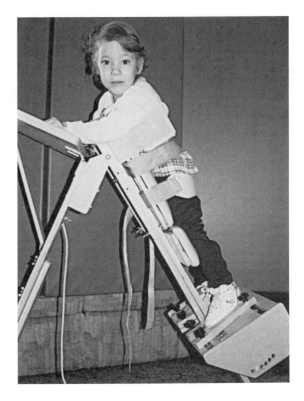

GUIDING HYPOTHESES

The next step in the HOAC model is to develop hypotheses about the causes of the client's problems. These hypotheses form the basis for intervention. According to Rothstein and Echternach, "No treatment should be administered that is not based on a hypothesis."[90] If the hypothesis is related to a cause that the therapist is not qualified or able to treat, then appropriate referral may be necessary.

REEVALUATION METHODOLOGY

Next, a procedure must be established to look at the success of the proposed intervention in meeting the goals. For children with special needs, federal laws provide the basic framework for assessment and reassessment, but more frequent or specific mechanisms are options.

INTERVENTION STRATEGIES AND TACTICS

According to the HOAC model, a strategy is defined as "the overall approach that will be adopted, whereas the tactics are the specific means of implementing the strategy."[90]

ANALYZING AND REFLECTING ON OUTCOMES

An important aspect of the HOAC model is to analyze and reflect on outcomes, working backward through each step of the model to determine if the various steps were correctly examined and carried out.

The goal to which Nicole's mother gave the highest priority will be used to illustrate how one would progress from the problem statement using the HOAC model.

I. Problem:

Inability to move independently for purposeful activity.

II. Goal:

Nicole will be able to purposefully ambulate forward (supported in an appropriately adapted and adjusted wheeled walker with trunk support) at least 10 feet in less than 5 minutes within 3 months.

III. Hypothesis:

It is hypothesized that the reason Nicole has not achieved any means of independent mobility to date is because there has never been a comprehensive intervention plan that includes

1. Adaptive equipment that is carefully selected, well adapted, and adjusted to provide the necessary postural support for upright mobility and
2. A behavior management program that is focused, incremental in its progression, appropriately reinforced, and consistently carried out at home and at school

IV. Reassessment:

If this hypothesis is true, then 3 months after implementing a comprehensive intervention plan with the elements described, Nicole should be able to achieve the stated goal. Working from a consultation model, the therapist would assess the appropriate implementation of intervention strategies on a weekly basis, talking with family members and school personnel and making adjustments in the program as necessary. Elements of the assessment would include the distance Nicole is able to walk, whether her function in typical environments improves as a result, and the meaning of the goal to Nicole and her caretakers.

V. Intervention Strategy:

Intervention will include several components: assistive technology and behavior modification in an indirect model of service delivery by the physical therapist. The equipment selected for Nicole is a front-leaning walker–gait trainer manufactured by Rifton. She is suspended over a wheeled frame with trunk support with freedom of movement at the hips and legs to allow reciprocal stepping. The walker comes with forearm supports to facilitate weight bearing in the upper extremity. With her arms strapped in a flexed position, flexor tone dominated throughout and Nicole was unable to stand even with maximal assist from the physical therapist (Fig. 4–12*A*). Instead, the forearm supports were removed, and she was allowed to use her arms to facilitate extension, permitting functional weight bearing (Fig. 4–12*B*). Nicole is accustomed to having a tray with all her adaptive equipment, and a tray was custom-fitted to the walker in an attempt to ease some apparent apprehension and give her a place to rest her arms, if needed (Fig. 4–12*C*). The walker provides trunk support, helps to reduce the weight Nicole must accept on her legs, and accentuates the translation of motor behavior to mobility—all with safety.

A structured behavioral program is developed based on the MOVE curriculum.[54] First, the task of walking is broken down into component tasks or skills: an ability to bear weight, to shift weight, and to flex one leg and swing it forward while maintaining weight on the other. Then a structured format is used to measure and score the various prompts that Nicole currently requires to walk with a walker. Finally, a process for reducing the prompts in an incremental manner is developed. This information is shared with the center-based staff and the parents and forms the basis for communication about specific, well-defined behaviors and how their attainment will be progressed over time. The structured program promotes consistency between environments and among caregivers, and change is both measurable and meaningful to all involved.

VI. Intervention Tactics:

The physical prompts required for Nicole to stand and walk are categorized, defined, and scored according to a system in the MOVE curriculum. Six categories of prompts are identified and scored (zero to 5) based on the amount of assistance required—from

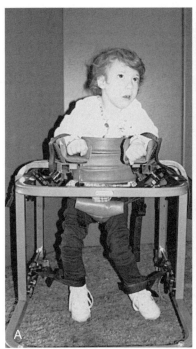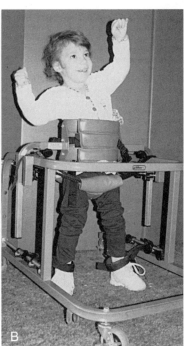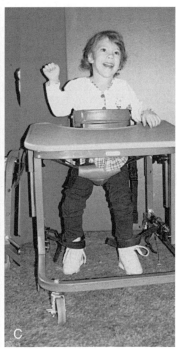

FIGURE 4–12. *A,* In the wheeled walker with her forearms strapped to the supports, Nicole's posture is dominated by flexor tone throughout and she is unable to bear weight even with a maximal assist from a therapist facilitating knee extension. The forearm supports work well for many children, but not for Nicole. *B,* Free of the forearm supports, Nicole uses her arms in almost pivot prone posture to facilitate extension throughout. She is happy and able to support full weight in stance. Reciprocal movement needed for stepping is difficult. *C,* Walker adapted with a tray (something Nicole is accustomed to on all her adaptive equipment) that gives her a place to rest her arms.

independent (zero) to greatest intervention (5). Nicole required prompts for walking as follows:

Category of Prompt	Type of Prompt	Score
Top-down prompt	Trunk level	3
Center-out prompt	Trunk	5
Body segment control	Hips	1
Amount of prompt	Requires support to maintain weight bearing	5
Type of prompt	Mechanical (i.e., walker)	5
Prompt position	Behind	5

These scores are transferred to a prompt reduction plan grid that establishes a common mode of communication, a systematic way to reduce prompts until independence is achieved, and a system for measuring progress.

This system is incorporated into a behavior program that establishes a schedule for frequent and consistent practice with meaningful reinforcement of desired behaviors on Nicole's part. In Nicole's situation, reinforcement is the encouragement and praise of her peers and caregivers because she is motivated by social reinforcement.

The program was designed to be carried out initially by educational staff at the center with the hope that the parents would agree to provide additional practice opportunities at home. The physical therapist monitored the program in an indirect service model, helping to solve problems and make adjustments as necessary.

VII. Analysis and Reflection on Outcomes:

If this program is successful, some monitors (reassessment at 6-, 9-, and 12-month intervals) will need to be put in place to ensure that there is not a natural regression in the functional use of newly acquired independent mobility. If the program is not successful, then working backward, one would look first at the assessment method chosen. Were the right parameters being assessed to measure functionally significant change? Were the tactics carried out correctly and on a consistent basis? Were the tactics appropriate to the strategy as established? Was the strategy effective in addressing the causes of the problems identified in the hypothesis? Was the equipment appropriately adapted? Would Nicole walk better with another person assisting instead of with a walker? Might that be at least a transitional stage? Was the reinforcement adequate to motivate her? Would Nicole benefit from a trial use of NMES to increase strength in the proximal leg muscles? Does the problem carry adequate significance for Nicole and those involved in her care to invest the energy required to address the problem? Would physical therapy provided in a direct model by a physical therapist or physical therapist assistant contribute to improved outcomes?

Other problems identified as having high priority for Nicole would be addressed in a similar way. It may seem to be a cumbersome process, but for a child with multiple disabilities, it is critical to focus the intervention, to address goals that are functional, to structure intervention so that there is consistency, and to plan a reassessment strategy so that documentation of outcomes justifies continued professional involvement.

CONCLUSION

Decision making for the development of care plans for the focus population is a challenging process, complicated by the complex interplay of the pathophysiology in multiple systems. Families of these children experience considerable stress, which might be described as a state of chronic sorrow and will tax their financial and personal resources. A long list of professionals and agencies involved in the care of the child challenges the systems of communication and the efficient, effective establishment of assessment and intervention plans. As physical therapists we find ourselves questioning the traditional neurofacilitation model, yet without clear guidance about how the motor control model applies to children with limited intelligence who may lack motivation to move. Successful interventions require consistent, structured programs, seemingly endless repetition, and, above all, patience. Health-related problems, too, often intervene to set back hard-won achievements, and gravity is a relentless and ever-present force whose impact increases as the child grows. Caring for and about this population demands extra insight, creativity, resourcefulness, and patience. The reward is a family with a reduced burden of care to enable greater enjoyment of their child in meaningful social activities.

RESOURCES

Many groups, both governmental and nongovernmental, have a significant impact on citizens in the United States affected either directly or indirectly by mental retardation. Several deserve mention as valuable resources for professionals and families:

Association for Retarded Citizens (National Headquarters, 500 East Border Street, Suite 300, Arlington, TX 76010), the largest national voluntary health organization, comprising more than 300,000 parents, educators, and professionals. Influential as a political lobby group for public policy issues. Telephone: 817-261-6003; web site: http://www.thearc.org.

American Association on Mental Retardation, previously the American Association on Mental Deficiency (444 North Capitol Street, NW, Suite 846, Washington, DC 20001), a multidisciplinary organization of professional practitioners and researchers. Responsible for the publication of the research journal *American Journal of Mental Deficiency; Mental Retardation*; the *AAMR Monograph Series*; and the *Manual on Terminology and Classification in Mental Retardation*. Telephone: 202-387-1968; web site: http://www.aamr.org.

Council for Exceptional Children (1920 Association Drive, Reston, VA 22091), comprising approximately 70,000 teachers. Has made significant contributions to the education of individuals with cognitive disabilities. Telephone: 703-620-3660; web site: http://www.cec.sped.org.

President's Committee on Mental Retardation (U.S. Department of Health and Human Services, Washington, DC 20201), acts in an advisory capacity to the President and the Secretary of Health and Human Services on matters relating to programs and services for persons with mental retardation. Comprising 21 citizen members, appointed by the President, and six public members, who meet quarterly. Annual reports and other publications are available to the public. Telephone: 202-619-0634.

REFERENCES

1. Humphrey H: *Quoted in* The Problem of Mental Retardation. President's Committee on Mental Retardation. DHEW Publication No. (OHDS) 79-21021. US Department of Health, Education, & Welfare, Washington, DC, 1979.
2. Baroff GS: Mental Retardation: Nature, Cause, and Management, 2nd ed. Hemisphere, New York, 1986.
3. Luckasson R, Coulter DL, Polloway EA, et al: Mental Retardation: Definition, Classification, and Systems of Supports. American Association on Mental Retardation, Washington, DC, 1992.
4. Association for Retarded Citizens Introduction to mental retardation. Available at: http://thearc.org/faqs/mrqa.html.
5. Grossman HJ (ed): Classification in Mental Retardation. American Association on Mental Deficiency, Washington, DC, 1983.
6. The Problem of Mental Retardation. President's Committee on Mental Retardation. DHEW Publication No. (OHDS) 79-21021. US Department of Health, Education, & Welfare, Washington, DC, 1979.
7. Weisz JR, Zigler E: Cognitive development in retarded and nonretarded persons: Piagetian tests of the similar sequence hypothesis. Psychol Bull 86:831, 1979.
8. Campbell SK: The child's development of functional movement. *In* Campbell SK, Vander Linden DW, Palisano RJ (eds): Physical Therapy for Children. WB Saunders, Philadelphia, 1994, p 7.
9. Zigler E, Balla D: Mental Retardation: The Developmental Difference Controversy. Lawrence Erlbaum, Hillsdale, NJ, 1982.

10. Menolascino FJ, McCann BM: Mental Health and Mental Retardation: Bridging the Gap. University Park, Baltimore, 1983.
11. Matson JL, Frame CL: Psychopathology among mentally retarded children and adolescents. *In* Kazdin AE (series ed): Clin Psychol Psychiatry Series 6:13, 1986.
12. Mulick JA, Kedesdy JH: Self-injurious behavior: Its treatment and normalization. Ment Retard 26:223, 1988.
13. National Institutes of Health: Treatment of destructive behaviors in persons with developmental disabilities. NIH Consens Statement Online 7(9):1–15, 1989 [cited May 20, 1996]. Available at: http://text.nlm.nih.gov/nih/edc/www/75txt.html.
14. Symons FJ, Thompson T: A review of self-injurious behavior and pain in persons with developmental disabilities. *In* Bray NW (ed): International Review of Research in Mental Retardation, vol 21. Academic, San Diego, 1997, p 69.
15. Baumeister AA: Origins and control of stereotyped movements. *In* Meyers CE (ed): Quality of Life in Severely and Profoundly Mentally Retarded People: Research Foundations for Improvement. American Association on Mental Deficiency, Washington, DC, 1978, p 353.
16. Short RJ: Stereotypical behaviors and handicapping conditions in infants and children. Top Early Child Special Ed 10:122, 1990.
17. MacLean W, Baumeister A: Observational analysis of the stereotyped mannerisms of a developmentally delayed infant. Appl Res Ment Retard 2:257, 1981.
18. Baranek GT, Foster LG, Berkson G: Tactile defensiveness and stereotyped behaviors. Am J Occup Ther 51:91, 1997.
19. Cermak SA, Daunhauer LA: Sensory processing in the postinstitutionalized child. Am J Occup Ther 51:600, 1997.
20. Lovaas IO, Newsom C, Hickman C: Self stimulatory behavior and perceptual reinforcement. J Appl Behav Anal 20:45, 1987.
21. Reisman JE: Using a sensory integrative approach to treat self injurious behavior in an adult with profound mental retardation. Am J Occup Ther 47:403, 1993.
22. Hutt C, Hutt SJ, Lee D, Ounstead C: Arousal and childhood autism. Nature 204:908, 1964.
23. Berkson G, Gutermuth L, Baranek GT: Relative prevalence and relations among stereotyped and similar behaviors. Am J Ment Retard 100:137, 1995.
24. Dunn W, Westman K: The Sensory Profile: The performance of a national sample of children without disabilities. Am J Occup Ther 51:25, 1997.
25. Dunn W: Performance of typical children on the Sensory Profile: An item analysis. Am J Occup Ther 48: 967, 1994.
26. Stevenson RE, Massey RJ, Schroer RJ, et al: Preventable fraction of mental retardation: Analysis based on individuals with severe mental retardation. Ment Retard 34:182, 1996.
27. Coulter DL: Prevention as a form of support: Implications for the new definition. Ment Retard 34:108, 1996.
28. Comptroller General of the United States: Preventing Mental Retardation. Publication HRD.77.37. General Accounting Office, Washington, DC, 1977.
29. President's Committee on Mental Retardation: A Presidential Forum—Citizens with Mental Retardation and Community Integration. Forum Proceedings. Department of Health and Human Services, Office of Human Development Services, Washington, DC, 1989.
30. Capute AJ, Shapiro BK, Palmer FB: Spectrum of developmental disabilities: Continuum of motor dysfunction. Orthop Clin North Am 12:3, 1981.
31. Conley RW: The Economics of Mental Retardation. John Hopkins, Baltimore, 1973.
32. Bruininks RH: Physical and motor development of retarded persons. *In* Ellis NR (ed): International Review of Research in Mental Retardation, vol. 7. Academic, New York, 1974, p 203.
33. Cleland CC, Powell HC, Talkington LW: Death of the profoundly retarded. Ment Retard 9:36, 1971.
34. Rempel GR, Colwell SO, Nelson RP: Growth in children with cerebral palsy fed via gastrostomy. Pediatrics 82:857, 1988.
35. Tecklin JS: Pulmonary disorders in infants and children and their physical therapy management. *In* Tecklin JS (ed): Pediatric Physical Therapy, 2nd ed. JB Lippincott, Philadelphia, 1994, p 249.
36. Fraser BA, Hensinger RN, Phelps JA: A Professional's Guide: Physical Management of Multiple Handicaps. Paul H Brookes, Baltimore, 1987.
37. Hoffer MM, Bullock M: The functional and social significance of orthopaedic rehabilitation of mentally retarded patients with cerebral palsy. Orthop Clin North Am 12:185, 1981.
38. Pettitt B: Surgery of the lower extremity in cerebral palsy: Considerations and approaches. Arch Phys Med Rehabil 57:443, 1976.

39. Lindsey RW, Drennan JC: Management of foot and knee deformities in the mentally retarded. Orthop Clin North Am 12:107, 1981.
40. Samilson RL: Orthopaedic surgery of the hips and spine in retarded cerebral palsy patients. Orthop Clin North Am 12:83, 1981.
41. Rinsky LA: Perspectives on surgery for scoliosis in mentally retarded patients. Orthop Clin North Am 12:113, 1981.
42. Askin GN, Hallett R, Hare N, Webb JK: The outcome of scoliosis surgery in the severely physically handicapped child: An objective and subjective assessment. Spine 22:44, 1997.
43. Anderson AL: Dental care for persons with mental retardation. *In* President's Committee on Mental Retardation: A Presidential Forum—Citizens with Mental Retardation and Community Integration. Forum Proceedings. Department of Health and Human Services, Office of Human Development Services, Washington, DC, 1989, p 187.
44. Gadow KD, Poling AD: Pharmacotherapy and Mental Retardation. Little, Brown, College-Hill, Boston, 1988.
45. Baldessarini RJ: Drugs and the treatment of psychiatric disorders. *In* Gilman AG, Rall TW, Nies AS, Taylor P (eds): The Pharmacological Basis of Therapeutics, 8th ed. Pergamon, Elmsford, NY, 1990, p 383.
46. Ault MM: Some educational implications for students with profound disabilities at risk for inadequate nutrition and the nontherapeutic effects of medication. Ment Retard 32:200, 1994.
47. Aman MG: Recent studies in psychopharmacology in mental retardation. *In* Bray NW (ed): International Review of Research in Mental Retardation, vol. 21. Academic, San Diego, 1997, p 113.
48. Richardson SA, Koller H, Matz M: Seizures and epilepsy in a mentally retarded population. Appl Res Ment Retard 1:123, 1981.
49. Ciccone CD: Pharmacology in Rehabilitation, 2nd ed. FA Davis, Philadelphia, 1996.
50. Baer MT, Kozlowski BW, Blyler EM, et al: Vitamin D, calcium and bone status in children with developmental delay in relation to anticonvulsant use and ambulatory status. Am J Clin Nutr 65:1042, 1997.
51. Piaget J: The Origins of Intelligence in Children. International Universities, Norton, NY, 1963.
52. Kahn JV: Relationship of Piaget's sensorimotor period to language acquisition of profoundly retarded children. Am J Ment Defic 79:640, 1975.
53. Uzgiris, Hunt: Uzgiris-Hunt Scales of Infant Psychological Development. University of Illinois Press, Urbana, Ill, 1978.
54. Bidabe L, Lollar JM: MOVE/Mobility Opportunities Via Education. MOVE International, Bakersfield, Calif, 1990.
55. Campbell SK, Wilhelm IJ: Anthropometric characteristics of young children with cerebral palsy. Pediatr Phys Ther 1:105, 1989.
56. Reilly S, Skuse D: Characteristics and management of feeding problems of young children with cerebral palsy. Dev Med Child Neurol 34:379, 1992.
57. Stevenson RD, Roberts CD, Vogtle L, et al: The effects of non-nutritional factors on growth in cerebral palsy. Dev Med Child Neurol 37: 124, 1995.
58. Stuberg WA: Bone density changes in non-ambulatory children following discontinuation of passive standing programs. Abstract. *In* Proceedings of American Academy of Cerebral Palsy and Developmental Medicine Conference, Louisville, Ky, Oct 10, 1991. American Academy of Cerebral Palsy and Developmental Medicine, Rosemont, Ill, 1991.
59. Gisel E, Patrick J: Identification of children with cerebral palsy unable to maintain a normal nutritional state. Lancet 1:283, 1988.
60. Shapiro BK, Green P, Krick J, et al: Growth of severely impaired children: Neurological versus nutritional factors. Dev Med Child Neurol 28:729, 1986.
61. Pollitt E: Developmental impact of nutrition on pregnancy, infancy, and childhood: Public health issues in the United States. In Ellis NR (ed): International Review of Research in Mental Retardation, vol 15. Academic, New York, 1988, p 33.
62. Lee J, Lyne ED: Pathologic fractures in severely handicapped children and young adults. Abstract. Paper No. 274. Presented at the annual meeting, Scientific Program, American Academy of Orthopaedic Surgeons, New Orleans, Feb 10, 1990. Available at: www.aaos.org/wordhtml/anmiit90/scipro/pp274.htm.
63. O'Toole MT (ed): Miller-Keane Encyclopedia and Dictionary of Medicine, Nursing, and Allied Health, 6th ed. WB Saunders, Philadelphia, 1997.
64. Harrell RF, Capp RH, Davis DR, et al: Can nutritional supplements help mentally retarded children: An exploratory study. Proc Natl Acad Sci USA 78:574, 1981.
65. Hitchings WD: Megavitamins and diet. *In* Feingold B, Bank C (eds): Developmental Disabilities of Early Childhood. Charles C Thomas, Springfield, Ill, 1978, p 92.

66. Cohen WI: Health care guidelines for individuals with Down syndrome. Down Syndrome Q 1:1, 1996.
67. Lakin KC, Prouty B, Smith G, Braddock D: Nixon goal surpassed two-fold. Ment Retard 34:67, 1996.
68. Conroy JW: The small ICF/MR program: Dimensions of quality and cost. Ment Retard 34:13, 1996.
69. Strauss D, Kastner TA: Comparative mortality of people with mental retardation in institutions and the community. Am J Ment Retard 101: 26, 1996.
70. Pub L No. 94-142. The Education for All Handicapped Children Act of 1975. 89 Stat. 773-796.
71. Pub L No. 99-457: Education of the Handicapped Act Amendments of 1986. 100 Stat. 1145-1177.
72. Pub L No. 102-119: Individuals with Disabilities Education Act of 1990. 105 Stat. 587-608.
73. Pub L No. 105-17: Individuals with Disabilities Education Act Amendments of 1997. 111 Stat. 37-157.
74. Sweeney JK, Heriza CB, Markowitz R: The changing profile of pediatric physical therapy: A 10-year analysis of clinical practice. Pediatr Phys Ther 6:113, 1994.
75. Heriza CB: Pediatric physical therapy: Reflections of the past and visions for the future. Pediatr Phys Ther 6:105, 1994.
76. Eyman RK, Miller C: Introduction: A demographic overview of severe and profound mental retardation. *In* Meyers CE (ed): Quality of Life in Severely and Profoundly Retarded People: Research Foundations for Improvement. American Association on Mental Retardation, Washington, DC, 1978, p ix.
77. Minnes P: Family stress associated with a developmentally handicapped child. *In* Bray NW (ed): International Review of Research in Mental Retardation, vol 15. Academic, New York, 1988, p 195.
78. Sparling JW, Kolobe TH, Ezzelle L: Family-centered intervention. *In* Campbell SK, Vander Linden DW, Palisano RJ (eds): Physical Therapy for Children. WB Saunders, Philadelphia, 1994, p 823.
79. McCubbin HI, Figley CR: Stress and the Family: Coping with Normative Transitions. Brunner/Mazel, New York, 1983.
80. Beckman PJ: Influence of selected child characteristics on stress in families of handicapped infants. Am J Ment Defic 88:150, 1983.
81. Barabas G, Matthews W, Zumoff P: Care-load for children and adults with severe cerebral palsy. Dev Med Child Neurol 34:25, 1992.
82. Wikler L, Wasow M, Hatfield E: Chronic sorrow revisited: Parents vs professional depiction of the adjustment of parents of mentally retarded children. Am J Orthopsychiatry 51:63, 1981.
83. Berndt J, Falconer A: Physical therapy in the educational setting. *In* Campbell SK (ed): Pediatric Neurologic Physical Therapy, 2nd ed. Churchill Livingstone, New York, 1992, p 361.
84. Bundy AC: Assessment and intervention in school-based practice: Answering questions and minimizing discrepancies. Phys Occup Ther Pediatr 15(2):69, 1995.
85. Effgen SK: The educational environment. *In* Campbell SK, Vander Linden DW, Palisano RJ (eds): Physical Therapy for Children. WB Saunders, Philadelphia, 1994, p 847.
86. Long T: Administrative issues. *In* Long TM, Cintas HL (eds): Handbook of Pediatric Physical Therapy. Williams & Wilkins, Baltimore, 1995, p 207.
87. Sparling J: Transdisciplinary approach with developmentally delayed children. Phys Occup Ther Pediatr 1(2):3, 1980.
88. Woodruff A, McGonigel MI: Early intervention team approaches: The transdisciplinary model. *In* Jordan JB, Gallagher JJ, Hutinger PL, et al (eds): Early Childhood Special Education: Birth to Three. Council for Exceptional Children, Reston, Va, 1988, p 166.
89. Rainforth B, York J, MacDonald C: Collaborative Teams for Students with Severe Disabilities. Paul H Brookes, Baltimore, 1992.
90. Rothstein JM, Echternach JL: Hypothesis-oriented algorithm for clinicians: A method for evaluation and treatment planning. Phys Ther 66:1388, 1986.
91. Echternach JL, Rothstein JM: Hypothesis-oriented algorithms. Phys Ther 69:559, 1989.
92. Law M, Baptiste S, McCall MA, et al: The Canadian Occupational Performance Measure: An outcome measure for occupational therapy. Can J Occup Ther 57:82, 1990.
93. Gould J: The use of the Vineland Social Maturity Scale, the Merrill-Palmer Scale of Mental Tests (non-verbal items) and the Reynell Developmental Language Scales with children in contact with the services for severe mental retardation. J Ment Defic Res 21:213, 1977.

94. Long TM: Measurement. *In* Long TM, Cintas HL (eds): Handbook of Pediatric Physical Therapy. Williams & Wilkins, Baltimore, 1995, p 55.

95. King-Thomas L, Hacker BJ (eds): A Therapist's Guide to Pediatric Assessment. Little, Brown, Boston, 1987.

96. Rothstein JM, Echternach JL: Primer on Measurement: An Introductory Guide to Measurement Issues. American Physical Therapy Association, Alexandria, Va, 1993.

97. Fewell RR, Glick MP: Observing play: An appropriate process for learning and assessment. Inf Young Child 5:35, 1993.

98. Casby MW: Symbolic play. I: A developmental framework. Infant-Toddler-Interv 1:219, 1991.

99. Linder TW: Transdisciplinary Play-Based Assessment. Paul H Brookes, Baltimore, 1990.

100. Linehan SA, Brady MP, Chi-en H: Ecological versus developmental assessment: Influences on instructional expectations. J Assoc Persons Severe Handicaps 16:146, 1991.

101. McCuller WR, Salzburg DL: The functional analysis of imitation. *In* Ellis NR (ed): International Review of Research in Mental Retardation, vol 11. Academic, New York, 1982, p 285.

102. Altman R, Ralkington LW, Cleland CC: Relative effectiveness of modeling and verbal instruction on severe retardates' gross motor performance. Psychol Rep 31:685, 1972.

103. Ritvo ER, Ornitz EM, La Franchi S: Frequency of repetitive behaviors in early infantile autism and its variants. Arch Gen Psychiatry 19:341, 1968.

104. Silverman FH: Communication for the Speechless. Prentice-Hall, Englewood Cliffs, NJ, 1980.

105. National Institutes of Health: Research Plan for the National Center for Medical Rehabilitation Research. NIH Publication No. 93-3509. National Institutes of Health, Bethesda, Md, 1993.

106. Pope AN, Tarlov AR (eds): Disability in America: Toward a National Agenda for Prevention. National Academy, Washington, DC, 1991.

107. Blasco PA: Primitive reflexes: Their contribution to the early detection of cerebral palsy. Clin Pediatr 33:388, 1994.

108. Capute AJ, Palmer FB, Shapiro BK, et al: Primitive Reflex Profile: Quantification of primitive reflexes in infancy. Dev Med Child Neurol 26:375, 1984.

109. Capute AJ, Accardo PJ, Vining EPG, et al: Primitive Reflex Profile. University Park, Baltimore, 1978.

110. Fetters L: Foundations for therapeutic intervention. *In* Campbell SK (ed): Pediatric Neurologic Physical Therapy, 2nd ed. Churchill Livingstone, New York, 1991, pp 19–32.

111. Westcott SL, Lowes LP, Richardson PK: Evaluation of postural stability in children: Current theories and assessment tools. Phys Ther 77:629, 1997.

112. Fiorentino MR: A Basis for Sensorimotor Development: Normal and Abnormal. Charles C Thomas, Springfield, Ill, 1981.

113. Chandler LS, Andrews MS, Swanson MW: Movement Assessment of Infants. Chandler, Andrews and Swanson, Rolling Bay, Wash, 1980.

114. Bohannon RW, Smith MB: Interrater reliability of a modified Ashworth scale of muscle spasticity. Phys Ther 69:225, 1989.

115. Connolly B: Testing in infants and children. *In* Hislop HJ, Montgomery J (eds): Daniels and Worthingham's Muscle Testing: Techniques of Manual Examination. WB Saunders, Philadelphia, 1995, p 235.

116. Russell DJ, Rosenbaum PL, Gowland C, et al: Gross Motor Function Measure. Gross Motor Measures Group, Hamilton, Ontario, 1990.

117. Russell DJ, Rosenbaum PL, Cadman DT: The Gross Motor Function Measure: A means to evaluate the effects of physical therapy. Dev Med Child Neurol 31:341, 1989.

118. Harris SR, Harthrun Smith L, Krukowski L: Goniometric reliability for a child with spastic quadriplegia. J Pediatr Orthop 5:348, 1985.

119. Stuberg WA, Fuchs RH, Miedaner JA: Reliability of goniometric measurements of children with cerebral palsy. Dev Med Child Neurol 30:657, 1988.

120. Cooke PH, Cole WG, Carey RP: Dislocation of the hip in cerebral palsy: Natural history and predictability. J Bone Joint Surg Br 71:441, 1989.

121. Scrutton D: Early management of hips in cerebral palsy. Dev Med Child Neurol 31:108, 1989.

122. Cusick BD, Stuberg WA: Assessment of lower extremity alignment in the transverse plane: Implication for management of children with neuromotor dysfunction. Phys Ther 72:3, 1992.

123. Sherrill C: Posture training as a means of normalization. Ment Retard 18:135, 1980.

124. Kendall HO, Kendall FP: Developing and maintaining good posture. Phys Ther 48:319, 1968.

125. Kitchener RF: Piaget's Theory of Knowledge: Genetic Epistemology and Scientific Reason. Yale University Press, New Haven, Conn, 1986.

126. Ayres AJ: Sensory Integration and Learning Disorders. Western Psychological Services, Los Angeles, 1976.

127. Fisher AG, Murray EA: Introduction to sensory integration theory. *In* Fisher AG, Murray EA, Bundy AC (eds): Sensory Integration: Theory and Practice. FA Davis, Philadelphia, 1991, p 3.

128. Montgomery PC: Assessment and treatment of the child with mental retardation: Guidelines for the public school therapist. Phys Ther 61:1265, 1981.

129. Ayres AJ: Sensory Integration and Praxis Tests. Western Psychological Services, Los Angeles, 1989.

130. Ayres AJ: Southern California Postrotary Nystagmus Test. Western Psychological Services, Los Angeles, 1975.

131. Hillegass EA: Cardiopulmonary assessment. *In* Hillegass EA, Sadowsky HS (eds): Essentials of Cardiopulmonary Physical Therapy. WB Saunders, Philadelphia, 1994, p 553.

132. Rothman JG: Effects of respiratory exercises on the vital capacity and forced expiratory volume in children with cerebral palsy. Phys Ther 58:421, 1978.

133. Watchie J: Cardiopulmonary Physical Therapy: A Clinical Manual. WB Saunders, Philadelphia, 1995.

134. Bjure J, Berg K: Dynamic and static lung volumes of school children with cerebral palsy. Acta Paediatr Scand Suppl 204:35, 1970.

135. Anwar F: Cognitive deficit and motor skill. *In* Ellis D (ed): Sensory Impairments in Mentally Handicapped People. College-Hill, San Diego, 1986, p 169.

136. Stout JL: Gait: Development and analysis. *In* Campbell SK, Vander Linden DW, Palisano RJ (eds): Physical Therapy for Children. WB Saunders, Philadelphia, 1994, p 79.

137. Thelen E, Ulrich BD, Jensen JL: The developmental origins of locomotion. *In* Woollacott MH, Shumway-Cook A (eds): Development of Posture and Gait Across the Life Span. University of South Carolina Press, Columbia, SC, 1989, p 25.

138. Illingworth RS: The Development of the Infant and Young Child, 5th ed. Churchill Livingstone, Philadelphia, 1974.

139. Shapiro BK, Accardo PJ, Capute AJ: Factors affecting walking in a profoundly retarded population. Dev Med Child Neurol 21:369, 1979.

140. Molnar GE, Gordon SU: Cerebral palsy: Predictive value of selected clinical signs for early prognostication of motor function. Arch Phys Med Rehabil 57:153, 1976.

141. Watt JM, Robertson CM, Grace MG: Early prognosis for ambulation of neonatal intensive care survivors with cerebral palsy. Dev Med Child Neurol 31:766, 1989.

142. Montgomery P, Gauger J: Sensory dysfunction in children who toe walk. Phys Ther 58:1195, 1978.

143. Tardieu C, Lespargot A, Tabary D, Bret M: Toe-walking in children with cerebral palsy: Contributions of contracture and excessive contraction of triceps surae muscle. Phys Ther 69:656, 1989.

144. Montgomery PC, Richter E: Sensorimotor Integration for the Developmentally Disabled Child: A Handbook. Western Psychological Services, Los Angeles, 1980.

145. Arvedson JC, Brodsky L: Pediatric Swallowing and Feeding: Assessment and Intervention. Communication/Therapy Skill Builders, a division of The Psychological Corporation, Harcourt Brace, San Antonio, Tex, 1993.

146. Morris SE, Klein MD: Pre-Feeding Skills: A Comprehensive Resource for Feeding Development. The Psychological Corporation, Communication/Therapy Skill Builders, a division of Harcourt Brace, San Antonio, Tex, 1987.

147. Tuchman DN, Walter RS: Disorders of Feeding and Swallowing in Infants and Children: Pathophysiology, Diagnosis and Treatment. Singular, San Diego, 1994.

148. Wolf LS, Glass RP: Feeding and Swallowing Disorders in Infancy: Assessment and Management. Communication/Therapy Skill Builders, a division of The Psychological Corporation, Harcourt Brace, San Antonio, Tex, 1992.

149. Lunnen KY: Children with severe and profound retardation. *In* Campbell SK (ed): Pediatric Neurologic Physical Therapy, 2nd ed. Churchill Livingstone, New York, 1991, p 251.

150. Barnard K: Nursing Child Assessment Feeding Scale. Nursing Child Assessment Satellite Training. University of Washington, School of Nursing, Child Development and Mental Retardation Center, Seattle, 1985.

151. Campbell M, Kelsey K: The PEACH survey: A nutrition screening tool for use in early intervention programs. J Am Diet Assoc 94:1156, 1994.

152. Pub L No. 100-407: Technology-Related Assistance for Individuals with Disabilities Act of 1998. 102 Stat. 1044.

153. Carlson SJ, Ramsey C: Assistive technology. *In* Campbell SK, Vander Linden DW, Palisano RJ (eds): Physical Therapy for Children. WB Saunders, Philadelphia, 1994, p 621.

154. Hutt ML, Gibby RG: The Mentally Retarded Child: Development, Training, and Education, 4th ed. Allyn & Bacon, Boston, 1979.
155. Sparrow SS, Balla DA, Cicchetti DV: Vineland Adaptive Behavior Scales. American Guidance Service, Circle Pines, Minn, 1984.
156. Haley SM, Faas RM, Carter WJ, et al: Pediatric Evaluation of Disability Inventory: Examiner's Manual. The Psychological Corporation, Communication/Therapy Skill Builders, a division of Harcourt Brace, San Antonio, Tex, 1989.
157. Palisano RJ, Campbell SK, Harris SR: Clinical decision-making in pediatric physical therapy. *In* Campbell SK, Vander Linden DW, Palisano RJ (eds): Physical Therapy for Children. WB Saunders, Philadelphia, 1994, p 183.
158. Bobath K, Bobath B: Diagnosis and assessment of cerebral palsy. *In* Pearson PH, Williams CE (eds): Physical Therapy Services in the Developmental Disabilities. Charles C Thomas, Springfield, Ill, 1972, p 31.
159. Semans S: The Bobath concept in treatment of neurological disorders: A neurodevelopmental treatment. Am J Phys Med 46:732, 1967.
160. Stockmeyer SA: An interpretation of the approach of Rood to the treatment of neuromuscular dysfunction. Am J Phys Med 46:900, 1967.
161. Stockmeyer SA: A sensorimotor approach to treatment. *In* Pearson PH, Williams CE (eds): Physical Therapy Services in the Developmental Disabilities. Charles C Thomas, Springfield, Ill, 1972, p 186.
162. Ostrosky KM: Facilitation versus motor control. Clin Manage 10: 34, 1990.
163. Norton Y: Neurodevelopment and sensory integration for the profoundly retarded multiply handicapped child. Am J Occup Ther 29:93, 1975.
164. Clark FA, Miller LR, Thomas JA, et al: A comparison of operant and sensory integrative methods on developmental parameters in profoundly retarded adults. Am J Occup Ther 32:86, 1978.
165. Ottenbacher K: Developmental implications of clinically applied vestibular stimulation: A review. Phys Ther 63:1, 1983.
166. Ottenbacher K, Short MA, Watson PJ: The effects of a clinically applied program of vestibular stimulation on the neuromotor performance of children with severe developmental disorders. Phys Occup Ther Pediatr 1(3):1, 1981.
167. Magrun WM, Ottenbacher K, McCue S, et al: Effects of vestibular stimulation on the spontaneous use of verbal language in developmentally delayed children. Am J Occup Ther 35:101, 1981.
168. Bright T, Bittick K, Fleeman B: Reduction of self-injurious behavior using sensory integrative techniques. Am J Occup Ther 35:167, 1981.
169. Evans RG: The reduction of hyperactive behavior in three profoundly retarded adolescents through increased stimulation. American Association for the Education of S & P Han Rev 4:259, 1979.
170. Arendt RE, MacLean WE, Baumeister AA: Critique of sensory integration therapy and its application in mental retardation. Am J Ment Retard 92:401, 1988.
171. Ottenbacher K: Research in sensory integration: Empirical perceptions and progress. *In* Fisher AG, Murray EA, Bundy AC (eds): Sensory Integration: Theory and Practice. FA Davis, Philadelphia, 1991, p 385.
172. Carr JH, Shepherd RB: The motor learning model for rehabilitation. *In* Carr JH, Shepherd RB (eds): Movement Science Foundations for Physical Therapy in Rehabilitation. Aspen, Rockville, Md, 1987, p 31.
173. Bradley NS: Motor control: Developmental aspects of motor control in skill acquisition. *In* Campbell SK, Vander Linden DW, Palisano RJ (eds): Physical Therapy for Children. WB Saunders, Philadelphia, 1994, p 39.
174. Shumway-Cook A, Woollacott MH: Motor Control: Theory and Practical Applications. Williams & Wilkins, Baltimore, 1995.
175. Horn EM, Warren SF, Jones HA: An experimental analysis of neurobehavioral motor intervention. Dev Med Child Neurol 37:697, 1995.
176. Atwater SW: Should the normal motor developmental sequence be used as a theoretical model in pediatric physical therapy? *In* Lister MJ (ed): Contemporary Management of Motor Control Problems: Proceedings of the II STEP Conference. Foundation for Physical Therapy, Alexandria, Va, 1991, p 89.
177. McEwen I: Mental retardation. *In* Campbell SK, Vander Linden DW, Palisano RJ (eds): Physical Therapy for Children. WB Saunders, Philadelphia, 1994, p 459.
178. Skinner BF: Science and Human Behavior. Macmillan, New York, 1953.
179. Whitman TL, Scibak JW, Reid DH: Behavior Modification with the Severely and Profoundly Retarded: Research and Application. Academic, New York, 1983.

180. Yule W, Carr J (eds): Behaviour Modification for People with Mental Handicaps, 2nd ed. Croom Helm, London, 1980.

181. Hill LD: Contributions of behavior modification to cerebral palsy habilitation. Phys Ther 65:341, 1985.

182. Gardner WI, Gracher JL: Use of behavioral therapies to enhance personal competency: A multimodal diagnostic and intervention model. *In* Bouras N (ed): Mental Health in Mental Retardation: Recent Advances and Practices. Cambridge University Press, Cambridge, 1994, p 205.

183. Bragg JH, Houser C, Schumaker J: Behavior modification in the treatment of children with cerebral palsy. Phys Ther 55:860, 1975.

184. Westervelt VD, Luiselli JK: Establishing standing and walking behavior in a physically handicapped, retarded child. Phys Ther 55:761, 1975.

185. Banks SP: Behavior therapy with a boy who had never learned to walk. Psychother Theory Res Pract 5:150, 1968.

186. Chandler LS, Adams MA: Multiply handicapped child motivated for ambulation through behavior modification. Case report. Phys Ther 52:399, 1972.

187. Hester SB: Effects of behavior modification on the standing and walking deficiencies of a profoundly retarded child. Case report. Phys Ther 61:807, 1980.

188. Kolderie ML: Behavior modification in the treatment of children with cerebral palsy. Phys Ther 51:1083, 1971.

189. Loynd J, Barclay A: A case study in developing ambulation in a profoundly retarded child. Behav Res Ther 8:207, 1970.

190. Miller H, Patton M, Henton K: Behavior modification in a profoundly retarded child: A case report. Behav Ther 2:375, 1971.

191. Rice HK, McDaniel MW, Denney SL: Operant conditioning techniques for use in the physical rehabilitation of mentally retarded patients. Phys Ther 48:342, 1968.

192. Garber NB: Operant procedures to eliminate drooling behavior in a cerebral palsied adolescent. Dev Med Child Neurol 13:641, 1971.

193. Daniels LE, Sparling JW, Reilly M, Humphry R: Use of assistive technology with young children with severe and profound disabilities. Infant-Toddler Interv 5:91, 1995.

194. Mann WC, Lane JP: Assistive Technology for Persons with Disabilities: The Role of Occupational Therapy. American Occupational Therapy Association, Rockville, Md, 1991.

195. Domaracki LS, Robinson-Dassel K, Hamilton DW, Goldstone F: Evaluation of biofeedback for improving head and trunk position in children with multiple, severe disabilities. Ped Phys Ther 2:192, 1990.

196. Bertoti DB, Gross AL: Evaluation of biofeedback seat insert for improving active sitting posture in children with cerebral palsy: A clinical report. Phys Ther 68:1109, 1988.

197. Ball TS, McCrady RE, Hard AD: Automated reinforcement of head posture in two cerebral palsied retarded children. Percept Mot Skills 40:619, 1975.

198. Silverstein L: Biofeedback with young cerebral palsied children. *In* Feingold B, Bank C (eds): Developmental Disabilities of Early Childhood. Charles C Thomas, Springfield, Ill, 1978, p 142.

199. Maloney FP, Kurtz PA: The use of a mercury switch head control device in profoundly retarded, multiply handicapped children. Phys Occup Ther Pediatr 2(4):11, 1982.

200. Leiper CI, Miller A, Lang J, et al: Sensory feedback for head control in cerebral palsy. Phys Ther 61:512, 1981.

201. Ball TS, Combs T, Rugh J, et al: Automated range of motion training with two cerebral palsied retarded young men. Ment Retard 15:47, 1977.

202. Skrotzky K, Gallenstein JS, Osternig LR: Effects of electromyographic feedback training on motor control in spastic cerebral palsy. Phys Ther 58:547, 1978.

203. Ball TS, McGrady RE: Automated finger praxis training with a cerebral palsied retarded adolescent. Ment Retard 13:41, 1975.

204. Frielander BZ, Kamin P, Hesse GW: Operant therapy for prehension disabilities in moderately and severely retarded young children. Train Sch Bull (Vinel) 71:101, 1974.

205. Nwaobi IM, Smith PD: Effect of adaptive seating on pulmonary function of children with cerebral palsy. Dev Med Child Neurol 28: 351, 1986.

206. Pierson SH, Katz DI, Tarsy D: Botulinum toxin A in the treatment of spasticity: Functional implications and patient selection. Arch Phys Med Rehabil 77:717, 1996.

207. Perske R, Clifton A, McLean B et al (eds): Mealtimes for Severely and Profoundly Handicapped Persons: New Concepts and Attitudes, 2nd ed. University Park, Baltimore, 1986.

208. Langley MB: A developmental approach to the use of toys for facilitation of environmental control. Phys Occup Ther Pediatr 10(2):83, 1990.

209. Presperin J: Seating systems: the therapist and rehabilitation engineering team. Phys Occup Ther Pediatr 10(2):17, 1990.
210. Miedaner JA: The effects of sitting positions on trunk extension for children with motor impairment. Pediatr Phys Ther 2:11, 1990.
211. Danquah SA: The effect of Danquah Communication System Boards on maladaptive behaviors among individuals with severe intellectual impairment and non-verbal communication skills. Int J Rehabil Res 19:143, 1996.
212. McEwen IR: Assistive positioning as a control parameter of social-communicative interactions between students with profound multiple disabilities and classroom staff. Phys Ther 72:634, 1992.
213. Wilson JM: Selection and use of adaptive equipment for children. Totline 6:4, 1980.
214. Stuberg WA: Considerations related to weight-bearing programs in children with developmental disabilities. Phys Ther 72:35, 1992.
215. Knutson LM, Clark DE: Orthotic devices for ambulation in children with cerebral palsy and myelomeningocele. Phys Ther 71:947, 1991.
216. Bertoti DB, Stanger M, Betz RR, et al: Percutaneous intramuscular functional electrical stimulation as an intervention choice for children with cerebral palsy. Pediatr Phys Ther 9:123, 1997.
217. Reed B: The physiology of neuromuscular electrical stimulation. Pediatr Phys Ther 9:96, 1997.
218. Pape KE: Therapeutic electrical stimulation (TES) for the treatment of disuse muscle atrophy in cerebral palsy. Pediatr Phys Ther 9:110, 1997.
219. Whitaker K: Self-care with TES. PT OT Today 4:8, 1996.
220. Comeaux P, Patterson N, Rubin M, Meiner R: Effect of neuromuscular electrical stimulation during gait in children with cerebral palsy. Pediatr Phys Ther 9:103, 1997.
221. Carmick J: Use of neuromuscular electrical stimulation and a dorsal wrist splint to improve the hand function of a child with spastic hemiparesis. Phys Ther 77:661, 1997.
222. Carmick J: Clinical use of neuromuscular electrical stimulation for children with cerebral palsy. Part I: Lower extremity. Phys Ther 73:505, 1993.
223. Carmick J: Clinical use of neuromuscular electrical stimulation for children with cerebral palsy. Part II: Upper extremity. Phys Ther 73:514, 1993.
224. Hazlewood ME, Brown JK, Rowe PJ, et al: The use of therapeutic electrical stimulation in the treatment of hemiplegic cerebral palsy. Dev Med Child Neurol 36:661, 1994.
225. Stanger M, Bertoti D (eds): Special Issue: An Overview of Electrical Stimulation for the Pediatric Population. Pediatr Phys Ther 9(3):1997.
226. Cloud HH: Expanding roles for dietitians working with persons with developmental disabilities. J Am Diet Assoc 97:129, 1997.

Chapter

5

Myelodysplasia (Spina Bifida)

M a r t h a   C .   G r a m , MS, PT

The term *myelodysplasia* encompasses a group of congenital defects of the spinal cord and, in some cases, the brain that vary widely in functional outcomes. The congenital defect is most commonly referred to as *spina bifida,* meaning "split spine."[1] Individuals within the group vary in terms of the degree of injury to the nervous system, genetic inheritance, and social and financial support to cope with the inherent problems associated with the defect. Each of these factors necessarily plays a part in the therapist's and the family's development of a habilitation plan for the affected individual.

The goal of this chapter is to provide the clinician with criteria to assist in making the decisions required to develop an appropriate habilitation plan for an individual child or adult with spina bifida. The chapter discusses the impairments common to children with spina bifida as a group and, more specifically, both the impairments and the functional limitations common to different lesion levels. Assessment methods and tools the therapist should consider using to develop an appropriate treatment plan are discussed, and treatment options for each lesion level are outlined. In addition, case studies illustrate the problems commonly faced by the clinician and the family. The final section of the chapter deals with secondary conditions that can develop as the child becomes an adult, some of which may be prevented if appropriate early care is provided to the individual.

Myelodysplasia is not unique to modern humans; it has been found in ancient mummies[2] and has been studied for years. Once thought to be equivalent to spinal cord injury in children, study has shown that this congenital defect has consequences even before birth, such as the development of clubfeet and hydrocephalus, which result in problems not associated with spinal cord injury acquired after birth.[2, 3]

Before the 1970s, many children born with spina bifida died from complications of hydrocephalus or kidney damage.[2, 4] In the late 1960s and early 1970s, however, recognition of the importance of early spinal lesion closure, the development of the shunt to control hydrocephalus, and better methods of emptying the bladder to prevent urinary reflux increased the survival rate of children with myelodysplasia.[4] Because of the poor survival rate of infants before the 1970s, few adults with spina bifida who are 40 to 50 years old are alive today. With the advent of improved control of hydrocephalus and the prevention of kidney damage, however, most infants born since 1970 have survived and have the potential for living far into adulthood.

With an increased survival rate, the need for improved habilitation methods for children and adults with spina bifida became apparent and has been an area of increased study in the past 20 years. As bracing and adaptive equipment appropriate for children with spina bifida are developed, debate concerning when and how to use this technology is the topic of ongoing discussion.[5, 6]

ETIOLOGY, PATHOLOGY, AND IMPAIRMENT
Etiology

Although spina bifida has been known for hundreds of years, its cause remains unclear but probably involves a combination of genetic and environmental factors.[4, 7] During pregnancy, spina bifida can be detected with a test for alpha-fetoprotein levels. High alpha-fetoprotein levels at 15 to 20 weeks' gestation can indicate the presence of spinal cord defects but can also indicate other major congenital defects, the presence of twins, fetal death, and various other complications.[8–12] It is therefore essential that the diagnosis of spina bifida by means of the alpha-fetoprotein level always be confirmed by a follow-up ultrasound examination. Research suggests that the prenatal anatomic spinal lesion level visualized by high-resolution ultrasonography can accurately predict the neuromotor level and functional motor outcome in the first years for infants diagnosed with spina bifida prenatally.[13] Early detection has led to improved parent counseling before delivery and to an increased number of deliveries of children with spina bifida by cesarean section. Delivery by cesarean section, in turn, improves neurologic outcomes and avoids damage to the mother and infant from the infant's enlarged head.[14] Data suggest that some of the damage to exposed neural elements of the spinal cord occurs in utero, further suggesting the possible need for surgical repair of the lesion in utero.[15]

Genetic links for spina bifida are not as direct as those for congenital defects such as muscular dystrophy, but its incidence does appear to be elevated for some groups relative to others. The lowest incidence has been reported for African blacks (1 in 10,000) and the highest for Celts (Irish-Scottish-Welsh, 1 in 80).[2] Hispanic populations have also been reported to have a high incidence. The incidence of myelodysplasia in the United States has been reported to be from 0.4 to 0.9 per 1000 births depending on the region of the country.[2] Environmental factors, such as alcohol or drug abuse, have been studied but are not well documented as possible etiologic factors.[2] Folic acid supplements have been shown in randomized controlled trials to prevent 50 to 70 percent of neural tube defects.[16] Because of these findings, the U.S. Public Health Service has recommended that all women capable of becoming pregnant consume 0.4 mg of folic acid per day,[17] and the U.S. Food and Drug Administration issued a rule on March 5, 1996, requiring the addition of folic acid to all enriched cereal grain products.[18]

Pathology and Impairment

Study of the embryology of neural tube and brain formation suggests that the neural tube defect probably occurs between 22 and 28 days of gestation (Fig. 5–1).[2, 4, 7] During this period, the spinal cord is forming by a process called *neurulation,* in which the ectoderm folds over the primitive spinal cord to form a tube. Failure of the ectoderm to complete this folding process can occur anywhere from spinal levels C1 to S2 and results in one of several types of spina bifida.

Two common types of myelodysplasia, meningocele and myelomeningocele, are named for the types of tissues involved in the defect. Figure 5–2 illustrates a meningocele, an incomplete closure somewhere along the spinal column, which has allowed the meninges lining the spinal canal and their spinal fluid to bulge out, forming an external "sac." This type of lesion generally does not disturb nerve conduction to muscles of the lower extremities because it does not include extruded neural elements. Figure 5–3 illustrates a myelomeningocele, the same type of incomplete closure of the spinal column, but in this lesion, neural elements as well as the meninges have protruded into the sac. The neural elements incorporated in the external sac may be complete and connected to innervated structures or may be malformed and disconnected. This second type of myelodysplasia is the type most commonly seen by physical therapists because lower extremity paralysis and sensory loss accompany the involvement of neural elements and habilitation for mobility is frequently needed. With the use of new microneurosurgical techniques for closure of the spinal defect, more neural elements can be preserved.[19, 20] The primary impairments caused by a loss of neural innervation to lower extremity and pelvic structures is thereby limited, and functional outcomes are improved. Table 5–1 summarizes the impairments, functional limitations, and disabilities that can be anticipated for children with spina bifida.

SECONDARY IMPAIRMENTS

The vertebral level at which the neural tube defect occurs determines the extent of neurologic damage and loss of muscle activity and determines what kind of challenges

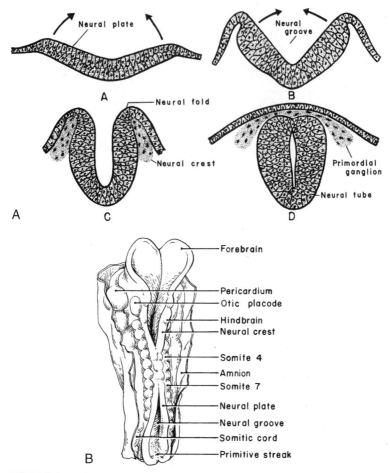

FIGURE 5–1. *A,* Cross-sections of the ectoderm of human embryos at successively later stages to illustrate the origin of the neural tube and neural crest, which forms the dorsal root ganglia and the sympathetic nerve ganglia. *B,* Dorsal view of a human embryo showing the closure of the neural tube between somites 4 and 7 and the open neural folds anterior and posterior to this. (*A* and *B,* From Villee CA: Biology, 5th ed. Philadelphia, Saunders College, 1995, p. 484.)

the parents and the child will have to meet for the child to attain mobility and independence in daily life.[21] Multiple body systems are affected by malformation of the neural tube and must be addressed to prevent secondary conditions from developing. The secondary conditions and functional abilities that the child acquires will depend both on the initial damage to the spine and brain and on the types of intervention that are available to the child from the medical team, the family, and society in general.

Brain and Spinal Cord

As mentioned earlier, one of the main causes of death in children with spina bifida before 1970 was hydrocephalus. Hydrocephalus results from excessive cerebrospinal fluid (CSF) in the ventricles of the brain. Uncontrolled hydrocephalus can cause the infant's ventricles to enlarge and the head to grow to a very large size, compromising brain development and sensorimotor function.[3, 22–24] Stein and Schut reported that 80 percent of the children with spina bifida that they studied developed hydrocephalus.[3] The Arnold-Chiari malformation, although not the only cause of hydrocephalus, is one of the primary causes.[2, 7, 25] In this condition, the circulation of CSF is blocked by a

Meningocele

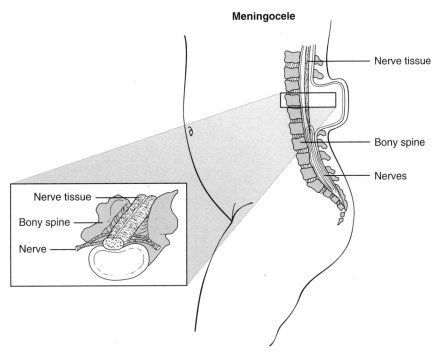

FIGURE 5–2. Meningocele, a form of myelodysplasia in which the sac contains meninges and spinal fluid but no neural elements. (Redrawn from Meyers GJ, Cerone SB, Olson AL: A Guide for Helping the Child with Spina Bifida. Springfield, Ill, Charles C Thomas, 1981, p 114. Courtesy of Charles C Thomas, Publisher, Ltd, Springfield, Ill.)

Myelomeningocele

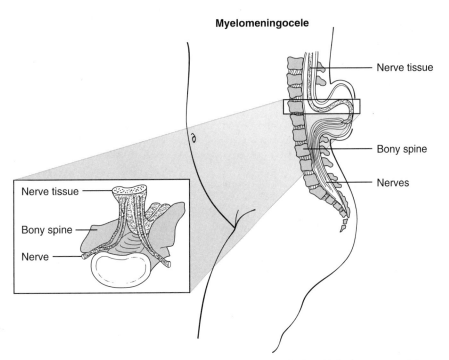

FIGURE 5–3. Myelomeningocele, a form of myelodysplasia in which the sac contains meninges, spinal fluid, and neural elements resulting in loss of neural innervation of structures below the level of the sac. (Redrawn from Meyers GJ, Cerone SB, Olson AL: A Guide for Helping the Child with Spina Bifida. Springfield, Ill, Charles C Thomas, 1981, p 115. Courtesy of Charles C Thomas, Publisher, Ltd, Springfield, Ill.)

Impairments, Functional Limitations, and Disabilities to Be Anticipated and Managed as Part of the Habilitation Plan for Persons with Spina Bifida

TABLE 5–1

Impairment	Functional Limitation	Disability
1. Disruption of nerve conduction below lesion level; loss of muscle function	1a. Reduced mobility and delay of motor milestones	1a. Reduced ability to keep up physically with peers; social isolation
	1b. Tendency to become obese	1b. Limited access to public areas not wheelchair accessible
2. Joint contractures due to muscle imbalance	2a. Limited ability to wear bracing or stand	2a. Difficulty reaching materials at home or work
	2b. Development of pressure sores due to bracing or long periods of sitting	2b. Loss of school or work time while healing
3. Decreased bone density related to decreased standing	3. Fractures, kyphosis, scoliosis requiring immobility	3. Possible requirement of time off from school or work, reducing learning time and job opportunities
4. Loss of sensation with reduced ability to respond to touch, pain, and temperature	4a. Decubitus ulcers requiring positioning limits (i.e., prone) or hospitalization	4a. Same as 2b and 3
	4b. Reduced ability to sense cold with increased risk of frostbite in cold weather	4b. Possible limitation of participation in outdoor activities
	4c. Reduced proprioception for balance in standing	4c. Reduced ability to walk and need for wheelchair-accessible entrances
5. Loss of bowel and bladder sphincter control; flaccid bladder; urinary reflux and kidney damage	5a. Incontinence and need for diapering or self-catheterization	5a. Social embarrassment and decreased interaction with peers
	5b. Urinary tract infections	5b. Requirement for medication and loss of school time; special bathroom facilities at school or work
6. CNS malformations: Arnold-Chiari malformation; hydrocephalus, often requiring shunt	6a. Shunt malfunctions and periods of illness	6a and b. Difficulty with learning; limited job opportunities; loss of school time due to shunt revisions; reduced time for learning
	6b. Visual perceptual problems	
	6c. "Cocktail party" speech	6c. Ineffective social interaction
7. Hydromyelia	7. Decreased muscle function or increased spasticity with loss of previously learned motor skills	7a. Time lost from school or work
		7b. Depression due to loss of skills

CNS, central nervous system.

downwardly displaced brainstem into the foramen magnum, which partially occludes the outlet for CSF to the spinal cord. To bypass the blockage, a shunt (plastic catheter) is surgically inserted into the lateral ventricles to drain excess fluid from the ventricles, generally into the peritoneal cavity. Because the shunt is a foreign body, it can become blocked by tissue overgrowth at either end or become twisted and fail to function. When this occurs, it must be surgically repaired or replaced. Signs of shunt failure may include headache, fever, altered speech, decreased visual acuity, increased spasticity in innervated muscles, and decreased school performance.[7]

In addition to hydrocephalus, the child with spina bifida may develop hydromyelia, in which increased CSF pressure causes enlargement of the spinal canal.[4] In some cases, increased pressure on the cord leads to increased tone in innervated muscles. Increased tone may also occur if the child develops a tethered cord. This may occur if adhesions develop around the lesion closure site or if bony spurs that protrude into the spinal canal develop. In either case, tearing of the spinal cord may occur as the child grows, producing either increased paralysis or increased muscle tone.[7, 20] A comparison of muscle activity found during initial assessment of the child's neural lesion level with current muscle strength gives the clinician data to determine if changes in muscle activity have occurred; such changes indicate that the child should be sent to the neurosurgeon for evaluation.

Cognition and Perception

Standardized testing of children with spina bifida (Wechsler Intelligence Scale for Children, Bender-Gestalt Test, Frostig Developmental Test of Visual Perception) has shown that cognitive deficits and visual perceptual problems are associated with spina bifida, particularly in children with hydrocephalus who have a shunt.[22, 24] Because the incidence of hydrocephalus is as high as 80 percent in children with spina bifida,[3] cognitive and visual perceptual problems need to be routinely assessed, particularly at the time of school placement. Tew and Laurence, using the Frostig scale, found that children with spina bifida who had shunts had difficulty with visual-motor organization, whereas those without hydrocephalus had normal perceptual abilities.[24] On reading and math tests, children with shunts had significantly lower scores than control subjects without spina bifida or peers with spina bifida who did not have shunts. The subjects' visual perceptual scores were found to be strongly correlated ($r = .82$, $P < .001$) with overall intelligence scores, making it unclear whether the low visual perceptual score was a separate issue or a reflection of overall lower intelligence. Therapists should keep in mind that a child with spina bifida may have visual perceptual difficulties that make the learning of motor sequences especially difficult.

Children with spina bifida may exhibit "cocktail party syndrome,"[23] in which the child has a good vocabulary but fails to use language with appropriate meaning. The child may "chatter" for social interaction without engaging in meaningful communication. This chatter may cause listeners who are unaware of this verbal characteristic to believe that such children are understanding more than they really are. Studies suggest that children with shunted hydrocephalus have delayed recall of recently acquired words and slowed acquisition of new words.[26] As with all the impairments and functional limitations described to this point, a child will exhibit some characteristics and not others, making careful individualized assessment essential to the development of an appropriate plan of care.

Physical Impairments

Constraints for the child with spina bifida in the development of gross motor skills and lower extremity function include (1) paralysis of lower extremity muscles, (2) the fact that the child lives in a gravity environment that demands muscular strength for support and movement of the body, and (3) the fact that the child is growing under these conditions. The child's spinal cord lesion level determines which muscles of the lower extremities are innervated, and, in turn, the pattern of muscle innervation determines what joint contractures may develop and what types of bracing may be needed to both prevent deformity and promote mobility.[21, 27] Contracture development can be an active process due to muscle imbalance, or it can be the result of the chronic positions of paralyzed limbs and the trunk in response to the pull of gravity. As a result, the higher the child's lesion, the more motor and contracture problems there are to anticipate and prevent if possible.

Other secondary problems that may occur with a loss of muscle power and decreased mobility include a diminished ability to physically keep up with and interact with peers, a tendency to use fewer calories because of diminished physical activity, and a resulting tendency to become obese. The reduced lower extremity bone density and the increased risk of fracture for a child with spina bifida have been associated with decreased weight bearing and with postsurgical complications.[28–32] Fractures have also been noted to occur most in those children with high-level lesions and extensive paralysis,[28, 31] who before the advent of standing frames and parapodiums had the least opportunity to be upright and weight bearing.

In addition to muscle loss, the child with spina bifida loses sensation to skin and joints below the lesion level.[7, 32] This loss of sensation to skin often results in decubitus ulcers from prolonged sitting, or in pressure areas or sores from rubbing of skin over environmental surfaces, such as rough ground, carpeting, or floor heating outlets, or from ill-fitting orthoses. Reduced muscle activity in the lower extremities decreases circulation in the legs, and a loss of sensation decreases awareness of cold, resulting in increased probability of frostbite in the toes.

Loss of joint sensation in the ankles, knees, or hips also reduces the normal sensory input from joints, which has been shown to be important for balance in standing.[33–35] This loss of joint sensation, combined with a loss of hip muscle activity for joint support and movement, greatly reduces the resources available to the child for the development of sitting or standing balance. Loss of joint sensation, in particular, makes the child more reliant on visual and vestibular inputs for the development of balance and restricts the ability to develop the more mature pattern of balance regulation that normally depends more on sensation from the ankles and hips than on vision.[33–35] Loss of muscular support at the hip and ankle, in turn, reduces the child's ability to dynamically adjust balance without the outside support of adaptive equipment (i.e., bracing, walker, corner chair) even when the child senses a loss of balance.

Bowel and Bladder

Because sphincter muscles are innervated by sacral-level nerves, a majority of children with spina bifida have bowel and bladder incontinence. Constipation is prevented by the use of stool softeners and a regular toilet schedule. Bladder incontinence is generally monitored using urine cultures and a yearly intravenous pyelogram to ensure that urinary tract infection and reflux do not occur and damage the kidneys.[4, 7, 36] Clean intermittent self-catheterization to fully empty the bladder and to prevent reflux is started when the child is mature enough to learn the procedure or is taught to the parents if reflux is a problem before the child is old enough to learn the procedure.[7, 36–38] Clean intermittent self-catheterization has been effective in reducing the number of urinary tract infections the child experiences over time and has reduced the problem of kidney damage due to reflux.[36, 37] The child's readiness for learning self-catheterization and the methods used to teach it are important criteria for the success of the program.[38] Children as young as 4 or 5 years of age have been able to learn the beginning procedures for self-catheterization, but true independence in the procedure may not occur until the child has a sense of time and can determine by reading a clock the time at which catheterization is needed each day. The catheterization program is usually initiated by the urologist and nursing staff of the specialty clinic in which the child is seen. Parents' and school nurses' questions about the child's catheterization program should be directed to the child's specialty clinic for answers to promote consistency in the method.

INTERDISCIPLINARY TEAM

Thorough assessment of the child is critical if the clinician is to make appropriate decisions while developing a physical habilitation plan for an individual child. Without sufficient information regarding the child's physical status, the family's goals, and the treatment plans of other members of the medical team, one team member might make decisions that are inappropriate or are in conflict with the goals of other members of the habilitation team. Because the child with spina bifida has many body systems that are affected by the spinal lesion and must be monitored by a variety of specialists, the best management is done through a specialty center.[39] The specialty center can promote opportunities for the many specialists involved in the patient's treatment to consult with one another and coordinate the necessary interventions. Research has shown that children not followed by a medical team develop more secondary impairments than those who have closely monitored care.[40] It is therefore important that any therapist from the community who sees the child for treatment be aware of and in contact with the child's specialty center. Because most children with spina bifida are managed medically by a team of specialists, it is important to be aware of assessments and recommendations of all team members. Both center and community personnel should share the results of their decision making in written communications.

A number of specialists are typically included in the clinic team. Most children are followed by a neurosurgeon for monitoring of head size and shunt function. The team also usually includes an orthopedist who monitors the need for splinting or bracing to prevent deformity or to assist with standing and mobility, or both, or who performs corrective surgery if contractures develop. The urologist provides monitoring of bladder and kidney function, medications for urinary tract infection, and surgical intervention if required. The nurse coordinator is a vital member of most specialty teams and is often a key component of urologic management by teaching children self-catheterization methods. This team member may be responsible for coordinating the patient's visits so that the number of trips to clinics is reasonable and maximizes the number of specialists seen at the most appropriate time. Pediatricians and physical therapists are part of some but not all clinical teams. The pediatrician monitors general health and in some clinics plays a major role in the coordination of care. Although the role of the physical therapist is vital to the treatment of children with spina bifida, not all teams have a therapist as a regular part of the team, instead relying on community therapists or therapists who rotate through the clinic to provide care. When a physical therapist is a part of the team, community therapists seeing the child will find the specialty center therapist to be helpful in communicating therapeutic needs to other members of the specialty team.

PHYSICAL THERAPY ASSESSMENT

Family Goals and Knowledge

An initial step in a physical therapy assessment should be an interview with the parents and the client if the client is younger than 18 years, or with the client alone if the client is older than 18 years. Parental and family involvement remain important for the older client, but the client must be the decision maker. Interviewing parents helps to identify the family's information needs, support structure, and goals. As the therapist gains understanding of what the parents and the family know and what they want for the child, the therapist is better able to develop a plan that helps to meet the family's goals. The physical therapist will not be able to supply all the information or knowledge that the family and child will need but should be aware of what the needs are and where the family may need to go for further information or consultation in order to empower them for effective decision making. In turn, the family will be more likely to understand and be active in the habilitation plan for facilitating the child's motor development and mobility.

Assessment of Impairment

Muscle Testing

As part of the therapist's initial assessment, the therapist needs to assess which muscles are intact and of grade 3 (fair) or better strength.[41] Muscle testing is an essential component of the assessment of the child with spina bifida because the number and types of innervated muscles the child retains significantly affect the plan for habilitation. Although the neurosurgeon assigns a lesion level to the child's condition, innervated muscles vary in strength. Although more specific muscle grades can rarely be assigned to muscles in an infant, muscles of grade 3 or better can be determined by observation of the infant in the supine, prone, and supported sitting positions. For example, with the child in the supine position, one can assess whether the child has grade 3 hip flexors by observing whether the child kicks spontaneously during a play session. Quadriceps muscle activity can be observed with the child in the supine or supported sitting position with the feet dangling by noting if the child is able to extend the knee against gravity. When an infant is in the prone position with the legs dangled over the therapist's lap, hip extensor activity can be observed as the infant raises the head or as an older infant reaches for a toy. The observant therapist can determine which major muscle groups are active by careful observation of the infant in play.

Muscles of grade 2 or less strength are more difficult to assess than those of grade 3, but muscles with minimal strength can have a deforming effect on the infant's limbs if ignored. Electrical stimulation was used in the clinic in which I worked for 8 years to identify innervation in muscles of grade 2 or less. This type of testing was found to be useful in anticipating what types of joint contracture might occur.

As the child reaches school age, more specific muscle testing can be done with more valid results across all grade levels because the child is able to assist by following simple instructions.

Range of Motion

Because imbalance in muscle power around any joint can result in the development of joint contractures,[42, 43] which ultimately affect the child's ability to perform daily motor activities, assessment of the range of motion (ROM) is essential. Assessment of the ROM does not require the degree of cooperation essential to valid muscle testing, so the infant's ROM can be tested with good accuracy. An initial record of the ROM is helpful in determining positioning, exercises, or orthoses needed to prevent deformity from developing or increasing. During passive handling of the infant's or child's limbs, the therapist has the opportunity to determine whether tone in innervated muscles is normal or increased by the degree of resistance to quick stretch. In most cases, the therapist will find normal tone in innervated muscle and flaccid tone in noninnervated muscle. Progression of joint deformities may indicate that the child spends too much time in a particular posture or may reveal an undetected muscle group of grade 2 or less strength. Deformities in flaccid lower extremities or those with unbalanced innervated muscles are difficult to remediate once they have developed, so measures to prevent or reduce the progression of deformity such as manual exercise, splinting, and positioning are important interventions to consider and implement at birth.[7, 42, 44] Specific contractures related to particular lesion levels are discussed later.

Sensation

In addition to assessment of muscle function and ROM, examination of skin sensation in the upper and lower limbs is needed. Skin sensation is difficult to determine in an infant or very young child. The response to a pinprick may be an effective means of assessing skin sensation but is not a good choice for a first assessment. It is often an appropriate caution to assume that the infant has a loss of skin sensation in most areas in which muscle loss is found. As the children reach 5 or 6 years of age, they will be able to be more specific regarding which areas of the lower body have retained sensations of touch, pain, or temperature.

The degree of skin sensation a child has guides the degree to which the therapist and the parents must monitor the infant for pressure sores from bracing and postures assumed daily. Eventually, however, this monitoring of skin should become the child's or young person's responsibility. This process can begin as early as when the children are sitting independently and can inspect their own feet and legs. At this time, the children need to become aware that their legs are a part of their body, despite the fact that they may not have the sensation that gives them this information. Parents can make skin inspection into a game, such as "Who can find a red mark?" This helps the children to become aware of their legs and to assist the parents in monitoring for possible sores before they become serious. As the children become older, they can take on more and more responsibility for checking their skin.

It is necessary for the family and the child to learn to inspect the skin daily in areas of anesthesia to make sure that pressure areas are not developing. It is also important to change a young child's position frequently during the day to prevent pressure areas that can develop into pressure sores and to prevent contracture development. Skin inspection can be used to determine if postures have been maintained for too long a period, because pressure marks in the form of red areas that remain overnight will develop. As children reach 4 or 5 years of age, those spending 50 percent or more of the day sitting should learn to do wheelchair pushups every 20 to 30 minutes to relieve pressure over the ischium for the prevention of decubitus ulcers. Wheelchair seats and chairs used daily should also be equipped with seat cushions designed to relieve pressure.[45, 46] The more sedentary a child is, the more important wheelchair pushups and appropriate seat cushions become, and the more ambulatory the child is, the more important skin inspection of the lower extremities and correctly fitting orthoses are for the prevention of pressure sores. For all children wearing orthoses, regular adjustments of the orthoses for a continued good fit is essential, particularly during growth spurts, to prevent pressure sores and to maximize appropriate function of the orthoses.

Functional Assessment

Motor Development and Function

Children with the same muscle innervation loss may differ in their development of basic gross motor skills as a result of multiple factors including innate personality, the degree of parental encouragement and involvement, and general health. It is therefore important in an initial assessment to determine the child's gross motor skills using an appropriate motor assessment tool. Although none of the current motor assessments for children were specifically designed for children with spina bifida, several can be used as an initial record of motor skills and comparison with norms for children without paralysis. Tests available for infants and young children include the Alberta Infant Motor Scale,[47] the Peabody Developmental Motor Scales,[48] and the Gross Motor Function Measure (GMFM).[49] Each of these tests provides the evaluator with information regarding the child's current gross motor skills, and all but the GMFM provide a comparison with gross motor skills of children of comparable age. For children with spina bifida, it is appropriate to do motor assessment with and without bracing to see in which areas bracing may improve, or in some cases impede, the child's abilities. As an example, the therapist may find that the child is unable to sit independently on the floor without propping when not in bracing but may be able to do so with bracing. This type of information can suggest to the therapist how and when the bracing should be used throughout the child's day or what additional equipment would assist the child to accomplish skill development goals. A gross motor assessment can also help determine when a child may be ready to begin standing and ambulation, which are discussed later. As the child reaches school age, the Pediatric Evaluation of Disability Inventory (PEDI)[50] may be useful for determining in which areas the child is independent and where significant assistance is given or needed for daily mobility, including transfers and community mobility, and for self-care. In addition, the cognitive and behavioral measures of the PEDI are useful to identify appropriate levels of play activity for use in therapy and to suggest areas for which occupational therapy, psychologic, or educational referrals are indicated. If the child has entered school, the psychologic and educational assessment will have been done by the school psychologist at entry, and that data may also be helpful to the therapist.

Balance Assessment

Many of the balance problems that children with spina bifida have become self-evident during the assessment of gross motor and functional motor skills using the motor tests just discussed. Formal assessment of balance, particularly in older children or young adults, may be helpful when determining the support needed for standing or sitting in a wheelchair, or for assessment of job performance needs. Two tests that might be useful, either as they exist or adapted for sitting, are the Functional Reach Test[51] and the Seated Postural Control Measure.[52] When these tests are administered, it must be kept in mind that lower extremity paralysis, particularly of hip extensors, has a large impact on the child's ability to control sitting or standing posture. Intervention to produce improvements in balance would then be expected to be in the form of finding means of compensations for the loss of muscle activity. Compensations might include bracing, walkers, or specific seat modification for the child's or adult's wheelchair.

The sum of these assessments in conjunction with information from other members of the medical team and from parents should give the therapist sufficient data to initiate a plan for physical habilitation. The assessments discussed provide the therapist with baseline data regarding muscle activity and sensation for the anticipation of contractures and pressure sores; the current level of motor skill and readiness for the development of new skills; areas of need for home programming and family education; and the need for orthoses or other technology to compensate for the loss of muscle activity. It is expected that the initial plan will require updates and reassessment on a regular basis as the child grows, develops motor abilities, and has changing needs for daily life activities.

PHYSICAL THERAPY
Neonatal Period and Early Infancy

The therapist who has the opportunity to be involved in the child's treatment plan from birth needs to be aware of the family's initial interaction with the medical team and the infant. Because the spinal defect is immediately apparent on delivery (and in many cases now even before delivery), the family of the child with spina bifida has little time to bond with the infant before they must make many surgical decisions. Usually within the first hours and certainly within the first few days, the parents are asked to give consent for closure of the spinal lesion. In some cases, the mother who delivers her infant in a rural or nonspecialty hospital may be separated from her infant for a period of time while the infant is transported to a tertiary care hospital. Decisions such as closure may have to be made with the infant in one hospital, the mother in a second, and the father torn by the decision to be with the infant or stay with his wife. All these early decisions often leave parents feeling traumatized. All medical staff, including the physical therapist, must keep this in mind when providing service. During the time that the infant is hospitalized, parents may also have to consider the placement of a shunt to relieve pressure on the infant's brain resulting from hydrocephalus. The infant's head and ventricle sizes are monitored from birth to determine whether hydrocephalus is present and, if so, whether it is progressing. If enlargement of the ventricles causes the head size to increase beyond the 90th percentile for age, a shunt may be recommended and inserted during the initial hospitalization. Reports have indicated that 80 to 90 percent of children with spina bifida who have hydrocephalus require shunting.[2, 4] Although not always as immediate a decision as that to close the spinal lesion, the process of deciding whether a shunt is needed begins early.

The therapist's role should also begin during the child's initial hospitalization. When the neurosurgeon following the infant has determined that the closure of the spinal lesion is stable, the therapist should be available to promote appropriate handling and positioning in the nursery to prevent the development of joint contractures. Education for both the parents and the hospital staff may be needed depending on the staff's experience. The parents may need encouragement to hold their infant by reassurance that they can do so without a risk of hurting the child further. The types of positioning the infant will need depend on the lesion level and the residual muscle power. Specific positioning needs for different lesion levels are discussed later, but in general, many infants have developed a flexed hip and knee posture and occasionally clubfeet as a result of their position in utero and their degree of paralysis. For infants without spina bifida, the flexed posture of the neonate resolves over time as the infant kicks and uses the hip and knee extensors. The infant with spina bifida, even one with a low lumbar or sacral lesion, frequently does not have the active hip extensor power needed to counteract the fetal flexed posture. This is especially true if the child has active hip flexors. It is then necessary to teach the family and hospital staff ROM exercises for hip and knee flexors and to provide guidelines for monitored prone positioning during the day. To fulfill the need for some extended time with gravity stretch to hip flexors, parents can use prone positioning during daytime periods when the child's breathing status can be monitored. ROM exercises for the ankles may also be recommended, unless the orthopedic surgeon prescribes early casting to resolve malalignment of the feet.

Splinting, such as abduction splints for hips or removable casts, may be ordered by the orthopedist. It is often helpful for the therapist to reinforce the orthopedist's instructions on how to put on and remove orthotic appliances and to answer questions the family may have regarding the orthoses' purpose. Because parents are frequently overwhelmed by the variety of problems and care instructions they receive, written instructions and repetition of education in ROM and positioning methods at each visit are helpful.

Therapeutic Needs by Level of Spinal Cord Lesion

Because the problems and needs of children with spina bifida are related to the level of their spinal lesion, in this section, for the purpose of describing therapeutic planning, children with spina bifida are divided into four groups according to their lesion level: (1) thoracic lesions, (2) high lumbar lesions (L1–L3), (3) low lumbar lesions (L4–L5), and (4) sacral lesions. Although children within each of the four groups vary, the basic needs and problems for habilitation are similar. Case histories are provided to illustrate the typical course of management. Table 5–2 outlines for the four groups the possible muscle function at each level, possible secondary impairments related to that muscle function, and the types of bracing that may be needed to prevent deformity and to promote mobility. Levels are arranged from the greatest muscle activity loss at the top of the chart to the least muscle activity loss at the bottom.

Thoracic Level Lesions

Muscle Function and Contractures to Be Prevented

Children with spinal cord lesions at T12 or above have no active muscles in the lower extremities and may have a loss of trunk musculature as well, depending on the level of the thoracic lesion. Because spinal nerve damage may or may not be exactly the same for both sides of the body, muscular imbalances between sides may also occur.

As a result of having no active muscular support in the lower extremities, the child's legs tend to respond to the pull of gravity by falling into external rotation (Fig. 5–4), whether the child is prone, supine, or sitting. Because external rotation of the legs

Possible Muscle Function, Possible Secondary Impairments, and Orthotics Needed for Children with Spina Bifida by Lesion Level

TABLE 5–2

Level	Possible Muscle Function*	Possible Secondary Impairments	Orthoses Needed

T6–T12	Upper trunk
	
	No lower extremity muscles
		Kyphoscoliosis
		
		Contractures:
		  Hip abduction
		  Hip external rotation
		
		Clubfeet
			TLSO
			
			AFO
			
			Night splint (leg wraps)
			
			Parapodium

L1–L3	Hip flexors Hip adductors Minimal knee extensors	Hip flexor contractures Hip dislocation Wind drift Scoliosis	Abduction splint Parapodium, early HKAFO, later
L4 L5	Knee extensors Ankle invertors/ dorsiflexors Hip abductors Minimal knee flexors and extensors	Hip flexor contractures Hip dislocation Lumbar lordosis Calcaneovarus	Night splint (abduction) HKAFO KAFO or AFO, later
S1–S2	Knee flexors Hip extensors Ankle evertors/ plantar flexors Toe flexors	Calcaneovarus Toe clawing Heel ulcers	AFO SMO, shoe inserts, or nothing
S3–S5	All muscle activity normal	None	None

*Each lesion level has all the muscle power described in the category or categories above it, in addition to that described in the lesion-level box.

From Badell A: Myelodysplasia. *In* Molnar GE (ed): Pediatric Rehabilitation, 2nd ed. Williams & Wilkins, Baltimore, 1992, p 222.

TLSO, thoracolumbosacral orthosis; AFO, ankle-foot orthosis; HKAFO, hip-knee-ankle-foot orthosis; KAFO, knee-ankle-foot orthosis; SMO, supramalleolar orthosis.

predominates in all postures, external rotation contractures with slight flexion of the knees can develop rapidly. In particular, the tensor fasciae latae muscles tend to shorten and are primary contributors to this problem. In addition, children with thoracic-level lesions have a high incidence of clubfeet at birth and are at high risk for the development of kyphoscoliosis.[4, 7, 31]

The prevention of contractures and deformities should be a part of the habilitation plan. The contractures described previously can limit the use of bracing or other mobility aids, can complicate dressing and transfers, and, in the case of kyphoscoliosis, can compromise sitting stability and the function of internal organs.[7, 53] The development of contractures can be minimized through daily passive ROM exercises, splinting, orthoses, or all of these. At birth, most infants with thoracic lesions do not have fixed contractures and can be put through full ROM exercises without discomfort or excessive pressure. To minimize the development of contractures, a few simple and inexpensive splinting strategies can prevent the infant's legs from falling into external rotation. One strategy

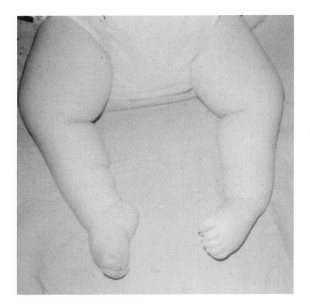

FIGURE 5–4. The typical externally rotated position of the legs of a child with a thoracic lesion as a result of flaccid paralysis and the pull of gravity. (Courtesy of the University of Rochester, Andrew J Kirsch Center, Rochester, NY.)

is to wrap the baby's legs together from hip to knee with a cloth diaper and pin it securely for overnight and naptimes. A second method is to put both of the child's legs into one pajama-bottom leg at night. This method works well with the older infant or child. A full night of correct positioning every 24 hours can maintain range and reduce the chance of contracture development. Lieber's studies on the constant stretch of muscles and joints indicate that the ROM can be maintained with as little as 15 minutes of constant stretch per day and improved with longer periods of time.[42]

The orthopedist may choose to correct foot deformities with serial casting or may suggest passive ROM exercises. When casting has been necessary, the child may need to wear ankle-foot orthoses (AFOs) to prevent recurrence of the contractures. Some clubfoot deformities also require surgery if they are primarily bony malalignments or do not respond to more conservative measures. The orthopedist will also be involved in management of the child's kyphoscoliosis if one develops. As with other forms of scoliosis, most physicians prescribe orthoses to prevent progression of the spinal curve and delay the need for spinal fusion until the child is older. In many cases, however, spinal fusion is required by the early teens. The current procedures for correction of the spinal curve include both an anterior (Dwyer or Zielke instrumentation) and a posterior (Harrington rod or Luque instrumentation) fusion spaced several weeks apart.[19, 53–55] A double procedure has been used because of the bony malformations of the vertebrae that already exist in the spine of the child with spina bifida and result in a need to stabilize anteriorly as well as posteriorly.

Because of a loss of sensation to the lower body, children with thoracic lesions are susceptible to pressure sores from many sources. Pressure sores may develop over the ischium from long periods of sitting, at the toes or knees if the child is allowed to crawl without shoes or protective covering for the legs, and over any part of the body that experiences excessive pressure from orthoses, for example, pressure over the kyphosis from a thoracolumbosacral orthosis or from poorly fitting standing braces. Too much time in any one position without change can be a problem, making skin checks and position changes important to emphasize in parent education.

Motor Development

Despite extensive muscle power loss, almost all children with spina bifida, including those with thoracic-level lesions, learn the basic motor skills of rolling, prone crawling, and moving to a sitting position. The timeline for the accomplishment of these basic motor skills may, however, extend well beyond the time period estimated to be normal for the average child who does not have a physical challenge.

Because of the immediate surgical interventions that are necessary to improve the child's survival and quality of life, parents may be reluctant to handle their newborn with spina bifida in the same ways they would an infant without spina bifida. There is often great concern that they will damage the infant's shunt or lesion site. Although some caution may be necessary during the healing period following the initial surgeries, most infants with spina bifida are born at full term and are reasonably sturdy. Parents need to be encouraged to pick up, hold, and position the child without more caution than would be necessary for any newborn. Observation of any mother's or father's handling of their baby reveals that a great deal of sensory stimulation is provided for the infant through walking with the child held in different positions, speaking or singing to the child who is held in various positions, holding the infant or young child in the air, or dancing with the child in the parent's arms. Because the child with a thoracic lesion will have limited self-mobility, it is important that the parent does not feel that activities that provide sensory stimulation through movement need to be eliminated for fear of damage to the child.

In addition to specific exercises to prevent contractures, parents need to be encouraged to provide "floor time" for the infant. The current use of infant seats, swings, backpacks, and frontpacks sometimes interferes with time on the floor. This time is critical for the infant to develop the postural patterns and control needed for rolling and prone crawling. Research in the area of motor development has demonstrated a link between the initiation of crawling and such perceptual skills as calibrating distances and depth perception.[56] Because research has also shown that visual perceptual skills are most deficient among children with thoracic-level lesions, self-mobility in the form of commando crawling becomes even more important. Rolling and commando crawling may be the only self-propulsion that the child with a thoracic lesion will accomplish without bracing or a wheelchair, so the opportunity to develop these skills is particularly important.

Development of the skill of sitting is often delayed in the child with a thoracic lesion. Most infants move into a sitting position initially by assuming a four-point posture and then dropping backward into the sitting position. The child with a thoracic lesion does not have the hip flexors or adductors needed to assist in maintaining a four-point posture as a precursor to sitting. In most cases, children with a thoracic lesion push backward from a prone-on-hands posture until they have pushed "through" their legs and into a sitting posture. Because the children have no hip extensor or adductor activity, which has been shown to be key in the development of sitting skills by stabilizing the pelvis,[57] sitting is maintained by propping both elbows on the thighs. Unfortunately, the need to prop to remain upright causes the child with a thoracic lesion to be unable to free one hand to reach for any length of time while sitting. The child is also frequently unable to use two hands together for toy manipulation other than what can be done while propping on two elbows. Floor seating such as a corner chair that provides trunk support, or equipment that provides both trunk support and mobility (e.g., a caster cart), can be helpful in providing the child an opportunity to use both hands together to explore and manipulate objects. Because visual perceptual problems and fine motor problems have been identified as significant for children with spina bifida,[58–60] every effort should be made to provide periods of time in which the child is well supported in the upright position so that two-hand manipulation can be accomplished. For the older child, ambulation bracing can serve the function of support for sitting on the floor as well as for walking. The Toronto or Rochester parapodium or the reciprocating gait orthosis (RGO) allows hip flexion and provides support to the pelvis and trunk in long sitting on the floor.[61, 62] Children often find that they are able to reach and use both hands together when sitting with the extra support of their ambulation braces.

Standing and ambulation are realistic goals for children with thoracic lesions, but primarily for exercise and movement within the home or schoolroom. The issue of whether children with thoracic lesions should stand or be exclusive wheelchair users has been studied by several researchers with varied conclusions.[63–66] The benefits of self-movement and weight bearing on the lower extremities to promote bone growth and to reduce the chance of decreased bone density and fracture have justified the use of both types of mobility.[28, 63] Standing also relieves pressure on the ischial tuberosities, a frequent site for the development of decubitus ulcers,[7, 19] and places it on the soles of the feet, which are designed for weight bearing. Standing in a well-fitting orthosis that provides standing with assistance for balance for several hours per day (not necessarily all at once) can also help to alleviate hip external rotation contractures.

For the child with a thoracic lesion, the standing posture can also be one of the positions in which the hands are free if bracing that provides assistance for balance is used.[61, 67] The different types of parapodiums do provide assistance with balance in standing and allow the child to use two hands together in standing. The RGO or other standard hip-knee-ankle-foot orthoses (HKAFOs) can free the hands only if used in conjunction with some type of standing box. Otherwise, the child must hold onto a walker or crutches to maintain an upright stance (Fig. 5–5).

For all children with thoracic-level lesions, a wheelchair will be needed for long-distance and outdoor travel. When a wheelchair is provided depends on the family's needs and goals, as well as the therapist's. Factors that may need to be considered include whether the child has become too large or too old to be comfortable in the more conventional strollers that are available, whether the child has sufficient maturity to propel a wheelchair without danger to the child or to others, and what type of vehicle the family has to transport the child's wheelchair. The child's wheelchair seatback must provide trunk support sufficient to allow hands-free sitting with and without bracing, and the chair must have seat cushions that allow transfers into and out of the chair and yet relieve pressure over the ischium to prevent decubitus ulcers, be lightweight for propelling, and be fitted appropriately initially yet possess the ability to expand with the child's growth over a period of several years. The wheelchair seat should also be wide enough or have removable thigh supports so that the child can use the chair with or without bracing.

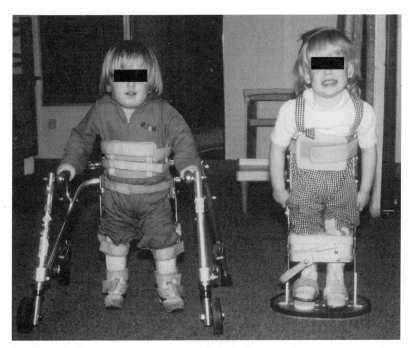

FIGURE 5–5. Two children with spina bifida in the standing position, one in a parapodium (right) and the other in a hip-knee-ankle-foot orthosis and a reverse Rollator walker. (Courtesy of the University of Rochester, Andrew J Kirsch Center, Rochester, NY.)

CASE STUDY

Michelle was seen initially in the nursery several hours after her birth. She was diagnosed with a lesion at T10–T12, with clubfeet and complete loss of muscle activity in the lower extremities. Her spinal lesion was repaired within 24 hours of birth. Her head size was recorded and ventricle size evaluated by magnetic resonance imaging. Although the ventricles were mildly enlarged, a shunt was not necessary in the first days of her life. Michelle's parents were with her daily in the nursery and available for consultation and teaching. As a part of the neurosurgeon's routine postsurgical protocol, Michelle was initially positioned with her hips slightly higher than her head using a roll under her hips. This positioning was discontinued 3 to 4 days after the surgical repair. The therapist met with the parents in the nursery within the first 5 days and discussed with them their understanding of Michelle's physical condition. This was the couple's third child, the other two being born without physical problems. The parents were anxious about Michelle's future but were ready to do anything they could to help her. Both parents expressed a concern that she would not walk or be able to do things for herself. The parents were given information concerning motor development and ideas of what they might expect in terms of orthoses, mobility, and self-care methods. They were also given information about the local Spina Bifida Association parent group and offered an opportunity to speak with the parent of a child with spina bifida selected from a list of volunteers.

After discussion and assessment of Michelle's lower extremities, it was determined that the first step toward physical mobility was to prevent the development of contractures. Michelle's lower extremities tended to fall into external rotation in both the prone and the supine position. Her hips and knees were determined to have full ROM, but both her feet were fixed in a position of plantar flexion and forefoot inversion. Both parents learned passive ROM exercises for Michelle's hips and knees, to be done daily with three of her diaper changes. Her parents also learned to wrap Michelle's legs together with a diaper for nighttime and naps. Michelle's clubfeet were casted by the orthopedist during the time she was hospitalized. Michelle's parents were also encouraged to pick her up and hold her as they had their other two children. The therapist saw the parents daily to review instructions and answer questions until Michelle was discharged to home.

Michelle was released from the hospital after 2 weeks with an appointment to return to the spina bifida clinic each week until casting for her clubfeet was complete. When casting was completed, appointments were made for monthly visits for the first year. At each appointment Michelle was scheduled to see the orthopedist for cast changes, and either the nurse coordinator, pediatrician, or neurosurgeon for head circumference measurement.

The therapist also saw the parents and Michelle at each clinic visit. During each visit, the therapist interviewed the family to determine what Michelle had been doing at home since the last visit and to see if the family had questions about her development or the activities that they had previously been given to do at home. The therapist then assessed Michelle's motor function in terms of her development of gross motor skills such as rolling, crawling, and sitting. Michelle's ROM was also reviewed and, along with her milestones, recorded in clinic notes. Suggestions were given to the family on how to assist Michelle in achieving the next motor stage, such as making sure that she had adequate time on the floor. As motor skills were achieved, the therapist gave the parents new motor activities to work on until the next visit, usually trying to limit the activities to one or two. The therapist's session with the family in this clinic followed the orthopedist's visit to further respond to any questions the family might have about Michelle's visit or the doctor's plan.

Within a few months it became apparent that Michelle's lower extremities were prone to fracture, as she developed two or three hairline fractures at once on several occasions during her first 6 months of life without any definable fall or injury. Nevertheless, motorically she developed head turning, arm waving, raising her head when prone, and rolling from the prone to the supine position and back. By 7 months of age, Michelle had begun prone crawling and was trying to push through her legs into the sitting position.

At 12 months of age, Michelle was sitting by propping on her legs with both elbows and was beginning to try to pull herself up from the floor at the couch in the family's home. Because Michelle was showing signs of wanting to be upright, it was decided that it was time for her to receive a parapodium for standing and beginning ambulation. Once she was fitted with the parapodium, Michelle's parents were given a "wearing" schedule to follow to help Michelle adjust to standing and she was given a parallel pusher (very elongated walker).[59] The parallel pusher gave her the opportunity to begin experimenting with moving inside the walker and pushing the walker back and forth. At the same time, Michelle became part of a group of children wearing parapodiums who met once monthly along with their parents for group instruction on how to use the parapodium and for participation in group motor activities such as rolling, crawling, falling into the parent's arms for practice of balance limits, standing, and ambulation. In addition to therapy instruction, this group gave the children's parents the opportunity to talk with one another about their children and to find out how other parents were managing similar situations. Michelle was also referred for individual physical therapy and occupational therapy at the local Easter Seals Center for weekly sessions to develop ambulation skills, as well as floor skills, in the brace.

During the first year, Michelle had setbacks in motor development as a result of hospitalizations for shunt placement and for surgical repair of her clubfeet. With daily standing, however, Michelle did not have the fracture problems noted before bracing with the parapodium. It was determined that when she sustained hairline fractures she healed more quickly and with greater callus formation if not casted but rather returned to the AFOs fabricated for her after foot surgery with the resumption of daily standing in the parapodium.

By 18 months of age Michelle was ambulating using the parallel pusher, and by 2.5 years she was ambulating in the parapodium without devices between pieces of furniture and on tile floors. By the age of 5 years, she was able to sit and stand from a chair in her parapodium, get up from the floor using the couch or a chair, and "swivel" walk without assistive devices for distances such as down the aisles of the local grocery store. Michelle received a manual wheelchair at 4 years of age and was transported to kindergarten in it. While at school, however, she wore her parapodium and ambulated around her classroom and school halls. Her motor progress was interrupted briefly by a shunt revision at 5 years of age. Although Michelle had short periods out of her parapodium for brace revisions, she was an active ambulator for most of her grade school years.

When she was approximately 11 years of age, Michelle's spine developed a curve of sufficient size that surgical fusion was required. After a double procedure, both anterior and posterior fusion, Michelle was in body casting for a number of months and out of her parapodium after surgery. The prolonged period of non–weight bearing as a result of hospitalizations and casting resulted in some additional leg fractures with residual deformities. These factors, combined with her age and increased size, resulted in increased effort for walking. As a result, Michelle and her family decided to discontinue the use of the parapodium, and she become a full-time wheelchair user.

During high school, Michelle remained mobile and active using her wheelchair. In addition to being a good student, she used her strength and energy as an active member of a local wheelchair track and field team sponsored by an adult with spina bifida. She was also part of the local teen group sponsored by the local Spina Bifida Association. Today, Michelle lives at home while attending a community college and uses her wheelchair for mobility.

REFLECTION ON PRACTICE

At the time of Michelle's birth, many of the current developmental motor tests were not available. Today, records of development in the first several years would be kept using tests like the Alberta Infant Motor Scale or the GMFM. These test results could then be shared with the parents to further help them understand the sequence of motor development and to provide anticipatory guidance regarding activities they might expect their child to develop next. As Michelle became older, the PEDI would have been a helpful tool to guide her parents and the school staff in determining in what daily skills they needed to provide assistance or in what areas they needed to allow Michelle to take care of the task herself.

Parental involvement was a critical factor in Michelle's excellent motor progress despite her extensive paralysis and fracture problems. Michelle's parents played a major role in her development of functional walking, dressing, and self-care skills, illustrating how important it is to provide teaching and support to parents. Michelle's parents' participation in the group therapy sessions not only benefited Michelle but encouraged a number of other parents and children as well. Because the stress caused by the birth of a child with spina bifida begins in the delivery room, group sessions of physical therapy can be helpful to parents who need to share with other parents, particularly in the first years of life.

Michelle's fragile bones and tendency to fracture complicated her management; these problems occur frequently in children with high lesions. In her case, weight bearing in the standing position was particularly important to develop bone density and to maintain proper skeletal alignment. To achieve this benefit, Michelle used her bracing for active walking, wearing it 4 to 5 hours per day in both standing and sitting. Adjustment of bracing in such cases is important as bones tend to mold to the shape of bracing worn that many hours. For example, if the patellar tendon–bearing supports of a brace become too low, the tibia can begin to dislocate posteriorly, or if the pelvic band or knee supports are not sufficiently wide, the lower leg can begin to develop valgus deformity. Careful monitoring of bracing by the therapist and the orthotist are important.

It becomes necessary, as it did in Michelle's case, to assist the child and family to make transitions to promote best function. At 11 years of age, when Michelle and her family decided that she would be a full-time wheelchair user, it was important for them to receive support and assistance in making that transition without feeling that the change in lifestyle represented failure. Michelle did make the transition well knowing that she had benefited from improved bone density and growth, a decreased fracture incidence, and confidence in performing a large number of transfer skills that she found useful as a full-time wheelchair user.

High Lumbar Lesions (L1–L3)

Muscle Function and Contractures to Be Prevented

Children with high lumbar spinal lesions have active hip flexors and adductors (L1–L2) but minimal knee extension activity (L3). The fact that children of this lesion level have some active musculature in the lower extremities is both a plus and a problem. The available active muscle power contributes to the development of motor skills but, on the negative side, increases the incidence of contractures at the hip. With activity in the hip flexors and adductors, the child with a high lumbar lesion lacks the problem of lower extremity external rotation because the child can bring the legs together and flex the hips. Unfortunately, the child does not have hip extensor or abductor activity to counteract the pulling forces of the active hip flexors and adductors. For this reason, the child with a high lumbar lesion tends to develop hip flexion contractures. To prevent the formation of contractures, both passive positioning for 30 or more minutes per day[42] and manual ROM exercises must begin at an early age and be done regularly. If hip flexion contractures do develop, the child will be forced to stand with excessive lumbar lordosis to maintain balance in standing and during walking. This hyperextended trunk posture reduces stability in standing and can result in back pain.

Children with high lumbar lesions also have a significant chance of developing femoral valgus[7, 19] and hip dislocation because of the unopposed hip adductor pull on the femur. Abduction splinting is often prescribed by the orthopedist early in infancy to promote the development of a sufficiently deep acetabulum to prevent dislocation of the hip.

Treatment of dislocated hips differs among orthopedists.[68] If the child is ambulatory and has one hip dislocated, most orthopedists opt for a varus osteotomy or another procedure to relocate the hip because the unlevel pelvis associated with a unilateral hip dislocation increases the chance that a scoliosis will develop or that an existing one will progress.[21] The incidence of resubluxation and problems with postimmobilization fractures,[28, 32] however, is such that the orthopedist sometimes elects not to relocate the hips when both are out or if the child is not or will not be a community ambulator. I have known children with spina bifida who, even with bilaterally dislocated hips, ambulate on a daily basis without pain.

The child with spina bifida may have different spinal lesion levels on each side of the spinal cord, producing a "wind drift" effect in which one leg becomes adducted while the other is abducted. This type of imbalance makes standing balance and ambulation difficult and can further increase the chances that the adducted hip will dislocate. Although each of these contractures can create significant problems for the child, early positioning, splinting, and manual ROM exercises can minimize their occurrence.

Motor Goals

The child with a high lumbar lesion can be expected to achieve the same basic motor skills as the child with a thoracic lesion. The presence of active hip flexors and adductors also provides the possibility that the child will be able to move from a prone to a four-point position. Whether the child is able to crawl on the hands and knees depends on the strength of the active hip flexors and to some degree on the child's personality. The highly active child will probably attempt to crawl at least for short distances. Even if the child is unable to crawl, the ability to attain the four-point position provides the potential for the child to drop into a sitting from a four-point position, rather than pushing through the legs as described for the child with a thoracic lesion. The ability to move to a four-point position can also promote pulling to kneeling at a couch, which gives the child an additional ability to explore the environment of the home. Most children at this lesion level, however, are not able to pull themselves to a standing position without bracing, but they may be able to pull themselves onto a chair or a couch. The child's ability to crawl independently and motor plan may also contribute to improved visual perceptual abilities, as described by Campos and associates for normal children as they begin to crawl.[56]

In sitting, the child with a high lumbar lesion has a greater ability to use two hands together to handle and explore toys than the child with a thoracic lesion because pelvic stability is improved by the activity of the hip adductors.[57] The child does not, however, have hip extensor activity to limit forward flexion and stabilize the pelvis and needs to prop with the arms for stability. The hip adductors may provide sufficient stability to allow the child to prop with one hand while reaching with the other and, in some cases, to raise both arms briefly. Nevertheless, devices that provide trunk support when sitting are useful to increase the degree of two-handed exploration the child can achieve.

The child with a high lumbar lesion has a greater potential for ambulation than the child with a thoracic lesion but will still use ambulation primarily within the home or schoolroom, for movement and exercise. The types of orthoses available for ambulation again include the parapodium and RGOs or HKAFOs. Because of a lack of active hip extension, three points of pressure (anterior chest, posteriorly at the hip, and anteriorly at the knee) are usually required to achieve an upright trunk posture when standing and walking.

Which orthotic device is best for children with this level lesion remains a topic of debate.[62-64] The child with a high lumbar lesion is more able to use RGOs and HKAFOs for ambulation than the child with a thoracic lesion because forward progression of individual limbs becomes easier with active hip flexion. Loss of proprioception from both knees and ankles continues to be a problem for children at this lesion level and compromises balance for standing and walking.[33-35] Considering muscle and propriocep-tive losses, the choice of bracing may depend not only on the child's muscle power but also on the child's type of personality. The active, assertive child may do well in the development of ambulation using separate leg bracing such as a standard HKAFO. The quieter, shy child, however, may find the challenge of standing without balance assistance from the bracing frightening. In that case, the child may benefit from the additional support and reduced need for balance a parapodium provides. If the RGO or HKAFO is the orthosis of choice, the child will need a walker for ambulation and probably a standing table or frame so that the child can wear the braces for longer periods of time and still be able to use two hands to play and explore when standing.

CASE STUDY

Jose was seen for the first time by the school therapist at 5 years of age as he entered kindergarten. Assessment to determine what services he would need in school included muscle testing, which indicated that he had a functional L1–L2 lesion level with grade 2+ hip flexors but minimal hip adductor muscle activity. His tight hamstrings and hip extensors made it difficult for him to sit on the floor in long sitting without propping backward on his hands. Jose's left foot had mild contractures producing plantar flexion and forefoot inversion tightness, but the foot was stretchable. An interview with Jose's mother using an interpreter revealed that Jose primarily crawled in the prone position on the floor at home and rarely sat on the floor, revealing the probable reason for this somewhat-unusual pattern of muscle tightness in noninnervated muscles.

The GMFM was used for assessment of Jose's basic gross motor skills. He was able to roll, prone crawl, and get to a sitting position with moderate assistance but then maintained the position only by propping backward. He was unable to move to a four-point or kneeling position or pull himself to a standing position in or out of braces. His overall score for the entire test was 40%, with the score diminishing from section A to E (Fig. 5–6).

Jose's RGOs were too small; the brace's hip and knee joints were located 1 to 1.5 inches below his anatomic hip and knee joints. As a result, Jose could stand while wearing his braces but could not sit in his wheelchair. He could, however, sit on the floor in his braces if his chest straps were unfastened. Jose's wheelchair seat was found to be too narrow for him to sit in while wearing his braces, even if the RGOs had fit. Because Jose could not sit wearing his RGOs, he was placed in them only for short walks, after which they were removed. This was done infrequently because of the amount of time involved in placing him in and taking him out of the braces. Jose had a reverse rolling walker and was secure enough to stand and walk for short distances with close adult supervision. Jose arrived at school each day in his wheelchair but was not able to push the chair independently for more than short distances within the classroom and was afraid to push himself outdoors.

A multidisciplinary conference was held at which Jose's assessments were shared and an Individual Educational Plan was written. Those who attended the meeting included school staff members, Jose's mother, an interpreter, and Jose's private therapist. The team members decided that in addition to other academic school goals Jose would work on the following goals for physical development: (1) increase his ability to wheel his own wheelchair without fatigue for longer distances within the school building and on the playground, (2) increase his hip ROM to gradually allow him to sit comfortably in his bracing on the floor during circle times, (3) improve his ability and comfort in walking in the classroom, and (4) develop his ability to transfer into and out of chairs from standing, including to and from his wheelchair, with less assistance. School physical therapy was included as part of Jose's school day. The service was to be 60 minutes of direct service per week, including consultation, and teaching Jose's one-to-one assistant how to place Jose in his bracing and to assist him in transfers and ambulation practice.

As follow-up, Jose's specialty clinic was contacted to request that his braces be enlarged or replaced so that they fit properly to allow him to sit in the wheelchair while wearing his braces. They were also asked to approve enlargement of the wheelchair seat to accommodate the bracing.

Over the school year, Jose had difficulty with attendance at school and with the process of having his braces repaired. The school social worker, the school physical therapist, and the bilingual teacher devoted many hours to interagency communication with the specialty clinic and private therapist to promote the acquisition of new braces and to help Jose's mother understand the importance of Jose's consistent attendance at school. Work on Jose's transfer goals was postponed until March of the school year, when new braces were completed and delivered, but he continued to stand and do some walking in the old braces. Once the bracing was replaced, Jose developed ambulation skills that allowed him to walk within his classroom and across the hall to

TESTING WITH AIDS/ORTHOSES

Indicate below with a check (✔) which aid/orthosis was used and in what dimension it was first applied. (There may be more than one.)

Aid	Dimension		Orthosis	Dimension	
Rollator/pusher	✔	D	Hip control	✔	AB,D
Walker	☐	___	Knee control	☐	___
H frame crutches	☐	___	Ankle-foot control	☐	___
Crutches	☐	___	Foot control	☐	___
Quad cane	☐	___	Shoes	☐	___
Cane	☐	___	None	☐	___
None	☐	___	Other	☐	___
Other	☐	___	(please specify)	☐	
(please specify)					

SUMMARY SCORE USING AIDS/ORTHOSES

DIMENSION	CALCULATION OF DIMENSION % SCORES	GOAL AREA (indicated with ✔ check)
A. Lying & rolling	$\frac{\text{Total Dimension A}}{51} = \frac{48}{51}$ x 100 = 94 %	A. ☐
B. Sitting	$\frac{\text{Total Dimension B}}{60} = \frac{45}{60}$ x 100 = 75 %	B. ✔
C. Crawing & kneeling	$\frac{\text{Total Dimension C}}{42} = \frac{14}{42}$ x 100 = 33 %	C. ✔
D. Standing	$\frac{\text{Total Dimension D}}{39} = \frac{1}{39}$ x 100 = 2 %	D. ✔
E. Walking, running & jumping	$\frac{\text{Total Dimension E}}{72} = \frac{}{72}$ x 100 = ___ %	E. ☐

TOTAL SCORE $= \dfrac{\%A + \%B + \%C + \%D + \%E}{\text{Total \# of dimensions}}$

$= \dfrac{94 + 75 + 33 + 2 + 0}{5} = \dfrac{204}{5} = 40$ %

GOAL TOTAL SCORE $= \dfrac{\text{Sum of \% scores for each dimension identified as a goal area}}{\text{\# Goal areas}}$

$= \underline{} = $ ___ %

FIGURE 5–6. The Gross Motor Function Measure (GMFM) score sheet used during Jose's school evaluation. *Illustration continued on following page*

CHECK (✓) THE APPROPRIATE SCORE:

Item	A: **LYING AND ROLLING**		SCORE			
1.	SUP: HEAD IN MIDLINE: TURNS HEAD WITH EXTREMITIES SYMMETRICAL	0☐	1☐	2☐	3✓	1.
2.	SUP: BRINGS HANDS TO MIDLINE, FINGERS ONE WITH THE OTHER	0☐	1☐	2☐	3✓	2.
3.	SUP: LIFTS HEAD 45°	0☐	1☐	2☐	3✓	3.
4.	SUP: FLEXES R HIP AND KNEE THROUGH FULL RANGE	0✓	1☐	2☐	3☐	4.
5.	SUP: FLEXES L HIP AND KNEE THROUGH FULL RANGE	0☐	1☐	2☐	3✓	5.
6.	SUP: REACHES OUT WITH R ARM, HAND CROSSES MIDLINE TOWARD TOY	0☐	1☐	2☐	3✓	6.
7.	SUP: REACHES OUT WITH L ARM, HAND CROSSES MIDLINE TOWARD TOY	0☐	1☐	2☐	3✓	7.
8.	SUP: ROLLS TO PR OVER R SIDE *In and out of bracing*	0☐	1☐	2☐	3✓	8.
9.	SUP: ROLLS TO PR OVER L SIDE *In and out of bracing*	0☐	1☐	2☐	3✓	9.
10.	PR: LIFTS HEAD UPRIGHT	0☐	1☐	2☐	3✓	10.
11.	PR ON FOREARMS: LIFTS HEAD UPRIGHT, ELBOWS EXT., CHEST RAISED	0☐	1☐	2☐	3✓	11.
12.	PR ON FOREARMS: WEIGHT ON R FOREARM, FULLY EXTENDS OPPOSITE ARM FORWARD	0☐	1☐	2☐	3✓	12.
13.	PR ON FOREARMS: WEIGHT ON L FOREARM, FULLY EXTENDS OPPOSITE ARM FORWARD	0☐	1☐	2☐	3✓	13.
14.	PR: ROLLS TO SUP OVER R SIDE *In and out of bracing*	0☐	1☐	2☐	3✓	14.
15.	PR: ROLLS TO SUP OVER L SIDE *In and out of bracing*	0☐	1☐	2☐	3✓	15.
16.	PR: PIVOTS TO R 90°USING EXTREMITIES	0☐	1☐	2☐	3✓	16.
17.	PR: PIVOTS TO L 90° USING EXTREMITIES	0☐	1☐	2☐	3✓	17.

TOTAL DIMENSION A | 48 |

Item	B: **SITTING**		SCORE			
18.	SUP, HANDS GRASPED BY EXAMINER: PULLS SELF TO SITTING WITH HEAD CONTROL	0☐	1☐	2☐	3✓	18.
19.	SUP: ROLLS TO R SIDE, ATTAINS SITTING	0☐	1☐	2✓	3☐	19.
20.	SUP: ROLLS TO L SIDE, ATTAINS SITTING	0☐	1☐	2✓	3☐	20.
21.	SIT ON MAT, SUPPORTED AT THORAX BY THERAPIST: LIFTS HEAD UPRIGHT, MAINTAINS 3 SECONDS	0☐	1☐	2☐	3✓	21.
22.	SIT ON MAT, SUPPORTED AT THORAX BY THERAPIST: LIFTS HEAD UPRIGHT, MAINTAINS 10 SECONDS	0☐	1☐	2☐	3✓	22.
23.	SIT ON MAT, ARM(S) PROPPING: MAINTAINS, 5 SECONDS	0☐	1☐	2☐	3✓	23.
24.	SIT ON MAT: MAINTAINS, ARMS FREE, 3 SECONDS	0☐	1✓	2☐	3☐	24.
25.	SIT ON MAT WITH SMALL TOY IN FRONT: LEANS FORWARD, TOUCHES TOY, RE-ERECTS WITHOUT ARM PROPPING	0☐	1☐	2✓	3☐	25.
26.	SIT ON MAT: TOUCHES TOY PLACED 45° BEHIND CHILD'S R SIDE, RETURNS TO START	0☐	1☐	2☐	3✓	26.
27.	SIT ON MAT: TOUCHES TOY PLACED 45° BEHIND CHILD'S L SIDE, RETURNS TO START	0☐	1☐	2☐	3✓	27.
28.	R SIDE SIT: MAINTAINS, ARMS FREE, 5 SECONDS	0☐	1☐	2☐	3✓	28.
29.	L SIDE SIT: MAINTAINS, ARMS FREE, 5 SECONDS *Out of braces*	0☐	1☐	2☐	3✓	29.
30.	SIT ON MAT: LOWERS TO PR WITH CONTROL	0☐	1☐	2☐	3✓	30.
31.	SIT ON MAT WITH FEET IN FRONT: ATTAINS 4 POINT OVER R SIDE	0☐	1☐	2✓	3☐	31.
32.	SIT ON MAT WITH FEET IN FRONT: ATTAINS 4 POINT OVER L SIDE	0☐	1☐	2✓	3☐	32.
33.	SIT ON MAT: PIVOTS 90°, WITHOUT ARMS ASSISTING	0☐	1✓	2☐	3☐	33.
34.	SIT ON BENCH: MAINTAINS, ARMS AND FEET FREE, 10 SECONDS	0☐	1☐	2☐	3✓	34.
35.	STD: ATTAINS SIT ON SMALL BENCH	0☐	1✓	2☐	3☐	35.
36.	ON THE FLOOR: ATTAINS SIT ON SMALL BENCH	0☐	1✓	2☐	3☐	36.
37.	ON THE FLOOR: ATTAINS SIT ON LARGE BENCH	0☐	1✓	2☐	3☐	37.

TOTAL DIMENSION B | 45 |

FIGURE 5–6 *Continued*

Item	C: **CRAWLING AND KNEELING**	SCORE				
38.	PR: CREEPS FORWARD 6'	0	1	2	3 ✓	38.
39.	4 POINT: MAINTAINS, WEIGHT ON HANDS AND KNEES, 10 SECONDS	0	1	2 ✓	3	39.
40.	4 POINT: ATTAINS SIT ARMS FREE	0	1	2 ✓	3	40.
41.	PR: ATTAINS 4 POINT, WEIGHT ON HANDS AND KNEES	0	1	2 ✓	3	41.
42.	4 POINT: REACHES FORWARD WITH R ARM, HAND ABOVE SHOULDER LEVEL	0	1	2 ✓	3	42.
43.	4 POINT: REACHES FORWARD WITH L ARM, HAND ABOVE SHOULDER LEVEL	0	1	2 ✓	3	43.
44.	4 POINT: CRAWLS OR HITCHES FORWARD 6'	0	1 ✓	2	3	44.
45.	4 POINT: CRAWLS RECIPROCALLY FORWARD 6'	0 ✓	1	2	3	45.
46.	4 POINT: CRAWLS UP 4 STEPS ON HANDS AND KNEES/FEET	0 ✓	1	2	3	46.
47.	4 POINT: CRAWLS BACKWARDS DOWN 4 STEPS ON HANDS AND KNEES/FEET *Slides*	0 ✓	1	2	3	47.
48.	SIT ON MAT: ATTAINS HIGH KN USING ARMS, MAINTAINS, ARMS FREE, 10 SECONDS	0 ✓	1	2	3	48.
49.	HIGH KN: ATTAINS HALF KN ON R KNEE USING ARMS, MAINTAINS, ARMS FREE, 10 SECONDS	0 ✓	1	2	3	49.
50.	HIGH KN: ATTAINS HALF KN ON L KNEE USING ARMS, MAINTAINS, ARMS FREE, 10 SECONDS	0 ✓	1	2	3	50.
51.	HIGH KN: KN WALKS FORWARD 10 STEPS, ARMS FREE	0 ✓	1	2	3	51.

TOTAL DIMENSION C `14`

Item	D: **STANDING** *In bracing only - with walker*	SCORE				
52.	ON THE FLOOR: PULLS TO STD AT LARGE BENCH *Emerging/Walker*	0	1 ✓	2	3	52.
53.	STD: MAINTAINS, ARMS FREE, 3 SECONDS	0 ✓	1	2	3	53.
54.	STD: HOLDING ON TO LARGE BENCH WITH ONE HAND, LIFTS R FOOT, 3 SECONDS	0 ✓	1	2	3	54.
55.	STD: HOLDING ON TO LARGE BENCH WITH ONE HAND, LIFTS L FOOT, 3 SECONDS	0 ✓	1	2	3	55.
56.	STD: MAINTAINS, ARMS FREE, 20 SECONDS	0 ✓	1	2	3	56.
57.	STD: LIFTS L FOOT, ARMS FREE, 10 SECONDS	0 ✓	1	2	3	57.
58.	STD: LIFTS R FOOT, ARMS FREE, 10 SECONDS	0 ✓	1	2	3	58.
59.	SIT ON SMALL BENCH: ATTAINS STD WITHOUT USING ARMS *Pulls to stand at walker*	0 ✓	1	2	3	59.
60.	HIGH KN: ATTAINS STD THROUGH HALF KN ON R KNEE, WITHOUT USING ARMS	0 ✓	1	2	3	60.
61.	HIGH KN: ATTAINS STD THROUGH HALF KN ON L KNEE, WITHOUT USING ARMS	0 ✓	1	2	3	61.
62.	STD: LOWERS TO SIT ON FLOOR WITH CONTROL, ARMS FREE *Lowers to chair from walker*	0 ✓	1	2	3	62.
63.	STD: ATTAINS SQUAT, ARMS FREE	0 ✓	1	2	3	63.
64.	STD: PICKS UP OBJECT FROM FLOOR, ARMS FREE, RETURNS TO STAND *Using chair or walker, reaches within 10" of floor*	0 ✓	1	2	3	64.

TOTAL DIMENSION D `1`

FIGURE 5–6 *Continued*

some of his English-as-a-second-language classes. He also began sitting on the floor in his braces, which slowly increased the range in his hips to 90 degrees of hip flexion, allowing him to sit without propping. Through daily practice at school, Jose became proficient in wheeling his chair to gym and to the bus, but he continued to be afraid of wheeling outside to the playground. In spring, daily outside play began, and the problem took on increased importance. It was noted that the sidewalk to the blacktopped play area was uneven with large gaps between concrete sections, which caused Jose's wheelchair to tip. His wheelchair was adjusted to make it more stable and less inclined to tip, and an inside route to a different door leading outside was used until the sidewalk could be repaired. Jose then became more willing to wheel his wheelchair outside.

It also became apparent that one of Jose's problems with school attendance was the fact that his single mother had difficulty getting him up a set of 10 stairs from her basement apartment to the bus. She had carried him up to his wheelchair when he was a small child, but now that he was getting larger, carrying him was becoming too difficult. The ideal solution was to move to a more accessible apartment, but this was not financially feasible. A home visit was made by the school therapy team, and the problem was dealt with by teaching the mother and Jose how to climb the stairs together using the stair rail and one crutch. Although Jose was not strong enough or coordinated enough to climb the stairs unassisted, with his mother's help he could do the push-up necessary to climb each step. School attendance then improved. Jose made progress toward his goals during the school year, but several of the ambulation and transfer skills were continued as goals into the next year as a result of the delay in obtaining new bracing. Jose is now in first grade and continues to work on transitions into and out of his wheelchair and up and down to the floor, and on ambulating the length of the school hallway.

REFLECTION ON PRACTICE

The fact that Jose's mother was single and Spanish-speaking made communication between herself and the persons caring for her son difficult. The specialty clinic Jose attended reported not always having an interpreter available when Jose arrived, in part because he frequently came unannounced or late. This caused Jose's mother to misunderstand many of the instructions for his care. It became clear that interagency communication was critical for Jose to receive the services that he required. The specialty clinic that Jose attended did not have as part of their clinic team a physical therapist who could make on-site recommendations regarding mobility devices. At the time of Jose's evaluation at school, he had not been seen in the clinic with his braces for a year. The specialty clinic was therefore not aware that problems with the braces were interfering with his mobility progress. The private physical therapist reported unsuccessful attempts to contact the clinic's nurse coordinator to resolve bracing problems, and it became necessary for both community therapists to work together to promote action on new braces. At 5 years of age, growth is so rapid that bracing needs to be inspected for adjustment a minimum of every 4 to 6 months. This problem might have been avoided if the specialty clinic had had a physical therapist on their staff to monitor such problems or at least to be more available to discuss them with the community therapist.

Knowledge of typical muscle innervation and the problems associated with patterns of muscle loss for a child with a high lumbar lesion helps the therapist anticipate what specific assessments need to done and some of the problems that should be avoided before they develop. With better communication with Jose's mother through consistent use of an interpreter, and through knowledge of the ways in which Jose moved and played at home (perhaps through home therapy rather than center-based therapy), some of the contractures described in this case could have been prevented before he reached the age of 5 years. Because children with spina bifida have muscle paralysis rather than muscle incoordination, equipment that substitutes for the lack of muscle activity or provides support to the children in daily functional activities becomes important to the children's success in mastering the environment in which they live. Compensation for muscle loss rather than improvement of muscle function, particularly in lower extremities, is often what is needed to maximize daily function. In addition, monitoring by the pediatric physical therapist to make sure that devices and orthoses continue to fit through growth spurts can be critical to the child's continued use of the device. The child's plan of care should designate who will take responsibility for tasks such as this, especially in situations involving multiple teams of professionals functioning in various sites. In many cases, a family member plays this role after being taught how to monitor significant signs.

Low Lumbar Lesions (L4, L5)

Muscle Function and Contractures to Be Prevented

It is expected that the child with low lumbar lesions will have more muscle function in the lower extremities than the child with higher lesion levels. It is therefore obvious that the child with a low lumbar lesion has all the muscle function described for the high lumbar level but has additional strength in knee extensors, and some dorsiflexion and hip abduction activity (L5). Although these children also tend to develop hip flexion contractures, the addition of hip abductor muscle activity tends to reduce the incidence of hip dislocation although not totally eliminate it. A hip abduction splint may be prescribed to promote the development of a well-formed acetabulum. Manual stretching of hip flexors and prone positioning for lengthening of the hip flexors are of value in preventing secondary contractures because the child with this lesion level does not have active hip extensor power to counteract the pull of the hip flexors. Lumbar lordosis is also a problem for the child with a low lumbar lesion. Because of the lack of active hip extension to stabilize the pelvis, the child tends to hyperextend the trunk to maintain sitting and standing balance. Hyperextension of the trunk and the resulting exaggerated lumbar lordosis can be reduced in the standing position if a chest pad is provided as part of the child's orthosis before hip flexion contractures can develop. Reduction of lumbar lordosis can diminish the possibility of lower back pain's developing as the child becomes older.

The child with an L5 lesion may require a chest strap to counteract the lack of hip extension initially but may have sufficient hip abduction and quadriceps muscle strength to ambulate with less bracing once growth is completed and an upright standing posture is established. A pelvic band is needed, however, as long as the child is walking because of weak or absent hip rotators that allow the child's legs to rotate inward or outward during walking. Over time this pattern can become fixed into a contracture. The child with a low lumbar lesion will be a household walker and may do some community walking as well. Because of increased walking and time in bracing it is especially important that the child's braces fit well and support the pelvis and trunk sufficiently to prevent secondary contractures such as those just discussed.[69]

Motor Goals

Children with low lumbar lesions achieve most, if not all, of the motor skills expected of typically developing children in the first 10 months of life, but at their own pace. Many children in this category crawl for exploration of their homes, pull themselves to a standing position, and walk holding on to furniture, sometimes even without bracing. Physical therapy may be most needed to promote mobility beyond pulling to a standing position. Children and their parents often need guidance on how much the child should wear the braces, what kind of walker is needed to promote ambulation, and how to promote the development of walking and movement transition skills.

Children with this lesion level are household ambulators and may be community ambulators but often need a wheelchair for long distances. Trips to the mall or zoo, or with peers who move at a much faster rate, may be limited if the child does not have a wheelchair. The wheelchair for this level lesion does not need to provide as much trunk support as required for children with thoracic lesions, but it should be lightweight, have seating that relieves pressure over the ischium because of possible anesthesia in that area, and be "growable" and durable.

Sacral-Level Lesions

Muscle Function and Contractures to Be Prevented (S1, S2)

The child with a sacral lesion has all the muscle groups previously described plus the hip extensors and ankle plantar flexors, which are lacking at other lesion levels. The stronger these muscle groups are, the greater the stability of the hips and the more normal the child's gait pattern will be. Imbalance of strength between everters and inverters of the foot, or between dorsiflexors and plantar flexors, however, can result in contractures for children with this lesion level. Because this group of children will use ambulation as a primary means of mobility, contractures and pressure sores of the feet are a major concern. Calcaneovarus, toe clawing, and dorsiflexion tightness can reduce stability in standing and result in pressure sores. The older, heavier child is particularly prone to decubitus ulcers of the heel, which can become serious. The foot position can be improved and the development of sores reduced through the use of AFOs, supramalleolar orthoses, or shoe inserts. Daily foot checks become especially important for this group of children as they become older and heavier, and the danger of the development of pressure sores increases because of increased body weight.

Motor Goals

This group of children should progress through the motor goals typical of the first year of life with minimal assistance but may do so at a slower rate than usual. Most children pull themselves to a standing position and walk but may need the assistance of the aforementioned bracing for foot stability and positioning, at least initially. Depending on the strength of the child's hip extensors and abductors, the gait pattern of this child may be of a Trendelenburg type, in which the child's trunk sways from side to side to compensate for the lack of hip stability. This is the only lesion level at which children generally do well with ambulation without assistive devices, such as walkers or crutches.

Children in this group may or may not need wheeled mobility for community ambulation. Their foot condition, general strength, lifestyle, and personality are all factors in the decision whether to purchase a wheelchair. Because individuals with sacral lesions may have foot sores that require a non–weight-bearing status for periods of time, sources for the rental or loan of a wheelchair are necessary. If foot problems are chronic, the purchase of a wheelchair may be advantageous.

General Guidelines to Promote Development of Gross Motor Skills

In the early years, regardless of the child's lesion level, it is important to help the child and the family develop play and daily routines that encourage the child to develop independence. Not only does the therapist need to provide suggestions on specific activities for each stage of motor development, but the therapist plays an important role in encouraging the family to engage in age-appropriate play with the child and to develop expectations for motor skill development from the child despite the initial trauma of learning about their child's problems. As the child becomes older and develops increasing ability to do daily activities independently, the therapist needs to help the family adjust to the child's changing need for assistance in such a way that they help the child continue to gain independence in mobility and transfers.

Development of Initial Mobility Skills

In the first 6 to 12 months of the child's life, as described for the child with a thoracic lesion, floor playtime is of particular importance for the development of basic mobility skills. If the child does not like being on the floor, it is important that the parents use the time on the floor as a social activity involving play with their child. To encourage mobility, parents should present toys designed for play with two hands in the supine position early but later should place toys slightly out of reach so that the child has to strive to move to reach the toy. The early trauma of the child's birth may influence parents to try to make things easy for their child, but the child with spina bifida needs reasonable challenges, just as any person does. Striving to obtain objects while playing on the floor is just one of the early components of developing the skills of rolling, prone crawling, and moving into a sitting position.

During the first year, when the child is crawling on the floor, parents should be alerted to the need to have the child's feet and legs covered so that skin abrasions can be minimized. The concept that the child has no sensation in the legs, feet, and buttocks is often difficult for the average adult to understand if they have not had a physical impairment themselves. This early parent education can help prevent the damage that can occur as a result of the children's insensitivity to heat sources of all kinds, or cold outdoors, and even from damage done by the infants who, out of curiosity, grab their own foot while supine (a normal infant motor activity) and bite their toe without any sensation of pain. Although the parents must take the initial responsibility for dressing the children to protect against injury, as the children reach 2 or 3 years of age and are developing independence in dressing tasks,[70] the parents should begin talking to the children about their legs' being a part of their body and showing them how to look at their legs to see if "redness" has appeared. By school age, the children should be able to inspect their own legs to alert their parents to problems. It may be late grade school or adolescent years, however, before children are able to accurately use a mirror to inspect for ischial pressure sores. This ability usually evolves with the children's development of self-catheterization skills.

Initiation of Ambulation and Transition Skills

When Should Bracing for Standing Begin? Between 12 to 14 months of age, children with spina bifida usually begin to demonstrate an interest in pulling themselves to a standing position. Parents should be alerted to watch for this stage as an indication that it may be time for their child to receive the orthoses needed for standing or ambulation. Although the child may not be a functional ambulator, the benefits of standing, as described in earlier sections, are worth the effort. One of the ways that the child with spina bifida indicates a readiness to stand is by prone crawling to a piece of furniture and making efforts to reach to pull up. If this natural urge to stand is ignored, a critical or transitional period in which the child is most able to learn to stand and ambulate, as described by Thelen and Ulrich,[71] may be lost. When presented with orthoses for assistance in standing at a later time, the child may have lost interest and may experience great difficulty in adjusting to braces and the upright position. In addition, as the child grows, the task becomes harder mechanically due to an increase in height of the center of mass. For example, I find that children placed in standing braces at 12 months are less frightened and more excited by standing than those who are placed in the standing position for the first time at 2 years of age, an age at which even the child without disability is developing the need for control.

Initial Steps in Adjusting to Wearing Braces. Once braces have been provided, the therapist should help the parent understand the time the child may need to spend in the braces to use them for daily activities. The therapist should be in conversation with parents concerning their daily routines and help them find times in the family's day when ambulation practice may be least stressful. Although the orthotist is the first person to show the parents how to put on the braces, the therapist will want to make this an area of teaching as well. The therapist may need to provide an initial method for putting the braces on but should guide the parents into methods of donning the braces that simulate what the children will need to do to put the braces on themselves. For instance, if the child will need to scoot into the bracing sitting on the floor, the parent should learn to place the bracing on the floor and move the child into it in the same way the child will use later. In this way, the parents model what the children will be expected to do as they become older. As with most self-care skills, the ability to put on bracing is an evolutionary process in which the parents model the method, and as the children mature they gradually take over portions of the task until they are able to do the whole task independently. Because of the complexity of this task, children with thoracic and high lumbar lesions with more complicated bracing are usually not be able to do this task independently until 5 years of age or later.

Development of Standing Balance. The therapist should be aware that the parents will be initially nervous about the child's standing in orthoses. It is important that the first orthotic device be provided along with a walker or other supportive device such as a standing table so that the child has an opportunity to stand for periods of time without the parents' or child's worrying about falling. At the same time, the best way to prevent an accidental fall is to initiate practice of falling into the therapist's or parent's arms (Fig. 5–7). In this way, the children learn the limits of their balance (which is different for parapodiums and HKAFOs) and both the parents' and children's fear of falling is diminished.

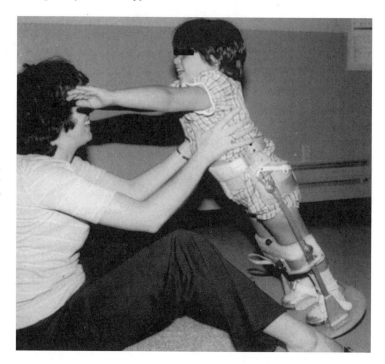

FIGURE 5–7. Child learning to fall forward, both to learn the limits of her standing balance and to reduce the fear of falling.

Development of Gait Pattern. Methods for the development of a gait pattern are slightly different depending on the type of braces chosen for the child. Gait patterns for the two most frequently used ambulation devices (parapodium and HKAFO) are somewhat different and require different approaches. Parapodiums usually require a side-to-side lean and rotation motion sometimes referred to as a swivel-walk (rather like skateboarding),[67] and the HKAFO usually requires a pattern of side-to-side weight shift and extension of the trunk to move one leg forward.[72] The use of either requires the use of a rollator walker or parallel pusher at first.[67] With practice and use, some children have the ability to walk without assistive devices using the parapodium, and some are able to move on to crutch walking using HKAFOs. A child's ability to ambulate for daily activities depends on the child's personality and level of muscle activity loss and the time per day that the child spends in the bracing. The time spent in bracing is maximized if the child is able to sit as well as stand in the braces.

Promoting Functional Use of Braces. To promote more functional use of braces, the therapist should teach the parent and child methods for the child to roll, crawl, and come to a sitting position in the braces, or the child will not be able to move on the floor or get up from the floor to stand without full assistance from an adult. An inability to move and sit on the floor in braces then limits the child's ability to explore and change position, which in turn leads to very limited use of the braces because of the need to put them on and take them off more often.

All children should also learn as many as possible independent methods of making the transition from standing to sitting and to the floor and back while in braces. Although work on transition from the floor to standing and into and out of chairs should begin shortly after the child is comfortable standing in the braces, independence is unusual before the child is at least 5 years of age. For children with a thoracic or high lumbar lesion, transfers from standing into a chair usually require a chair with arms of optimal height. The children frequently need to use the arms of the chair to pull themselves backward until they are resting against the seat of the chair (Fig. 5–8). The children then disengage their hip locks and pull themselves into the chair. It is important that hip locks for any orthotic device be easy to engage and disengage. Otherwise, the children have no chance of becoming independent in this activity. The child with a low lumbar

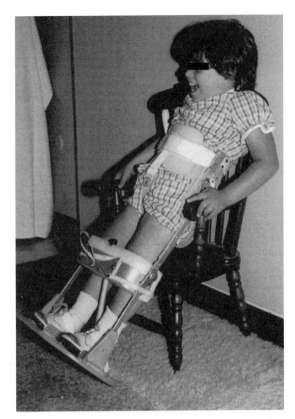

FIGURE 5–8. Child with a thoracic lesion who has pulled herself backward into a chair from a standing position and is now pulling on the side loop to unlock the hip locks of her parapodium to allow her to sit.

or sacral lesion may not need hip locks on the bracing, which may enable the child to move into and out of a chair using the same technique as any other child.

Getting up from the floor is also an important skill. The child with a thoracic or high lumbar lesion has to learn a jackknife method (Fig. 5–9) of coming to a standing position or moving to the floor whether in RGOs or in a parapodium. The hip lock function and the correct fit of the orthoses are again key to the success or failure of the child in learning this motor skill. Although children with high lesions may not become independent in getting up from the floor, this method of bringing the child to a standing position increases the child's arm strength and is less stressful on the parent than a full body lift. The child with a low lumbar or sacral lesion may be able to use a half-kneel to move to a standing position as is expected in the nonparalyzed child.

Both sitting into and getting out of a chair and getting up and down from the floor are skills that facilitate independence in exploration and changes of position at both home and school. Each is developed by assisting the child at first and then gradually withdrawing assistance as the child can take over portions of the skill. The therapist has a key role in helping the parent determine when and how to assist and when to withdraw assistance from portions of the activity. These two skills, like donning bracing, may not be fully developed until the child is 5 years of age or older because of the degree of motor planning, strength, and coordination they require. In addition, children with visual perceptual problems may require many repetitions of the same motor sequence before it is learned. Once the child has learned a motor task, however, it is usually retained and used as an important skill in the child's repertoire for independence and mobility.

For children with high lesions, wheelchair transfer without braces needs to be done as a sliding transfer in the sitting position. This method of transfer is important to develop particularly for movement from the wheelchair to the bed and from the wheelchair to the tub or toilet seat. It is important for the therapist to discourage the parent from lifting and carrying the child like an infant as the child reaches 3 to 4 years of age, but instead to use transfer methods that encourage the child to do part of the task

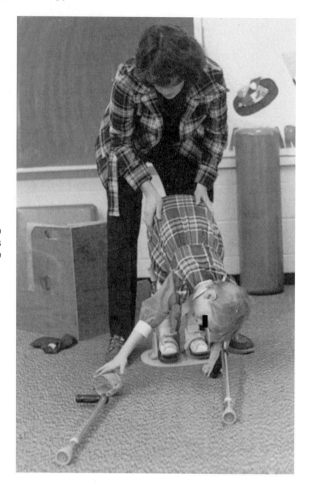

FIGURE 5–9. Jackknife method of getting down to or up from the floor using crutches. The child usually uses furniture to assist in getting up when first learning to use this method.

and the parent to assist. It is the therapist's role to explore with the parents information on times during the day when transfers are required and to assist them in developing methods of transfer that are assisted rather than lifting transfers. The PEDI transfer scale can be used to track progress in this area.

Referral to Occupational Therapy

In addition to work on gross motor skills, which are typically within the realm of the physical therapist, many children with spina bifida need assistance with fine motor, self-care, activities-of-daily-living, and perceptual-motor development. Because the child is often thought to have "good upper extremities," referral for occupational therapy may not be made. Nevertheless, it is important that the child be assessed for age-appropriate development in these areas and provided with treatment by the occupational therapist if the examination results indicate a need. Because the physical therapist typically sees the child first, it may fall to the physical therapist to screen for fine motor and perceptual-motor deficits and to refer the child for occupational therapy.

Preparation for School

As the children reach 3 years of age, they become eligible for preschool screening. Children with lesions higher than the sacral level are usually found eligible for early-childhood classes because of delayed gross or fine motor function, visual perceptual deficits, and language delays. Parents need counsel as to whether to enroll their child in special early-childhood programs and may turn to the physical therapist for advice. Because of the child's reduced ability to access neighborhood friends in their homes or on playgrounds, participation in an early-childhood program can be important in terms of opportunity for social interaction with peers and an opportunity to separate from the family to practice and gain confidence in social, physical, and communication skills outside the home. Early-childhood programs sponsored by the local school district frequently provide speech and language, occupational therapy, and physical therapy services to assist the teacher in providing an appropriate individualized program for the child.

In some cases, the child may do well if enrolled in a community preschool program either as an alternative or in addition to the early-childhood program. In this case, the parent may need to be more of an advocate for the child, as the staff members of a community preschool may not have had prior experience with a child with spina bifida and do not usually have the therapeutic support services that are provided by school district programs. Most preschool-age children with spina bifida are still wearing diapers for continence management and are in the process of learning dressing, feeding, and mobility skills.[70] The school must be aware of the child's special needs and be ready to learn ways to accommodate those needs. Private therapists who have worked with the child from an early age can be helpful in the education of the staff through both personal consultation and written reports. The therapist needs to assist the parents in learning how to be assertive advocates for their child's needs while at the same time understanding that most school teams care about their children and try to provide an appropriate program.

From kindergarten to the senior year of high school, public school is available for all children in the United States. Parents are a part of the team that will determine what type of school program will be needed to meet their child's educational needs and need to stay involved in their child's school program to actively promote communication between medical caregivers and the school staff. When entering school the child has an initial assessment that consists of a psychologic assessment, a medical interview, a social assessment, hearing and vision screening, and assessments by therapists as deemed necessary by the intake team. Parent participation in the assessment process includes providing information regarding who the child's medical caregivers are, therapists' reports, and past history. With this information, the school staff, in conjunction with the parents, are able to develop a school plan that best meets the child's needs.

Many children with spina bifida now attend their community schools with the support of school therapists, school nurses, and special educators as resource teachers.[73] The school physical therapist should be the team member who provides assistance to the school staff for methods of movement around the classroom and school building, and for continued development of transfers into and out of chairs as appropriate to participate in school activities, or from the wheelchair to the toilet or mat for catheterization programs. The therapist may also have a role in promoting the child's participation in physical education (PE) if the school has not had previous experience with a child with physical limits or does not have a teacher with adapted PE experience. Because of the time that the child spends in school, the school therapist may be the person who observes the child's movement ability most often and may be the appropriate person to assist with equipment selection and updates.

Transition to Adulthood

As the child with spina bifida moves into the teen and adult years, issues of prevention of inappropriate weight gain and promoting continued physical activity in support of lifelong health-related physical fitness become important. As children with spina bifida reach adolescence, they experience growth and hormonal changes that are common to the average adolescent. During this period of significant growth and hormonal change, the adolescents may experience fatigue and loss of interest in walking, even when they have previously been active walkers.[74–77] Surgical interventions at this age, such as spinal fusion for scoliosis management, may also result in discontinuation of ambulation.

The transition to high school, with frequent changes of classes within a large building, may also result in the need to depend more on a wheelchair for mobility and lead to a more sedentary lifestyle. Several studies have looked at the energy cost associated with walking using braces and wheelchairs and have concluded that walking with bracing or wheeling a wheelchair has higher energy costs than normal gait.[77–82] This increased energy output for mobility can reduce the energy available for participation in the academic demands of school[79] and must be considered when the method of mobility for school is determined. At the same time, a lack of physical activity can result in weight gain and decreased cardiovascular conditioning, which in turn results in increased difficulty with walking or pushing a wheelchair, and more weight gain. If the high school that the adolescent attends is not attuned to the student's need for continued physical activity through PE classes or is new to inclusion with no provisions for adapted PE, the adolescent with spina bifida may not even have the amount of daily activity afforded to students without paralysis through their PE classes. The family, private therapist, and school therapist should work together to promote appropriate participation in physical activity during the school day as well as outside the school day in the form of leisure activities. Although many more are needed, wheelchair athletic teams and other recreational opportunities designed for persons with mobility impairments are more available through park district programs than ever before. All options should be explored and the adolescent encouraged to participate in selected activities on a weekly basis.

The decision to become a full-time wheelchair user should not make the child, family, or therapists feel that they have failed, as the benefits gained from years of ambulation continue to be useful for wheelchair mobility.[64] For example, ambulation has improved bone growth and bone density during growth years, facilitated the development of a sense of balance, and utilized transfer skills, all of which continue to be useful in wheelchair mobility. In some cases, the adolescent may want to have some type of equipment or bracing for standing at home, particularly if ischial decubitus ulcers become an issue, even though they have chosen to be wheelchair mobile.

Employment opportunities and social involvement are of primary importance to the adult. Programs through state agencies such as the Department of Rehabilitation Services can help persons with spina bifida train for and find employment after high school. These programs also assist persons with disabilities to obtain the technology and the personal services (personal care assistant) that may be needed for employment. To access job and social opportunities, many adults with spina bifida can learn to drive using hand controls. Programs for driving assessment and training are usually available through large rehabilitation centers and on occasion through school systems. For those who are not able to drive, wheelchair-accessible transportation systems are available in most metropolitan areas. When prior arrangements are made, these systems can provide door-to-door transportation to work or leisure activities for the person with limited mobility and one personal care assistant.

Community park districts and the local chapter of the Spina Bifida Association of America frequently have programs and publications designed for children and adults. The association, located at 4590 MacArthur Boulevard NW, Suite 250, Washington, DC 20007-4226, can provide the client with a publication list that includes information on medical issues, advocacy, sexuality, and social development. This list also includes a clinic directory for the United States that indicates which specialty clinics have developed services for adults with spina bifida. Although many persons with spina bifida develop their own social groups, programs sponsored by local chapters of the association can be a useful way to meet other people with similar issues and to find support. It is therefore important that the therapist have knowledge of this and other resources in the community that may be helpful to their clients with spina bifida.

In a symposium that studied the problem of preventing secondary conditions for persons with spina bifida and cerebral palsy specifically in the areas of physical, psychologic, and social health, recommendations were made for young adults with spina bifida and for health care professionals.[83] Preventable secondary conditions have been shown to be a costly portion of care provided to adults with spina bifida.[84] Recommendations for ways young adults can prevent secondary conditions included the following:

1. To prevent secondary physical conditions, young adults are encouraged to monitor and control their own health, specifically to question caregivers and keep a record of their own health condition and treatments. In addition, young adults should promote good health by monitoring their own diet and by developing a pattern of regular exercise and sport activity. They are also encouraged to learn more about their own health by serving as a resource person for specialty clinics.

2. To prevent secondary psychologic conditions, young adults are encouraged to communicate with each other, parents, and professionals to find out more about recognizing feelings of depression or isolation, methods of coping with these feelings, and managing sexual roles and functioning. Young adults are encouraged to be assertive in taking time for themselves, to require privacy and respect for their own body, and to request information on topics needed. They are encouraged to learn about people in the community who can help with psychologic problems, such as psychologists, social workers, and counseling services in schools and local mental health associations.

3. To prevent secondary social conditions young adults are encouraged to participate in peer support groups, both for their own and others' sake. Groups suggested in which young persons can both participate and be mentors include the Adolescent Vocational Readiness Center in Washington, DC (202-884-3203) and the Association for Children with Learning Disabilities, Council for Exceptional Children.

Recommendations to health care professionals from this symposium included many that are applicable to physical therapists. A number of the recommendations centered on the concept that therapists should educate clients and families in the types of technologies available through the organization of demonstration showrooms and technology fairs such as Ability Expo and then respect families' choices. As discussed earlier, the symposium emphasized the importance of not viewing alternatives to ambulation and a change of mobility methods over the years as failure. In addition, health care professionals are encouraged to promote peer counseling, to explore clients' experiences with what types of technology work for them, and to consider both functional performance and the prevention of secondary conditions when recommending seating or other technology.

In the journey from childhood to adulthood the child with spina bifida has many physical obstacles and psychologic challenges to overcome, but with appropriate medical intervention and habilitation planning, and with the support of the family, friends, and community resources, the child with spina bifida also has great potential to have a full and purposeful life.

REFERENCES

1. Myers GJ, Cerone SB, Olson AL: A Guide for Helping the Child with Spina Bifida. Charles C Thomas, Springfield, Ill, 1981.
2. Shurtleff DB, Lemire R, Warkany J: Embryology, etiology and epidemiology. *In* Shurtleff DB (ed): Myelodysplasia and Exstrophies: Significance, Prevention, and Treatment. Grune & Stratton, Orlando, Fla, 1986, p 39.
3. Stein SC, Schut L: Hydrocephalus in myelomeningocele. Childs Brain 5:413, 1979.
4. Badell A: Myelodysplasia. *In* Molnar GE (ed): Pediatric Rehabilitation, 2nd ed. Williams & Wilkins, Baltimore, 1992, p 222.
5. Stallard J, Major RE, Patrick JH: The use of the orthotic research and locomotor assessment unit (ORLAU) parawalker by adult myelomeningocele patients: A seven year retrospective study—Preliminary results. Eur J Pediatr Surg 5:24, 1995.
6. Park BK, Song HR, Vankoski SJ, et al: Gait electromyography in children with myelomeningocele at the sacral level. Arch Phys Med Rehabil 78:471, 1997.
7. Hinderer KA, Hinderer SR, Shurtleff DB: Myelodysplasia. *In* Campbell SK, Vander Linden

DW, Palisano RJ (eds): Physical Therapy for Children. WB Saunders, Philadelphia, 1994, p 571.

8. Macri JN, Haddow JE, Weiss RR: Screening for neural tube defects in the United States. Am J Obstet Gynecol 133:119, 1979.

9. Haddow JE, Marci JN: Prenatal screening for neural tube defects. JAMA 242:515, 1979.

10. Bennett MJ, Blau K, Johnson RD, et al: Some problems of alpha-fetoprotein screening. Lancet 2:1296, 1978.

11. Crandall BF, Hanson FW, Tennant F, et al: Alpha-fetoprotein levels in amniotic fluid between 11 and 15 weeks. Am J Obstet Gynecol 160:1204, 1989.

12. Milunsky A, Jick SS, Bruell CL, et al: Predictive values, relative risks, and overall benefit of high and low maternal serum alpha-fetoprotein screening in singleton pregnancies: New epidemiologic data. Am J Obstet Gynecol 161:291, 1989.

13. Coniglio SJ, Anderson SM, Ferguson JE: Functional motor outcomes in children with myelomeningocele: Correlation with anatomic level on prenatal ultrasound. Dev Med Child Neurol 38:675, 1996.

14. Shurtleff DB, Luthy DA, Nyberg DA, et al: The outcome of fetal myelomeningocele brought to term. Eur J Pediatr Surg 4:25, 1994.

15. Meuli M, Meulisimmen C, Hutchins GM, et al: The spinal cord lesion in human fetuses with myelomeningocele—Implications for fetal surgery. J Pediatr Surg 32:448, 1997.

16. Klien NW, Oakley GP, Erickson JD, et al: Folic acid and prevention of spina bifida. JAMA 275:1636, 1996.

17. Centers for Disease Control and Prevention: Recommendations for the use of folic acid to reduce the number of cases of spina bifida and other neural tube defects. Morb Mortal Wkly Rep 41(RR-14):1, 1992.

18. Food and Drug Administration: Food standards: Amendment of standards of identity for enriched grain products require addition of folic acid. 61 Federal Register 8781, 1996.

19. Garber JB: Myelodysplasia. *In* Campbell SK (ed): Pediatric Neurologic Physical Therapy, 2nd ed. Churchill Livingstone, New York, 1991, p 169.

20. McLone DG: Technique for closure of myelomeningocele. Childs Brain 6:65, 1980.

21. Carstens C, Rohweder J, Berghof R: Orthotic treatment and walking ability of patients with myelomeningocele—Analysis of influencing factors. Z Orthop Ihre Grenzgeb 133:214, 1995.

22. Miller E, Sethi L: The effect of hydrocephalus on perception. Dev Med Child Neurol Suppl 13:77, 1971.

23. Tew B: The Cocktail Party Syndrome in children with hydrocephalus and spina bifida. Br J Disord Commun 14:89, 1979.

24. Tew B, Laurence KM: The effects of hydrocephalus on intelligence, visual perception and school attainment. Dev Med Child Neurol Suppl 17:129, 1975.

25. Carmel PW: The Arnold Chiari malformation. *In* McLaurin RL, Epstein F (eds): Pediatric Neurosurgery: Surgery of the Developing Nervous System. New York, Grune & Stratton, 1982.

26. Yeates KO, Enrile BG, Loss N, et al: Verbal learning and memory in children with myelomeningocele. J Pediatr Psychol 20:801, 1995.

27. Graham HK: Three dimensional gait analysis in spina bifida. J Pediatr Orthop 16:786, 1996.

28. Lock TR, Aronson DD: Fractures in patients who have myelomeningocele. J Bone Joint Surg Am 71:1153, 1989.

29. Rosenstein BD, Greene WB, Herrington RT, et al: Bone density in myelomeningocele: The effects of ambulatory status and other factors. Dev Med Child Neurol 29:486, 1987.

30. Stuberg WA: Considerations related to weight-bearing programs in children with developmental disabilities. Phys Ther 72:35, 1992.

31. Mazur JM, Shurtleff DB, Menelaus M, et al: Orthopaedic management of high-level spina bifida. J Bone Joint Surg Am 71:56, 1989.

32. Townsend PF, Cowell HR, Steg NL: Lower extremity fractures simulating infection in myelomeningocele. Clin Orthop 144:255, 1979.

33. Butterworth G, Hicks L: Visual proprioception and postural ability in infancy—A developmental study. Perception 6:255, 1977.

34. Shumway-Cook A, Horak F, Black O: A critical examination of vestibular function in motor-impaired learning disabled children. J Pediatr Otorhinolaryngol 14:21, 1987.

35. Williams H, McClenaghan B, Ward D, et al: Sensory-motor control and balance: A behavioral perspective. *In* Whiting HA, Wade MG (eds): Themes in Motor Development. NATO Advanced Study Institute on "Motor Skill Acquisition in Children," Maastricht, Netherlands, 1985, p 247.

36. Hannigan KF: Teaching intermittent self-catheterization to young children with myelodysplasia. Dev Med Child Neurol 21:365, 1979.

37. Enrile BG, Crooks KK: Clean intermittent catheterization for home management in children with myelomeningocele. Clin Pediatr 19:743, 1980.

38. Segal ES, Deatrick JA, Hagelgans NA: The determinants of successful self-catheterization programs in children with myelomeningocele. J Pediatr Nurs 10(2):82, 1995.

39. Begeer JH, Staalschreinemachers AL: The benefits of team treatment and control of adult patients with spinal dysraphism. Eur J Pediatr Surg 6:15, 1996.

40. Salomao JF, Leibinger RD, Carvalho JG, et al: Ambulatory follow-up of patients with myelomeningocele in a pediatric hospital. Arq Neuropsiquiatr 53:444, 1995.

41. Kendall FP, McCreary EK, Provance PG: Muscle Testing and Function, 3rd ed. Williams & Wilkins, Baltimore, 1993.

42. Lieber RL: Skeletal Muscle Structure and Function. Williams & Wilkins, Baltimore, 1992.

43. Karol LA: Orthopedic management in myelomeningocele. Neurosurg Clin North Am 6:259, 1995.

44. Menelaus MB: The Orthopedic Management of Spina Bifida Cystica, 2nd ed. Churchill Livingstone, Edinburgh, 1980.

45. Stewart SFC, Eng M, Palmieri BS, et al: Wheelchair cushion effect on skin temperature, heat flux, and relative humidity. Arch Phys Med Rehabil 61:229, 1980.

46. McFadyen GM, Stoner DL: Polyurethene foam wheelchair cushions: Retention of supportive properties. Arch Phys Med Rehabil 61:234, 1980.

47. Piper MC, Darrah J: Motor Assessment of the Developing Infant. WB Saunders, Philadelphia, 1994.

48. Folio MR, Fewell RR: Peabody Developmental Motor Scales and Activity Cards. DLM Teaching Resources, Allen, Tex, 1983.

49. Russell D, Rosenbaum P, Gowland C, et al: Gross Motor Function Measure, 2nd ed. McMaster University, Gross Motor Measures Group, Hamilton, Ontario, 1993.

50. Haley SM, Coster WJ, Ludlow LH, et al: Pediatric Evaluation of Disability Inventory (PEDI). Communication/Therapy Skill Builders, San Antonio, Tex, 1996.

51. Duncan PW, Weiner DK, Chandler J, et al: Functional Reach: A new clinical measure of balance. J Gerontol 45(6):192, 1990.

52. Story M, Fife S: Seated Postural Control Measure. Sunny Hill Hospital for Children, Vancouver, BC, 1992.

53. Allen BL, Ferguson RL: The operative treatment of myelomeningocele spinal deformity—1979. Orthop Clin North Am 10:845, 1979.

54. Ward WT, Wenger DR, Roach JW: Surgical correction of myelomeningocele scoliosis: A critical appraisal of various spinal instrumentation systems. J Pediatr Orthop 9:262, 1989.

55. Sarwark JF: Spina bifida. Pediatr Clin North Am 43:1151, 1996.

56. Campos JJ, Bertenthal BI, Kermoian R: Early experience and emotional development: The emergence of wariness of heights. Psyschol Sci 3:61, 1992.

57. Harbourne RT, Giuliani C, MacNeela J: A kinematic and electromyographic analysis of the development of sitting posture in infants. Dev Psychol 26:51, 1991.

58. Grimm RA: Hand function and tactile perception in a sample of children with myelomeningocele. Am J Occup Ther 30:234, 1976.

59. Sand PL, Taylor N, Hill M, et al: Hand function in children with myelomeningocele. Am J Occup Ther 28:87, 1974.

60. Mazur JM, Menelaus MB, Hudson I, et al: Hand function in patients with spina bifida cystica. J Pediatr Orthop 6:42, 1986.

61. Gram M, Kinnen E, Brown J: Parapodium redesigned for sitting. Phys Ther 61:657, 1981.

62. Knutson LM, Clark DE: Orthotic devices for ambulation in children with cerebral palsy and myelomeningocele. Phys Ther 71:947, 1991.

63. Mazur JM, Shurtleff D, Menelaus M: Orthopaedic management of high-level spina bifida. J Bone Joint Surg Am 71:55, 1989.

64. Liptak GS, Shurtleff DB, Bloss JW, et al: Mobility aids for children with high-level myelomeningocele: Parapodium versus wheelchair. Dev Med Child Neurol 34:787, 1992.

65. Hebert EB: Comparative study of the effects of three mobility devices used by children with meningomyelocele. Dev Disabil 10(2):1, 1987.

66. Hoffer MM, Feiwell E, Perry R, et al: Functional ambulation in patients with myelomeningocele. J Bone Joint Surg Am 55:137, 1973.

67. Gram M: The Parapodium: Adjunct to the Habilitation of the Paraplegic Child. MM Therapeutics, Woodridge, Ill, 1991.

68. Sherk HH, Uppal GS, Lane G, et al: Treatment versus non-treatment of hip dislocation in ambulatory patients with myelomeningocele. Dev Med Child Neurol 33:491, 1991.

69. Lusskin R: The influence of errors in bracing upon deformity of the lower extremity. Arch Phys Med Rehabil 47:520, 1966.

70. Sousa JC, Telzrow RW, Holm RA, et al: Developmental guidelines for children with myelo-dysplasia. Phys Ther 63:21, 1983.
71. Thelen E, Ulrich BD: Hidden skills: A dynamic systems analysis of treadmill stepping during the first year. Monogr Soc Res Child Dev No 223, 56(1), 1991.
72. Kahn-D'Angelo L: The reciprocating-gait orthosis for children with myelodysplasia. Phys Occup Ther Pediatr 9(2):107, 1989.
73. Lord J, Varzos N, Behrman B, et al: Implications of mainstream classrooms for adolescents with spina bifida. Dev Med Child Neurol 32:20, 1990.
74. Stout JL: Gait: Development and analysis. *In* Campbell SK, Vander Linden DW, Palisano RJ (eds): Physical Therapy for Children. WB Saunders, Philadelphia, 1994, p 79.
75. Glaser RM, Sawka MN, Wilde SW, et al: Energy cost and cardiopulmonary responses for wheelchair locomotion and walking on tile and on carpet. Paraplegia 19:220, 1981.
76. Hildebrandt G, Voight ED, Bahn D, et al: Energy costs of propelling a wheelchair at various speeds: Cardiac response and effect on steering accuracy. Arch Phys Med Rehabil 51:131, 1970.
77. Evans EP, Tew B: Energy expenditure and movement among children with myelomeningocele. Spina Bifida Ther Int J 4(2):43, 1982.
78. Findley TW, Agre JC, Habeck RV, et al: Ambulation in the adolescent with myelomeningocele. I: Early childhood predictors. Arch Phys Med Rehabil 68:518, 1987.
79. Franks CA, Palisano RJ, Darbee JC: The effect of walking with an assistive device and using a wheelchair on school performance in students with myelomeningocele. Phys Ther 71:570, 1991.
80. Gaff JE, Robinson JM, Parker PM: Walking ability of 14 to 17 year-old teenagers with spina bifida—A physiological study. Physiotherapy 70:473, 1984.
81. Cuddeford TJ, Freeling RP, Thomas SS, et al: Energy consumption in children with myelomeningocele—A comparison between reciprocating gait orthosis and hip-knee-ankle-foot orthosis ambulators. Dev Med Child Neurol 39:239, 1997.
82. Katz DE, Haideri N, Song K, et al: Comparative study of conventional hip-knee-ankle-foot orthoses versus reciprocating-gait orthosis for children with high level paraparesis. J Pediatr Orthop 17:377, 1997.
83. Lollar DJ (ed): Preventing Secondary Conditions Associated with Spina Bifida or Cerebral Palsy. Spina Bifida Association of America, Washington, DC, 1994.
84. Kinsman SL, Doehring MC: The cost of preventable conditions in adults with spina bifida. Eur J Pediatr Surg 6:17, 1996.

Chapter

6

Brachial Plexus Injury

Roberta B. Shepherd, EdD, MA, DipPhty, FACP

Although both the occurrence and the severity of brachial plexus injury in the neonate have been reduced by improved obstetric techniques, as Eng[1] has pointed out, the current incidence is not negligible, and the resultant handicap can be very severe.[2] The relatively small number of such infants seen by therapists constitutes a problem in terms of establishing optimal intervention strategies, as there has been little investigation of new and more effective ways of ensuring the maximum possible recovery of function. There have, however, been advances in the application of microsurgical techniques in reconstructing damaged peripheral nerves in infants with brachial plexus lesions. Some advocate intervention very early in infancy; however, this remains controversial. Unfortunately, early physical treatment of infants with brachial plexus injury is still seen largely as constituting passive movements to prevent soft tissue contractures.[3] A major role of physical therapy, whether for infants or children, is the stimulation of muscle activity and training of effective functional movement.[2, 4]

Advances in the broad area of movement science provide the physical therapist with an increased understanding of the development and biomechanics of reaching and grasping[5, 6] and of the need for task-related training of muscle activity and movement.[4, 7, 8] Furthermore, with modern technology, it is now reasonable to expect physical therapists to test the effectiveness of motor training using, for example, biomechanical data derived from videotape recordings.

Brachial plexus injuries are usually classified under three headings: pure Erb's or upper-plexus type (involving C5 and C6, sometimes C7), Klumpke's or lower-plexus type (C7, C8, and T1), and whole-arm type (C5 to T1). Exact localization of the anatomic lesion is often difficult, however,[9, 10] and many infants demonstrate a mixed upper and lower type. Considerable variation in the type of lesion occurs, ranging from a mild edema affecting one or two roots to total avulsion of the entire plexus. Involvement is usually unilateral, and the results of the lesion are always immediately recognizable.

ETIOLOGY AND INCIDENCE

Injury to the brachial plexus in infants occurs most commonly as a result of a difficult birth.[3, 11] The factors implicated include high birth weight; prolonged maternal labor; a sedated, hypotonic, and therefore vulnerable infant; a heavily sedated mother; traction in a breech presentation or rotation of the head in a cephalic presentation; and a difficult cesarean extraction. It has been suggested that another possible cause of injury to the plexus may be an abnormal uterine posture leading to a pressure neuropathy.[12] It is known that some infants with brachial plexus impairment experience uneventful cesarean section or no mechanical difficulty with birth.[13]

During the birth process, the trauma that injures the plexus may also injure the facial nerve, causing a mild facial paralysis.[1] Other complications include fractures of the clavicle or humerus; traction to the cervical cord with signs of upper motoneuron lesion; subluxation of the shoulder; and torticollis. Many infants also experience a period of intrapartum asphyxia.[12] The phrenic nerve (C4) may also be injured, causing an ipsilateral hemiparalysis of the diaphragm. Eng reported on an infant with a peripheral radial nerve lesion in addition to bilateral Erb's paralysis.[1]

235

Trauma to the shoulder region other than birth injury may also result in injury to the brachial plexus, although this is not common. Such trauma may include pressure from a body cast,[14] falls involving traction and hyperabduction of the shoulder, and pressure from the neck seal of a continuous positive airway pressure head box.[15]

The lower plexus may be injured as a result of pressure from congenital abnormalities such as cervical rib, abnormal thoracic vertebrae, or shortened scalenus anticus muscle. An unusual neuritis of the brachial plexus, called *paralytic brachial neuritis*, which is of unknown cause, has been described by Magee and DeJong.[16]

Although the incidence of severe brachial plexus injury is considered to have declined because of improved obstetric management of difficult labor, there is considerable variability, some reports indicating that the overall incidence has not declined.[11] Adler and Patterson reported that the incidence declined from 1.56 to 0.38 per 1000 live births between the years 1938 and 1962.[10] Others report incidences ranging from 0.6 to 3 per 1000 births.[12, 17–20]

PATHOLOGY

To understand the mechanism of injury, it is necessary to study the anatomy of the brachial plexus and its relationship to its surrounding structures. The reader is referred to the many anatomy texts available. Figure 6–1 illustrates diagrammatically the three main trunks of the plexus. Anatomic findings have been reported to differ markedly in children born in breech presentations compared with those delivered in cephalic presentations. Breech deliveries result in more localized C5–C6 lesions, whereas cephalic presentations result in total lesions with a greater likelihood of rupture.[12]

Stretch to the plexus may result in two anatomically different lesions with different morbidities. The nerve may be partially or totally ruptured beyond the vertebral foramen, causing a neuroma at the damaged site from expanding axons and Schwann cells. Alternatively, spinal nerve rootlets may be avulsed from the spinal cord.[12] In theory, any force that alters the anatomic relationship between neck, shoulder, and arm may result in injury to the plexus. The plexus is attached by fascia to the first rib medially and to the coracoid process of the scapula laterally. Lateral movement of the head with

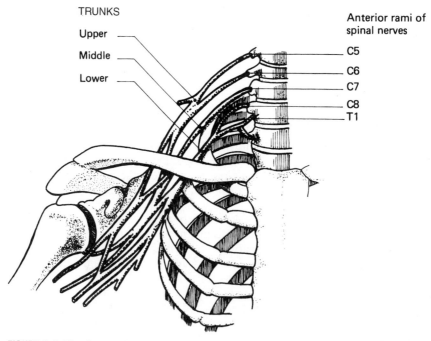

FIGURE 6–1. The three main trunks of the brachial plexus.

depression of the shoulder girdle can stretch the nerves and compress them against the first ribs. Forced abduction (hyperabduction) of the shoulder with traction on the arm stretches the nerves and compresses them under the coracoid process. The former causes injury to the upper plexus, the latter to the lower plexus. When the trauma is severe and stretch reaches a certain force, complete avulsion of the nerves results.

Stretching of the nerve roots or trunk of the plexus may result in injuries ranging from swelling of the neural sheath with blocking of nerve impulses to hemorrhage and scar formation and to axonal rupture with wide separation of fragments.[21] The nerve roots may be completely avulsed from the cord. A combination of these lesions is common and is reflected in the findings from electromyography (EMG).[21] If avulsion occurs there is hemorrhage into the subarachnoid space, and the presence of blood in the cerebrospinal fluid is an indication of more serious injury. Some investigators recommend the use of somatosensory cerebral-evoked potentials for specific diagnosis of dorsal root avulsion.[22, 23] The presence of Horner's syndrome (deficient sweating, recession of the eyeball into the orbit, abnormal pupillary contraction, and ptosis) indicates an intraspinal avulsion of the root of T1 with involvement of the sympathetic fibers.

Regeneration of nerves is unlikely after complete axonal rupture. However, most brachial plexus lesions are less severe, and in these cases, recovery occurs owing to resolution of edema and hemorrhage or to regrowth of nerve fibers down the sheath. In the latter case, recovery is slow because of the distance over which regenerating axons must grow. Regrowth, if it occurs, proceeds at approximately 1 mm per day. In the upper-arm type, this regeneration is usually complete by 4 to 5 months, in the whole-arm type, by 7 to 9 months.[21]

Eng describes serial EMG studies that depict the evolution of the disorder.[1] The lesion is indicated by decreased voluntary motor unit activity and the presence of denervation potentials in the form of fibrillation and sharp wave potentials. Regeneration is signified by the appearance of small polyphasic motor units. As recovery progresses, there is an increase in the number of motor units recorded, a decrease in denervation potentials, and eventually a return of excitability of the nerves to electric stimuli. Degenerative changes in muscles are indicated by absent motor unit activity and a paucity of denervation potentials plus nonconduction.

In adults, denervation of a muscle is followed by changes in the contractile properties of that muscle. A denervated muscle atrophies, with shrinkage of individual muscle cells and thickening of endomysium, perimysium, and epimysium. Studies by Stefanova-Uzunova and colleagues suggest that if denervation occurs at birth, there is also impairment of the normal developmental changes in the contractile properties of muscle that normally occurs postnatally.[24]

DIFFERENTIAL DIAGNOSIS AND PROGNOSIS

The other principal causes of upper limb paralysis in infancy that need to be excluded are upper motoneuron lesions (lesions of the cervical cord or brain) and lower motoneuron lesions (lesions of the anterior horn cell) such as occur in poliomyelitis. Although the clinical appearances of the upper limb in hemiplegia and in brachial plexus paralysis may be similar in terms of the arm's posture and the absence of movement in either the whole arm or certain muscle groups, hemiplegia can usually be easily differentiated by careful analysis of lower limb function and by the testing of reflexes. In upper motoneuron lesions, tendon reflexes are present and hyperactive in both limbs on the affected side or in all four limbs. In addition, there may be sustained ankle clonus and a persistent Babinski sign. A spinal cord lesion is also characterized by sensory abnormalities over the trunk and involvement of the bladder.

Poliomyelitis may be confused with the whole-arm type of brachial plexus lesion but can usually be differentiated by the typical clinical picture and by the presence of intact sensation.

Most cases of brachial nerve injury have a favorable prognosis,[3, 25, 26] with 90% of patients making a complete recovery.[12] It is not the extensiveness of the involvement but the severity of the involvement (i.e., the degree of neural damage) that gives the clue to the prognosis. Eng reported that EMG findings on the extent of the involvement did not correlate with the rate of recovery.[1] For example, an extensive paralysis that is merely a neurapraxic lesion may recover completely, whereas a lesion of only C5 and C6, if complete axonal rupture is involved, may not recover at all.

Without recovery of limb function, the infant is at risk of developing bony deformities and soft tissue contractures[27] due to muscle imbalance and abnormal stress. There is considerable interest in developing reliable predictors of recovery so that the necessity for early surgical intervention can be evaluated. It has been suggested that active elbow flexion together with extension of the elbow, wrist, thumb, and fingers at 3 months of age may be the best predictors of recovery at 12 months.[26]

PHYSICAL THERAPY ASSESSMENT

Assessment is necessary as an aid to diagnosis, as a record of progress, and, by providing a detailed analysis of function, as an important stage in the clinical problem-solving process. An important part of the physical therapy examination is the analysis of motor performance, the objective of which is to gain the most complete picture possible of the infant's current status, the impairments underlying dysfunction (i.e., the status of individual muscle activations), and the problems that may arise in the future. For analysis of motor function to be sufficiently thorough, the therapist needs an understanding of the muscle function required for the performance of everyday movements, particularly reaching to grasp. In the case of infants, the therapist must also understand the development of motor control that occurs as the infant's brain matures and it becomes possible to practice increasingly complex motor tasks.

Muscle activation can be analyzed by observation and palpation of muscle during active movement. EMG, however, enables a more accurate picture of a muscle's ability to contract. Motor performance is analyzed by observation of the infant's attempts at movement (particularly reaching toward an object) during interactions with parents. A record is kept of EMG recordings; muscle activation can be recorded on a muscle chart, and motor performance can be documented on videotape for future comparisons.

Sensory loss may not correspond to the extent of motor loss. Sensory testing is not possible with any degree of accuracy in young infants, and the problem is compounded by the muscle paralysis. The response to a pinprick can be tested, using the infant's appearance of discomfort as a guide, and the result can be recorded on a body chart. O'Riain describes a wrinkle test that may be helpful.[28] The fingers are immersed in water at 40°C for 30 minutes. Normal skin wrinkles, but denervated skin does not. Wrinkling returns as the skin is reinnervated. In older children, two-point discrimination can be tested using an esthesiometer, and other standard tests can be performed.[29]

Analysis of Motor Function

The presence of movement is assessed by *observation* of the following:

1. Spontaneous movement and posture as the infant lies in the supine and prone positions and is moved around, cuddled, and talked to
2. Motor behavior during testing of reflexes and reactions, particularly the Moro reflex, the placing reaction of the hands, the Galant (trunk incurvation) reflex, the neck-righting reaction, and the parachute reaction

Observation gives some indication of muscle activity, which can be graded and recorded on a chart as, for example,

0 = absent
1 = present, but lacking full range of movement
2 = present throughout a full range of movement

This chart is upgraded at subsequent visits, the therapist always searching actively for the presence of muscle contraction in different parts of the range and different relationships to gravity because a muscle may twitch under certain conditions but not others.

Although it is usual in the literature to see a list of the typically denervated muscles in the various types of lesions, the therapist should take care not to assume weakness and paralysis in certain muscles and normal function in others. Careful analysis of motor function frequently reveals a mixed lesion. In addition, as time passes, a lack of use of the limb results in disuse weakness of other muscles not involved in the original lesion.

Several authors describe the use of EMG *assessment*.[21, 29] Eng suggests that EMG is useful in topographically delineating the extent and severity of the injury and in giving information about the expected recovery.[1] EMG would also provide the therapist with the information needed in planning treatment, as EMG signs of return usually precede clinical evidence of function by several weeks. Serial EMG studies are begun within the first 2 weeks after birth and are repeated at 6- to 8-week intervals for as long as indicated.

Decreased denervation potentials and the appearance of reinnervation potentials may predate subjective clinical evidence by several weeks. The appearance of these EMG findings should therefore be followed immediately by intensified therapy to stimulate activity in these muscles. EMG information would enable the therapist and the parents to concentrate on the eliciting of motor activity in particular muscles and the training of functional movements at a time when the therapist may not otherwise be able to recognize the first signs of motor activity. Although excessive fatigue should be avoided, specific motor training at this point in recovery may be crucial to the infant's ability to make the most of neural recovery. Therefore, EMG should probably be used more extensively than at present in order to guide the motor training program.

Range of motion is analyzed using simple videotape analyses under standardized conditions. *Grip strength* is measured using a force transducer, a grip force dynamometer, or a special piece of apparatus involving a rubber bulb connected to a manometer.[29] *Functional motor performance* can be measured using standardized videotaping, which allows several measures to be taken, ranging from the simple (number of reaches to an object in a set period of time) to the complex (kinematic analysis of reaching to grasp). In older children, reliable tests of function such as the nine-hole peg test are used.

Patterns of Muscle Dysfunction

In the *upper-plexus type*, the dysfunction may involve the rhomboids, levator scapulae, serratus anterior, deltoid, supraspinatus, infraspinatus, biceps brachii, brachioradialis, brachialis, supinator, and long extensors of the wrist, fingers, and thumb (Fig. 6–2).

In the *lower-plexus type*, dysfunction involves the intrinsic muscles of the hand and the extensors and flexors of the wrist and fingers. Many infants demonstrate some mixture of upper- and lower-type dysfunction.

In the upper- and lower-plexus types, behavioral (altered movement patterns) and structural (soft tissue length changes) adaptations arise as a result of the paralysis or weakness of certain muscles, the unopposed activity of other muscles, and the resultant muscle imbalance. These adaptations result in persistent movement substitutions (Fig. 6–3), abnormal posturing of the arm (see Fig. 6–2), posterior displacement of the humeral epiphysis and posterior radial dislocation (Fig. 6–4), and eventually, skeletal deformity and poor bone growth.

The resting position of the arm is normally at the side. After brachial plexus injury, this position, the paralysis or weakness of the shoulder abductors and flexors and of the scapular retractors and protractors, and the overactivity of the unopposed shoulder adductors and medial rotators eventually result in soft tissue contracture of those muscles held at their shortened length. Elbow flexion contracture has been reported to be common even in children with force-generating capacity in the elbow extensors.[32] This brief

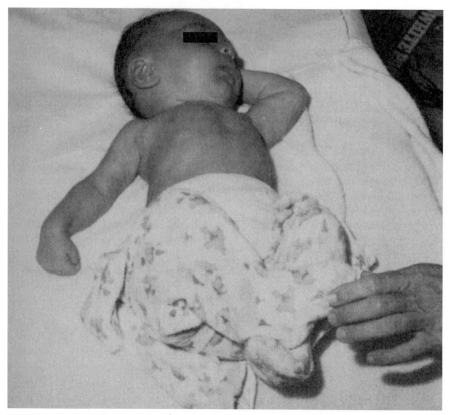

FIGURE 6–2. Infant 4 weeks of age with partial paralysis of the right arm.

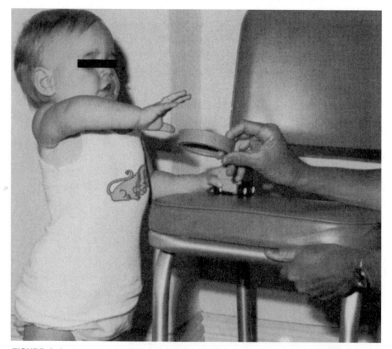

FIGURE 6–3. Infant 13 months of age showing an adaptive motor pattern of the arm and trunk; that is, movement that reflects the action of innervated musculature, encouraged in this case by the position of the toy and the ease with which it can be grasped with the forearm in pronation.

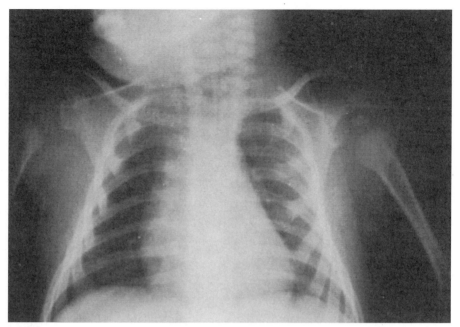

FIGURE 6–4. Radiograph of an infant showing dislocation of the right glenohumeral joint.

report reflects a common finding in clinical practice with both adults and children, particularly in association with a brain lesion, that the prevailing posture of the upper limb is with the elbow flexed.

Paralysis of the rhomboideus muscle, together with the unopposed activity and eventual contracture of the muscles that link the humerus to the scapula (subscapularis, teres minor, latissimus dorsi), causes the scapula to adhere to the humerus, and any flexion or abduction movement of the arm is accomplished in a 1:1 ratio instead of the normal 6:1 humeroscapular relationship in the first 30 degrees of movement.

Abnormal movement of the arm reflects the structural and functional muscle imbalance and resultant substitution of movements that reflect the action of unaffected musculature.[33] The typical posturing of the neonate with the upper-plexus type of paralysis (adducted, medially rotated shoulder, extended and pronated forearm, flexed wrist) gives way to an elevated, slightly abducted, medially rotated, and pronated arm as some muscle activity returns and as the infant makes adaptive movements in attempts to reach out with the arm.

It is common to see abnormal combinations of movement components, for example, the combination of wrist flexion and forearm pronation with finger extension for grasping. These altered movement patterns are similar to those seen as part of the motor dysfunction resulting from central nervous system lesions. It is likely, however, that these abnormal movements are the result of the infant's attempts at reaching in the most biomechanically advantageous way given the state of muscle innervation and muscle length. These substitutions may be reasonably effective in the short term and will be persistently repeated by the infant and become well learned.

Some investigators refer to these adaptive movements as *synkinetic movements* or *associated movements*. Contractions of the biceps brachii and deltoid muscles have been noted to occur in conjunction with inspiratory movement.[34, 35] Esslen found synchronous motor unit potentials in different muscles supplied by the same nerve.[36] De Grandis and colleagues described a 13-year-old girl who was incapable of extending her fingers without flexing the forearm and wrist and a 15-year-old girl whose strong finger flexion was associated with flexion of the forearm and wrist.[37] These authors concluded that there is simultaneous innervation by the same motoneurons of one or more "motor subunits" in different muscles. They also suggested that an inability to perform some movements may be due to simultaneous contraction of antagonistic muscles and not to a lack of muscle strength. Tada and associates, in their study of rats, discussed disordered recovery and suggested that functionally different neurons as well as the correct neurons participate in the regeneration of the disrupted nerves.[38]

In the *whole-plexus type* of muscle dysfunction there may be no apparent muscle activity in the limb. Major problems are caused by the dependent position of the arm with the resultant stretch of soft tissues, together with a lack of muscle activity with which to preserve the integrity of the glenohumeral joint. This may result in subluxation and dislocation of the joint.

Other problems that may result from muscle paralysis are *learned nonuse*, a delay in achieving certain motor milestones such as independent sitting, and an inability to perform two-handed actions in addition to those actions involving only the affected limb.

Analysis of Respiratory Function

Phrenic nerve paralysis, resulting in decreased movement of the ipsilateral thorax with respiratory distress and cyanosis, may mimic diaphragmatic hernia.[39]

Hemiparalysis of the diaphragm should be suspected whenever there are persistent physical and radiographic findings of atelectasis and unilateral diaphragmatic elevation. However, examination of diaphragmatic function using EMG and fluoroscopy should be carried out for all infants with the upper- or whole-plexus type of paralysis. When EMG is unavailable, assessment involves observation of thoracic and abdominal movement in order to detect motor asymmetry.

PHYSICAL THERAPY

The infant should rest for the first few days to allow hemorrhage and edema to resolve. Physical treatment then begins, with the major objectives being to ensure the optimal conditions for recovery of motor function, to provide the environmental conditions and the motivation necessary to enable muscles to resume function as soon as sufficient neural regeneration has taken place, and to train motor control by the practice of actions such as reaching to objects.

To ensure the optimal conditions for recovery, one should minimize the problems of soft tissue contracture; disorganization of movements at the shoulder and shoulder girdle joints; learned nonuse of the limb; and adaptive movement habits (substitutions). To ensure that optimal functional recovery will follow neural regeneration, therapy includes specific training of functional movement once the affected muscles are reinnervated and capable of contraction. If recovery does not occur, the objectives of physical therapy change to provide for the specific training that will be necessary after microsurgery to repair nerves[40] or surgery to transplant muscles or arthrodese joints.

The role of physical therapy extends, therefore, beyond the maintenance of soft tissue length and the stimulation of movement; it includes preventing and minimizing disorganized movement of the limb, training task-related motor control, and preventing learned nonuse of the limb. In addition, the physical therapist trains the parents to carry out exercises at home. Treatment follows from a detailed analysis of the impairment and the adaptation, together with an up-to-date understanding of the need for specificity of muscle stimulation and task-related motor training, and the biomechanics of, in particular, reaching to interact with objects. The significance of the growing area of movement science to physical therapy in rehabilitation has been pointed out by Carr and Shepherd[41] and others and is also relevant to movement-disabled infants and children.[4] The effects of each step in therapy should be subject to measurement to ensure that unproductive methods are discarded and new methods are introduced when necessary.

Motor Training

A program of specific motor training should begin within the first 2 weeks of the infant's life. Although there can be no activity in muscles that are not innervated, this early motor training probably serves several purposes: to stimulate activity in muscles whose nerve supply is only temporarily disconnected; to enable muscles to be activated as soon as nerve regeneration has taken place; and to prevent, or minimize, soft tissue contracture, nonuse, and the habituation of ineffective substitution movements.

Motor training should be specific, in that particular actions such as reaching to a goal are trained. The infant's actions are carefully monitored, the therapist using guidance and feedback to ensure that the infant moves as effectively as possible, that is, activates the appropriate muscles for the movement. In the selection of the muscles on which to focus attention, it may be helpful to consider that certain of the involved muscles are particularly essential for reaching to grasp an object, for example, the abductors, flexors, and lateral rotators of the shoulder; together with the scapular rotators, retractors, and protractors; the supinators of the forearm; the wrist extensors and radial deviators; and the palmar abductor of the thumb. Of course, this is not to suggest that these are the only muscles to be trained, but only to point out that there is an urgent need to train these muscles as early as recovery allows, before learned substitution of nonparalyzed muscles and shortening of soft tissues make it difficult for recovering muscles to demonstrate their optimal activity. (See the later case study.)

Training begins under the best possible conditions for each muscle, taking into account leverage, the relationship of the limb to gravity (Figs. 6–5 and 6–6), the fact that an eccentric contraction can often be elicited before a concentric contraction (Fig. 6–7), and the need for optimal alignment to encourage the required muscle action (Fig. 6–8). Hence, the therapist must actively search for the presence of muscle contraction, checking different sectors of the movement range and different relationships of the limb to gravity and trying to elicit eccentric as well as concentric activity if concentric activity is not present.

Unless the therapist elicits these activities, the earliest manifestations of recovery of motor activity in particular muscles may pass unnoticed. In the earliest stage of recovery, a muscle may not be able to contract under conditions of leverage that require more force generation than the muscle is capable of, and the task may have to be modified to be achievable. For example, the deltoid may not be strong enough to raise the arm from the side but may be able to hold the arm and lower it a few degrees from a horizontal position when the patient is sitting (see Fig. 6–7) or hold it in a vertical position when the patient is lying (see Fig. 6–6). Similarly, the wrist extensors may not be able to contract strongly enough to lift the hand from a position of wrist flexion

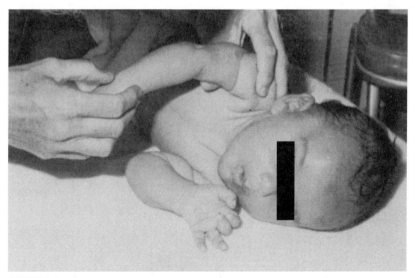

FIGURE 6–5. Infant 4 weeks of age. Attempting to elicit activity in the deltoid muscle by encouraging the infant to take his hand to his face. This would require the muscle to work both concentrically and as a fixator.

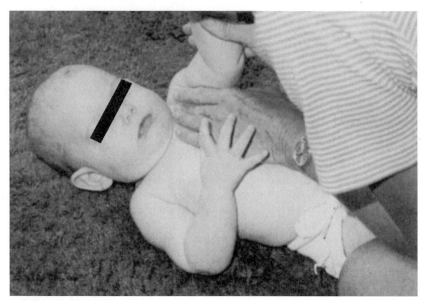

FIGURE 6–6. Infant 4½ months of age. Encouraging activity in the deltoid muscle by holding the patient's arm in flexion as he reaches up to touch the therapist's face.

concentrically, but they may be able to contract eccentrically from a position in which they are shortened, or the radial extensor may be able to contract to radially deviate or lift the wrist from the table.

Motor training continues for as long as recovery is still occurring. It may be that nerves have the potential for recovery for a relatively long period of time. Gatcheva reports EMG evidence of reinnervation and the return of nerve conduction for 6 to 8 years after brachial plexus injury and suggests that it is essential to continue rehabilitation for many years.[42] Gatcheva's observation is contrary to the usual opinion that recovery takes place within the first 2 years. His observations, however, are supported by those of Krichevets and colleagues[43] (see the later case study). The therapist should continue

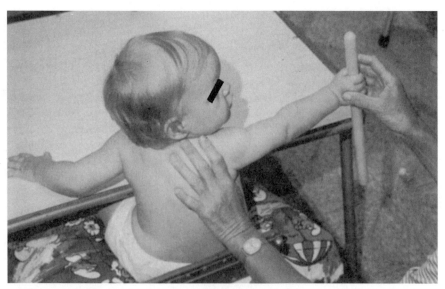

FIGURE 6–7. Infant 13 months of age. Attempting to elicit eccentric deltoid activity in the inner range. The therapist guides scapula movement with her left hand.

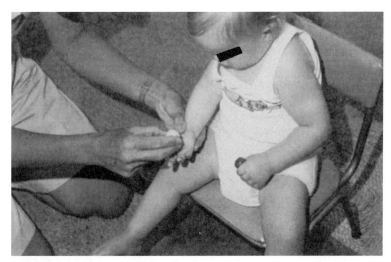

FIGURE 6–8. Infant 13 months of age. Encouraging grasp and release with the forearm in supination. She spontaneously grasps and releases only in pronation.

with periods of intensive motor training, following protocols designed by the therapist, with EMG used to provide guidance on recovery.

Support through the upper limb when the patient is prone and sitting, combined with reaching to grasp, are two actions to concentrate on in training infants and children in upper extremity use because these are principal functions of the upper limb to be developed for effective everyday life. From research by von Hofsten, it is now evident that reaching occurs as a meaningful action considerably earlier than was once thought.[5, 44] The clinical implication is that training in reaching can begin in early infancy. From von Hofsten's work, it appears that certain factors are important to elicit reaching in very young infants: (1) the infant may use the arm more effectively sitting in a semireclined and supported posture in a chair; (2) the object used to elicit the action should be irresistible in its form and color and should be graspable (von Hofsten used a fishing lure minus hook); and (3) the object is more easily detected if it moves across the infant's field of vision at a distance of 5 to 7 inches, rather than being stationary. As the infant matures and more complex reaching games can be played, the object can be placed to encourage flexion and external rotation of the shoulder during reaching and to discourage internal rotation and abduction.

Practice

Object-mediated guidance is usually essential during practice (Figs. 6–9 and 6–10) so that the desired muscle activity can be encouraged and adaptive movements prevented. For example, if the therapist attempts to elicit motor activity by encouraging reaching and other movements without appropriate guidance (see Fig. 6–3), the infant, who will tend to use the stronger muscles or those that have the greatest mechanical or functional advantage, will practice adaptive movements, and these substitutions will be repeated and become learned. Manual guidance needs to be used carefully because the movement will be more likely to be learned if the infant is free to make the movement and not restricted or controlled by the therapist. Object-mediated guidance, in which the therapist presents a toy that by its position in space and its shape requires a certain approach, is potentially more effective (see Fig. 6–18).

Once substitution movements have become a constant part of the infant's repertoire, it may be difficult for them to be "unlearned," at least not until the child is old enough to concentrate for longer periods on motor training and practice. In certain cases, muscles with the potential to recover may fail to develop maximal function because of the early establishment of adaptive movement habits. For this reason, a simple method

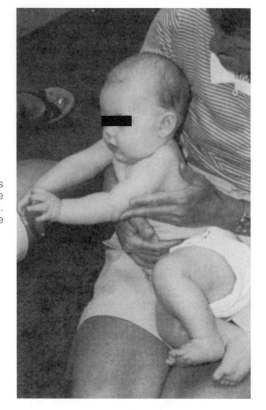

FIGURE 6–9. Manual guidance to ensure that the infant reaches forward in flexion and external rotation. Without guidance he would hold the shoulder in some abduction and internal rotation. The object he reaches for should be one that "forces" some supination.

of identifying the earliest manifestations of muscle activity by EMG should be used so that the therapist and the parents have notice of muscle reinnervation and can concentrate their attention on organizing practice to ensure the best possible recovery of function. Of course, when there has been severe disruption of the nerve supply, there may be no recovery of function, no matter how skilled the therapist and the parents.

Fitts and colleagues have pointed out that the first stage in motor learning is *cognitive*; that is, the beginner tries to "understand" the overall idea of the task and what it demands. The second stage is *associative*, a period of continuous adjustment and reorganization of motor behavior in which components are tried out and put together, and the third stage, the *autonomous* or automatic stage, is characterized by coordinated execution of the task, requiring little cognitive control and suffering less from distractions.[45, 46] Although there is an increasing lack of conscious awareness during this stage, learning does not cease. It is generally assumed that movement in infants can be stimulated only at an automatic level by play or by *facilitation* of movement. However, even small babies are able to *learn* motor patterns by seeking a goal and by reacting to feedback generated by successful attainment of that goal and reinforced by the therapist and the parents. An advantage of training interaction with desirable objects is that the infant also gets feedback about the successful (or not) outcome of the action. The tasks practiced need to be varied frequently to keep up motivation and to take account of the infant's relatively short attention span.

It is therefore necessary to think of many tasks for the infant to practice that involve the required muscle action. It is likely that the motor training of infants would be more effective if it concentrated on stimulating the infants' awareness of what he or she must do in order to achieve a goal (e.g., grasp a toy) rather than simply on eliciting an automatic response. During training, the infant should not merely practice (and repeat) what can already be done, because this will usually be an adaptive movement reflecting muscle imbalance. As muscles regain the capacity to contract and generate force, the necessary movement patterns need to be "forced." An interesting example of

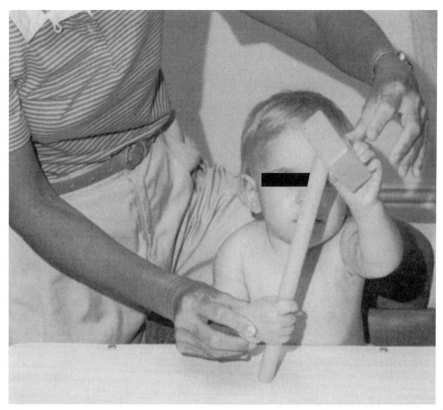

FIGURE 6–10. A game to encourage supination of the right forearm and to ensure the appropriate forearm alignment for grasping.

how this can be done comes from a single case study reported from Moscow.[43] As the authors point out, if an activity is interesting and if attention is directed at the outcome rather than at the disability, children (and infants) appear to be able to use their limbs more easily.

CASE STUDY

A 13-year-old boy, Alex, who had had Erb's palsy since birth, demonstrated an apparently immobile upper limb. His arm hung by his side with a depressed shoulder girdle, extended elbow and wrist, pronated forearm, and flexed fingers. Although he had an almost full passive range of motion, he had virtually no active movement. He could use adaptive ("trick") movements such as trunk movement to lift his arm onto a table.

The goal of helping him to achieve "well-controlled" arm movement required the solving of two problems: first, to stop the use of the adaptive motor behavior ("pathologic motor stereotypes") that he had developed in response to his impairments; second, to "restore strength to the main muscle groups of the arm, beginning with the external upper arm rotator muscles."

A training device that involved a computer and specially designed controls was developed. The computer screen conveyed audiovisual information during a game that required Alex to be accurate in the control of certain spatial and temporal movement parameters. The game took about 1 hour and was played 2 or 3 times a week. The apparatus was designed to enable certain movements of the shoulder or elbow, or both, to result in a desired movement of a sighting beam on the screen. (Placing the beam over a submarine resulted in an explosion and the destruction of the submarine.) For example, to move the handle up, he had to move his arm forward and upward; to move the handle to the right required external rotation of the shoulder joint. Adaptive movements were discouraged and made difficult by the construction of the device. In several days, Alex switched from trying to use the established adaptive movements to the movements wanted at this stage by the investigators.

At the conclusion of the study (no length of time was provided), Alex was able to raise his arm almost to the horizontal position without adaptive movements. Training is continuing.

ANALYSIS

This report illustrates very well the importance of preventing the replacement of adaptive motor patterns for the patterns of movement required for successful task performance. The result appears to illustrate a point made by others that the repetitive use of adaptive movements can become so well learned, so habitual, that they may be used even when the potential to move differently is present.[33, 47]

From the text of the article, it appears that not only did Alex have to *unlearn* adaptive movement patterns, but he also had to work to eliminate unnecessary muscle activity (called *hypertonus* by the authors). The authors comment that such a technique capitalized on the boy's motivation to succeed; that he concentrated on the outcome of his movements rather than on the actions themselves. A similar outcome has also been reported from a study of children with cerebral palsy,[48] who were able to increase their range of active forearm supination more during a task in which supination was required to beat a drum (a concrete task) than in another that involved attempting to supinate as far as possible (an abstract task).

Physical therapists can learn important lessons from such studies. Physical therapy for individuals with movement impairments typically consists of the patient's being moved by the therapist or responding to therapist-induced movement; when exercise is active and self-initiated, it often consists of uninteresting exercises or abstract tasks. This situation prevails despite proposals that physical therapy could instead involve motivating, enabling, and forcing self-initiated tasks directed toward attaining desirable goals and involve considerable practice *without* the therapist present. Such proposals were first made more than a decade ago.

Verbal Feedback and Reinforcement

The infant's effective attempts at using the arm are rewarded so that feedback is an inducement to a successful repetition. *Verbal feedback* of successful performance, with reinforcement from the tone of voice, a smile, and a general attitude of pleasure, seems to have meaning even for small infants, who usually strive to repeat the performance. The appropriate selection of objects and tasks, the necessary guidance that ensures that the infant is as successful as possible, and verbal feedback mean that training sessions are fun and motivating for the infant.

Behavior therapy is a more formalized method of ensuring maximal learning of the desired motor behavior. Behavior therapy involves positive reinforcement by smiling and saying, "Good," or by giving actual rewards, and by shaping or reinforcing successive approximations of the desired behavior. For example, if the child will not concentrate on practicing a particular activity, the child is rewarded for practicing for 2 minutes, then for 3 minutes, and so on.

Treatment of Movement Disorganization

Disorganization of scapulohumeral movement is frequently a serious problem evident in the older infant and child (Fig. 6–11). Early therapy not only should aim to prevent adaptive shortening of muscles, such as the subscapularis, that link the scapula and the humerus but also should aim to stimulate the rhomboids and serratus anterior muscles

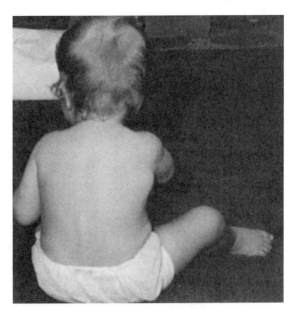

FIGURE 6–11. Note the abnormal relationship between the scapula and the humerus on the right side. The scapula is protracted and moves with the humerus.

to contract. Passive movement that ensures the normal range of shoulder abduction and flexion will have no real effect if the muscles that retract, protract, and rotate the scapula are inactive or weak. Figures 6–12 and 6–13 show two ways of ensuring that the scapular retractors have the maximal opportunity to contract. However, once contraction with the arm by the side is possible, these muscles should be encouraged to contract with the arm progressively more and more abducted. Training the serratus anterior muscle is more difficult, but the therapist can stabilize the scapula against the thoracic wall while the infant takes weight through the hands. Therapy aims to train a more normal relationship both between the protractors and retractors themselves and between these muscles and the muscles for which they act as stabilizers and synergists.

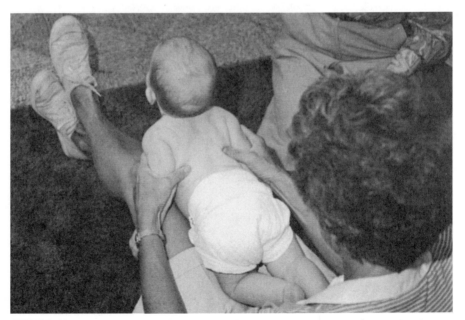

FIGURE 6–12. Infant 4½ months of age. An activity to encourage the scapula retractors to contract.

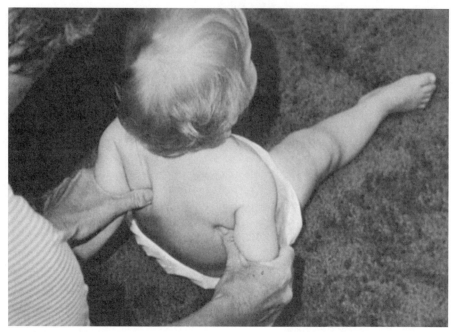

FIGURE 6–13. Another method of encouraging the scapular retractors to contract. The infant's weight is shifted backward onto her hands.

Attempts are made to elicit activity in the supinators of the forearm, when these are weak or paralyzed, as early as possible in infancy. Unfortunately, infants in the early months can accomplish much of what they want to do with the forearm in a pronated position (Fig. 6–14), so specific ways of training active supination need to be instituted by the therapist (Figs. 6–15 and 6–16). Active supination is easier to elicit if the elbow and arm are stabilized to prevent other movements (see Fig. 6–15). The elbow-flexed

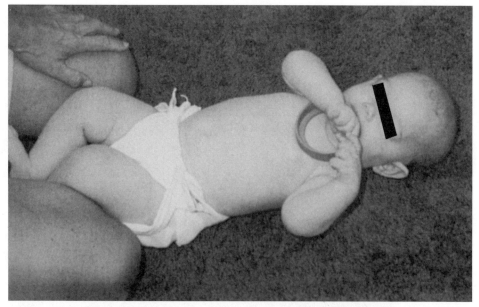

FIGURE 6–14. Note the inappropriate alignment of wrist and forearm. If the infant continues practicing without control of the wrist and forearm position, this posturing may become habitual even though recovery of affected muscles takes place.

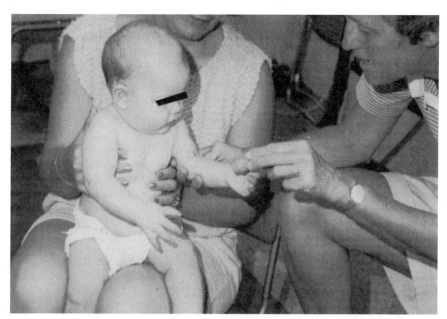

FIGURE 6–15. Holding the elbow in flexion probably makes it easier to activate supination of the forearm.

position also favors the contraction of the biceps brachii, which is the most efficient supinating muscle in this position. Not only is supination more difficult to localize with the elbow extended, but muscle activity is also less likely to be elicited, as the supinator muscle needs to be of good strength to act in this position. The therapist should be aware that forced passive supination of the forearm when the pronators are contracted may reinforce the tendency toward dislocation of the radius.[21] Passive movements are in

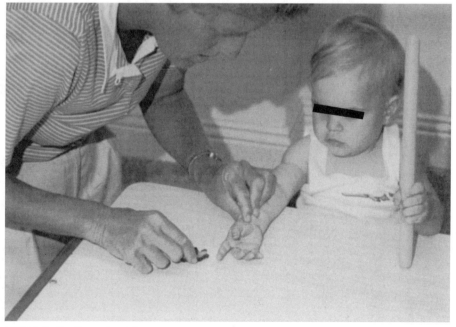

FIGURE 6–16. Once the infant has some active supination, this movement should also be encouraged with the elbow extended.

any case of no value, as the infant will persist in using the hand in the pronated position, and passive movement will not stimulate active contraction of the supinators. Practicing beating a drum has been shown to be an effective means of gaining maximal supination effort from a child.[48] Some other ways to stimulate specific motor activity are illustrated in Figures 6–17 to 6–19.

Biofeedback

Biofeedback, or sensory feedback therapy, is potentially a means of reinforcing the required motor behavior in infants and children. The development of biofeedback devices will eventually progress to the stage at which they are simple and accurate enough to give an irresistible signal to an infant, which will be motivation for further practice.

Orthoses

If during training sessions the infant's movements are not guided and "forced" by a therapist or a parent, it is possible that potential improvement in recovering muscles will not take place. Potential improvement may also be inhibited if abnormal alignment of a joint (or joints) is maintained outside therapy sessions, encouraging the infant to practice only the adaptive movement.

Splinting or strapping can therefore be used to prevent excessive use of unopposed or relatively unopposed muscles until the child can be trained to contract only those muscles necessary for a movement and to eliminate activity in others not required for the movement. In this way, innervated but weak muscles can be forced to contract, the further development of movement substitutions may be prevented, and the child may have a better chance of regaining functional use of the limb.[2, 49]

To make it possible for the appropriate muscle activity to be practiced, the child or infant may wear a small, light splint for a significant part of the day. For example, an infant with paralysis of the palmar abductor of the thumb may need a small molded-

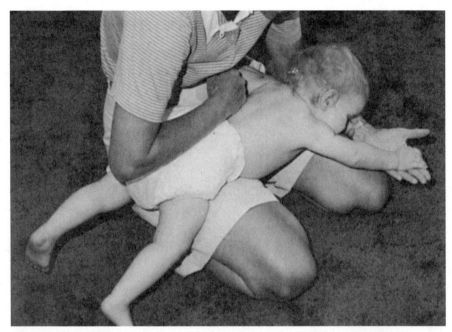

FIGURE 6–17. Training deltoid muscle and scapular retractors. The therapist is eliciting eccentric contractions by encouraging the infant to lower her hand toward the therapist's hand, a clapping game. Beating a drum is another game.

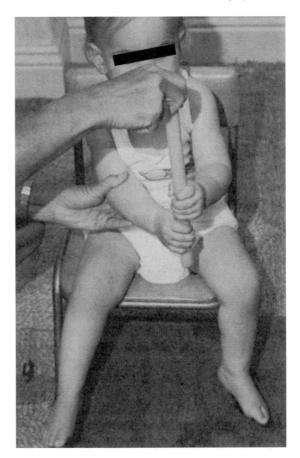

FIGURE 6–18. Practicing grasp and release and shoulder flexion by placing hand over hand. The therapist guides the movement by preventing shoulder abduction.

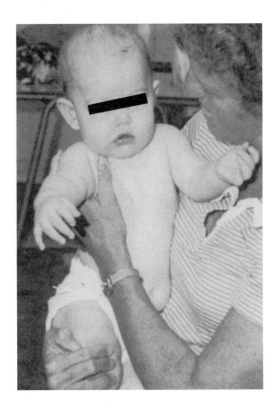

FIGURE 6–19. If the parents hold the infant like this, the tendency to abduct instead of flex the shoulder is controlled and the movement of flexion is encouraged.

plastic splint to hold the thumb in palmar abduction, but this should be worn only for periods of the day to help in using the hand effectively and should not interfere with what appropriate movement the infant has. Similarly, a small wrist splint may be worn for part of the day to encourage activity in the wrist extensors with the hand in the necessary alignment. Dynamic splinting may be useful to reinforce wrist extension in infants with a C7 paralysis.[1]

With increased maturity and ability and inclination to interact with the environment, the infants will practice what they like, whether the movement is a substitution or not, and at this stage the provision of an orthotic device may be effective in forcing nonadaptive practice and in encouraging the use of the limb. If a splint is used, it is designed so that it does not discourage or impede the movement wanted. Training to stimulate activity in particular muscles in the older infant can be combined with the use of a training device (see the earlier case study), which will also make training sessions enjoyable and enable appropriate home practice.

Electrical Stimulation

The use of electrical stimulation is controversial, and its efficacy has not been adequately tested in children. However, there has been at least one report of the effective use of functional electrical stimulation in promoting the regaining of activation of shoulder muscles in a flaccid upper limb after a stroke.[50] Eng and colleagues suggested that the use of electric current of sufficient intensity to cause a maximal muscle contraction under isometric conditions may prevent the wasting of denervated muscle and loss of awareness of the affected limb.[1, 21] Liberson and Terzis also suggested that there is considerable clinical evidence that electrical stimulation of denervated muscle fibers prevents muscle atrophy.[51] However, they are critical of typical physical therapy practice, which they consider grossly inadequate in terms of, for example, the length of time allotted to muscle stimulation. In contrast, functional electrical stimulation has been shown to be effective when approximately 6 hours per day of stimulation is given. These authors have developed a "slow pulse stimulator" that they believe overcomes many of the problems associated with manually operated galvanic stimulation. Functional electrical stimulation can be begun as soon as active muscle contraction can be obtained, with emphasis at this time on active training of the limb.

Soft Tissue Contracture

Passive Movements

Many authors stress the importance of passive movements in preventing soft tissue contracture, particularly scapulohumeral adhesion.[1, 4] Passive movements must, however, be done gently to avoid damage to the unprotected shoulder joint. Zancolli comments that forceful manipulation is one of the factors that contributes to an alteration in the anatomy of the glenohumeral joint.[52] Although it is important to prevent contracture of the muscles that link the scapula to the humerus, the normal relationship between the scapula and the humerus, and the necessity for controlled scapular movement as the glenohumeral joint is abducted or flexed,[53] must be taken into account. The scapula should not be manually restrained once the humerus is moved beyond 30 degrees of range. Elevation of the arm without rotation of the scapula and without lateral rotation at the glenohumeral joint can traumatize the glenohumeral joint by causing the humerus to impinge on the immobile acromion process. Abduction or flexion of the arm should therefore not take place without external rotation, which should be assisted if necessary.

Particular care is also taken in teaching the infant's parents how to do passive movements. Parents should receive instruction in the anatomy of the shoulder so that they understand the movements they must do and the importance of keeping within the normal range. They should understand the anatomic reasons why they must be careful not to overmobilize and why they must be gentle. They should be warned not to proceed with any movement that causes the infant to cry. Without this knowledge, a parent may severely injure the infant's arm.

Soft tissue contracture, however, will ultimately be prevented only if activity recovers in the affected muscles. Passive movements will not lead to the restoration of active function. Training therefore concentrates not only on ensuring the optimal position and alignment of joints, but most particularly on the stimulation of active contraction at their lengthened range of those muscles resting persistently at a shortened length.

Splinting

Splinting, particularly when it involves the shoulder, remains a controversial issue.[9–11] Although some investigators have recommended it, evidence exists that several of the problems that arise in these infants may be directly related to the type of splinting used.

In the upper-plexus type, some have suggested that the arm be held in abduction and lateral rotation by pinning the sleeve to the pillow or by a "Statue of Liberty" splint, or held in abduction and midrotation by an abduction splint. In subsequent articles, some of these investigators, as well as others,[9, 11, 39, 54–56] have pointed out, however, that splinting the arm in this position may lead to "overmobility" of the glenohumeral joint, and that this positioning may be a factor that contributes to abnormality in the glenohumeral joint, even to anterior dislocation.[21] Although there seems to be sufficient evidence to discontinue the use of the types of shoulder splinting listed previously, when paralysis affects the entire limb it should be possible for therapists, orthotists, and bioengineers to design a means of supporting the humerus in the glenohumeral cavity that will not discourage use of the limb and will not predispose to joint dysfunction.

Neglect of the Arm, or Learned Nonuse

Neglect of a paralyzed arm is relatively common in hemiplegic infants and children and in adults after stroke.[4, 41] It is also likely to occur in infants with brachial plexus lesions and may be an important contributing factor to the failure to develop motor control. If initial attempts to use the arm result in failure, the infant may cease trying. Nonuse may also be a factor in preventing the recovery of muscle function that could potentially have occurred as a result of nerve regeneration. Several reports in the literature mention infants with good return of muscle function who nevertheless ignored the arm and refused to use it.[1, 39] Wickstrom attributed this neglect to the lack of development of "functional cerebral motor patterns of coordination."[9] Zalis and colleagues suggested that transitory interruption of peripheral nerve pathways at birth prevented the establishment of normal patterns of movement and the organization of body image.[57] Taub has described what he calls *learned nonuse*, which is demonstrated by monkeys after either deafferentation or brain lesion, and which is primarily due, according to Taub, to a learning phenomenon.[58] The animals learn *not* to use the affected limb because they can perform in a satisfactory manner with the remaining limbs and no motivating factor exists to encourage them to use the affected limb. This habitual nonuse persists so that even when the limb becomes potentially useful, the animal does not seem aware of this possibility. Others have described similar findings.[59] Investigations have shown promising results for intact limb constraint together with intensive task-related training in increasing arm use after stroke.[60] Consequently, motor training procedures for infants with brachial plexus lesions should include constraint of the unaffected arm (Fig. 6–20). One study of two hemiplegic infants involved constraint of the intact arm during training sessions for short periods during the day.[61] After 6 months of training, both children were able to successfully use the previously paretic arm and hand. Constraint of the intact limb plus intensive training ("forced" use) has been proposed elsewhere for infants, children, and adults with motor disorders affecting one upper limb.[4, 62]

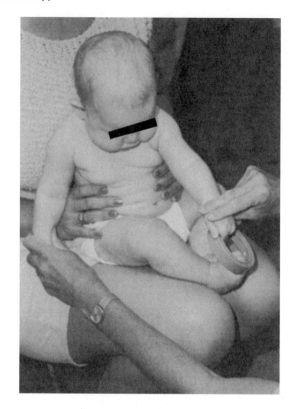

FIGURE 6–20. The unaffected limb can be constrained during training sessions. However, the arm should be constrained within a well-fitting vest or bandaged to the upper body.

Sensory Unawareness

In treatment, specific attempts should be made to stimulate sensory awareness, but these can probably only be effective once the infant is old enough to play sensory games, such as locating certain objects in sand, localizing touch stimuli, and recognizing and naming common objects while blindfolded. When the child is older, two-point discrimination and stereognosis guessing games can be used in an attempt to improve awareness. A study of individuals after stroke demonstrates that practice of particular sensory experiences can result in improved awareness of those sensations.[63]

Abnormal Respiratory Function

When diaphragmatic paralysis exists, respiration can be aided by oxygen with continuous positive airway pressure or continuous negative pressure.[64, 65] If the nerve lesion is a neurapraxia, there is eventual recovery of diaphragmatic function, but during the period of paralysis, it is important to prevent respiratory problems such as atelectasis. Positioning with the paralyzed side underneath should be avoided. Postural drainage in the prone position at a 45-degree angle should be carried out at home for short periods during the day with the objective of preventing retention of secretions in the relatively immobile parts of the lung.

SURGICAL TREATMENT

Between 8 and 20 percent of children with brachial plexus lesions are reported to require surgical intervention.[12, 26] Surgery is not usually performed in infancy, although some investigators suggest that with certain lesions, surgical intervention may help in the removal of hematomas or the neurolysis of adhesions,[14] and others suggest early surgical exploration and repair by nerve graft.[66] In the older child, surgery to stabilize joints, tendon transplantation, and soft tissue elongation are performed with the objective of gaining some improvement in function.[67, 68] Zancolli describes surgical techniques aimed at improving function and cosmesis of the shoulder.[52]

CONCLUSION

Brachial plexus injury at birth may, in a small proportion of children, result in considerable disability involving muscle paralysis and weakness, soft tissue contracture, loss of sensation, and sympathetic changes. The major loss of function is the infant's inability to reach out and to use the hand effectively. Therapists should question whether existing treatment procedures are optimal in view of increased knowledge of movement dynamics, the adaptability of the system, and the use of technology to drive learning and performance. More effective ways of training motor control and of preventing habitual substitution movements and learned nonuse of the limb need to be developed and applied to infants and children with neural impairments.

REFERENCES

1. Eng GD: Brachial plexus palsy in newborn infants. Pediatrics 48:18, 1971.
2. Sjoberg I, Erichs K, Bjerre I: Cause and effect of obstetric (neonatal) brachial plexus palsy. Acta Paediatr Scand 77:357, 1988.
3. Draznin E, Maloney FP, Brammell C: Functional strapping for incomplete Erb palsy: A case report. Arch Phys Med Rehabil 65:731, 1984.
4. Shepherd RB: Physiotherapy in Paediatrics, 3rd ed. Butterworth-Heinemann, Oxford, 1995.
5. Von Hofsten C: Development of visually directed reaching: The approach phase. J Hum Movement Stud 5:160, 1979.
6. Jeannerod M: The timing of natural prehension movements. J Motor Behav 16:235, 1984.
7. Carr JH, Shepherd RB (eds): Movement Science. Foundations for Physical Therapy in Rehabilitation. Aspen, Rockville, Md, 1987.
8. Rutherford OM, Jones DA: The role of learning and coordination in strength training. Eur J Appl Physiol 55:100, 1986.
9. Wickstrom J: Birth injuries of the brachial plexus: Treatment of defects of the shoulder. Clin Orthop 23:187, 1962.
10. Adler JB, Patterson RL: Erb's palsy: Long-term results of treatment in eighty-eight cases. J Bone Joint Surg Am 49:1052, 1967.
11. Johnson EW, Alexander MA, Koenig WC: Infantile Erb's palsy (Smellie's palsy). Arch Phys Med Rehabil 58:175, 1977.
12. Ubachs JMH, Slooff ACJ, Peeters LLH: Obstetric antecedents of surgically treated obstetric brachial plexus injuries. Br J Obstet Gynaecol 102:813, 1995.
13. Jennet RJ, Tarby TJ, Kreininck CJ: Brachial plexus palsy: An old problem revisited. Am J Obstet Gynecol 166:1673, 1992.
14. Swaiman KF, Wright FS: Neuromuscular Diseases of Infancy and Childhood. Charles C Thomas, Springfield, Ill, 1970.
15. Turner T, Evans J, Brown JK: Monoparesis. Complication of constant positive airways pressure. Arch Dis Child 50:128, 1975.
16. Magee KR, DeJong RN: Paralytic brachial neuritis. JAMA 174:1258, 1960.
17. Jackson ST, Hoffer MM, Parrish N: Brachial plexus palsy in the newborn. J Bone Joint Surg Am 70:1217, 1988.
18. Greenwald AG, Schute PC, Shively JL: Brachial plexus birth palsy: A 10-year report on the incidence and prognosis. J Pediatr Orthop 4:689, 1984.
19. Specht EE: Brachial plexus palsy in the newborn. Clin Orthop 75:32, 1975.
20. Davis DH, Onofrio BM, MacCarty CS: Brachial plexus injuries. Mayo Clin Proc 53:799, 1978.
21. Eng GD, Koch B, Smokvina MD: Brachial plexus palsy in neonates and children. Arch Phys Med Rehabil 59:458, 1978.
22. Zverina E, Kredba J: Somatosensory cerebral evoked potentials in diagnosing brachial plexus injuries. Scand J Rehabil Med 19:47, 1977.
23. Landi A, Copeland SA, Wynn Parry CB, et al: The role of somatosensory evoked potentials and nerve conduction studies in the surgical management of brachial plexus injuries. J Bone Joint Surg Br 62:492, 1980.
24. Stefanova-Uzunova M, Stamatova L, Gatev V: Dynamic properties of partially denervated

muscle in children with brachial plexus birth palsy. J Neurol Neurosurg Psychiatry 44:497, 1981.

25. Al-Qatter MM, Clarke HM, Curtis CG: The prognostic value of concurrent clavicular fractures in newborns with obstetric brachial plexus palsy. J Hand Surg Br 19:729, 1994.

26. Michelow BJ, Clarke HM, Curtis CG, et al: The natural history of obstetrical brachial plexus palsy. Plast Reconstr Surg 93:675, 1994.

27. Tachdjian MO: Pediatric Orthopedics, 2nd ed. WB Saunders, Philadelphia, 1990.

28. O'Riain S: New and simple test of nerve function in the hand. BMJ 3:615, 1973.

29. Sundholm LK, Eliasson A-C, Forssberg H: Obstetric brachial plexus injuries: Assessment protocol and functional outcome at age 5 years. Dev Med Child Neurol 40:4, 1998.

30. Bufalini C, Pescatori G: Posterior cervical electromyography in the diagnosis and prognosis of brachial plexus injuries. J Bone Joint Surg Br 51:627, 1969.

31. Leffert RD: Brachial plexus injuries. N Engl J Med 291:1059, 1974.

32. Ballinger SG, Hoffer MM: Elbow flexion contracture in Erb's palsy. J Child Neurol 9:209, 1994.

33. Shepherd RB, Carr JH: Commentary: "Normal" is not the issue: It is "effective" goal attainment that counts. Behav Brain Sci 19:72, 1996.

34. Gjorup L: Obstetrical lesion of the brachial plexus. Acta Neurol Scand Suppl 18:9, 1966.

35. Robinson PK: Associated movements between limb and respiratory muscles as a sequel to brachial plexus birth injury. Johns Hopkins Med J 89:21, 1951.

36. Esslen E: Electromyographic findings on two types of misdirection of regenerating axons. Electroencephalogr Clin Neurophysiol 12:738, 1960.

37. De Grandis D, Fiaschi A, Michieli G, et al: Anomalous reinnervation as a sequel to obstetric brachial plexus palsy. J Neurol Sci 1:127, 1979.

38. Tada K, Ohshita S, Yonenobu K, et al: Experimental study of spinal nerve repair after plexus brachialis injury in newborn rats: A horseradish peroxidase study. Exp Neurol 2:301, 1979.

39. Rose FC (ed): Paediatric Neurology. Blackwell Scientific, Oxford, 1979.

40. Boome RS, Kaye JC: Obstetric traction injuries of the brachial plexus. J Bone Joint Surg Br 70:571, 1988.

41. Carr JH, Shepherd RB: A Motor Relearning Programme for Stroke, 2nd ed. Heinemann, London, 1987.

42. Gatcheva J: Early diagnosis and long term management of obstetric paralysis. Int Rehabil Med 3:126, 1979.

43. Krichevets AN, Sirotkina EB, Yevsevicheva IV, Zeldin LM: Computer games as a means of movement rehabilitation. Disabil Rehabil 17:100, 1995.

44. Von Hofsten C: Eye-hand coordination in the newborn. Dev Psychol 18:450, 1982.

45. Fitts PM: Perceptual motor skill learning. *In* Melton AE (ed): Categories of Human Learning. Academic, San Diego, 1964.

46. Fitts PM, Posner MI: Human Performance. Prentice-Hall, London, 1973.

47. Shepherd RB: Adaptive motor behaviour in response to perturbations of balance. Physio Theory Practice 8:137, 1992.

48. Van der Weel FR, van der Meer ALH, Lee DN: Effect of task on movement control in cerebral palsy: Implications for assessment and therapy. Dev Med Child Neurol 33:429, 1991.

49. Perry J, Hsu J, Barber L, Hoffer MM: Orthoses in patients with brachial plexus injuries. Arch Phys Med Rehabil 55:134, 1974.

50. Faghri PD, Rodgers MM, Glaser RM, et al: The effects of functional stimulation on shoulder pain in hemiplegic stroke patients. Arch Phys Med Rehabil 75:73, 1994.

51. Liberson WT, Terzis JK: Some novel techniques of clinical electrophysiology applied to the management of brachial plexus palsy. Electromyogr Clin Neurophysiol 27:371, 1987.

52. Zancolli EA: Classification and management of the shoulder in birth palsy. Orthop Clin North Am 12:433, 1981.

53. Cailliet R: The Shoulder in Hemiplegia. FA Davis, Philadelphia, 1980.

54. Carter S, Gold AP: Neurology of Infancy and Childhood. Appleton-Century-Crofts, East Norwalk, Conn, 1974.

55. Schut L: Nerve injuries in children. Surg Clin North Am 52:1307, 1972.

56. Aitken J: Deformity of elbow joint as sequel to Erb's obstetrical paralysis. J Bone Joint Surg Br 34:352, 1952.

57. Zalis OS, Zalis AW, Barron KD, et al: Motor patterning following transitory sensorymotor deprivation. Arch Neurol 13:487, 1965.

58. Taub E: Somato-sensory deafferentation research with monkeys: Implications for rehabilitation medicine. *In* Ince LP (ed): Behavioural Psychology in Rehabilitation Medicine: Clinical Applications. Williams & Wilkins, Baltimore, 1980, p 371.

59. Yu J: Functional recovery with and without training following brain damage in experimental animals: A review. Arch Phys Med Rehabil 57:38, 1976.

60. Taub E, Miller NE, Novak TA, et al: A technique for improving chronic motor deficit after stroke. Arch Phys Med Rehabil 74:347, 1993.

61. Schwartzman RJ: Rehabilitation of infantile hemiplegia. Am J Phys Med 53:75, 1974.

62. Carr JH, Shepherd RB: Neurological Rehabilitation: Optimising Motor Performance. Butterworth-Heinemann, Oxford, 1998.

63. Yekutiel M, Guttman E: A controlled trial of the retraining of the sensory function of the hand in stroke patients. J Neurol Neurosurg Psychiatry 56:241, 1993.

64. Bucci G, Marzetti G, Picece-Bucci S, et al: Phrenic nerve palsy treated by continuous positive pressure breathing by nasal cannula. Arch Dis Child 49:230, 1974.

65. Weisman L, Woodall J, Merenstein G: Constant negative pressure in the treatment of diaphragmatic paralysis secondary to birth injury. Birth Defects 12:297, 1976.

66. Gilbert A, Khouri N, Cartioz H: Exploration chirurgicale du plexus brachial dans la paralysic obstetricale. Rev Chir Orthop 66:33, 1980.

67. Hoffer MM, Wickenden R, Roper B: Brachial plexus birth palsies: Results of tendon transfers to the rotator cuff. J Bone Joint Surg Am 60:691, 1978.

68. Manske PR, McCarroll HR, Hale R: Biceps tendon rerouting and percutaneous osteoclasis in the treatment of supination deformity in obstetrical palsy. J Hand Surg 5:153, 1980.

The Infant at Risk for Developmental Disability

Suzann K. Campbell, PT, PhD, FAPTA

The advent of high-technology neonatal care has produced the miracle of increased survival of infants who 2 decades ago would have been considered nonviable. Although 90 percent mortality rates were formerly common for babies born weighing less than 1000 g, today 40 to 60 percent of these infants survive.[1, 2] Yet these immature survivors, and others with complicated medical problems in the perinatal period, continue to have high rates of developmental morbidity such as cerebral palsy (CP), developmental delay, and learning and behavioral disabilities.[3] Morbidity rates ranging from 10 to 80 percent for various conditions and outcomes have supported the role of physical therapists in special care nursery settings and in monitoring programs for developmental follow-up of infants at high risk for disability.

GUIDES TO DECISION MAKING

Evidence-based decision making by the physical therapist serving infants at risk for developmental disabilities can be guided by a number of reference sources:

1. The American Physical Therapy Association (APTA) Section on Pediatrics statements on competencies for the physical therapist in the neonatal intensive care unit (NICU)[4] and in early intervention (EI) settings[5]
2. Federal and state guidelines for the provision of services to infants at risk for developmental disabilities[6]
3. The consumer-generated Principles for Family-Centered Neonatal Care[7]
4. Research reports on

    a. Characteristics of infants at risk for developmental disabilities and their families
    b. Assessment tools with diagnostic or predictive validity for developmental outcome
    c. Efficacious interventions to foster optimal development of these infants

5. Cumulative risk indices or formally structured critical pathways[8] for follow-up of developmental progress in infants at risk for developmental disabilities

ROLES AND COMPETENCIES

The therapist may provide services in the special care nursery itself, as a member of a developmental follow-up team in an outpatient clinic, as a member of an EI team in a community-based school or EI center, in home-based practice, or in a pediatric rehabilitation facility. According to the Section on Pediatrics guidelines, roles in each of these types of settings require advanced skills in pediatric physical therapy.[4] The APTA competency document indicates that prior experience in assessing the development of normal infants and in treating infants with disabilities is needed before practicing in the

NICU. The generalist or new graduate should not provide NICU services without supervision. Recommended means of obtaining the skills needed for competency in the NICU environment include a mentored experience under the supervision of a therapist experienced in the management of infants at risk for or with diagnosed developmental disabilities.[9] Such training was not found to be typical of actual practice in a survey conducted by Rapport just before the APTA competency statement was published.[10]

Rapport's study of NICU practice reported that the typical therapist's roles include (1) consultation on environmental modifications and follow-up developmental assessment, (2) screening of infants for risk and the need for longitudinal evaluation of developmental progress, (3) assessment of sensorimotor development, (4) family education and anticipatory guidance, (5) inservice education for nurses, and (6) direct treatment using interventions to promote age-appropriate and optimal development.[10] In 1988 when Rapport's data were collected, 30 percent of therapists reported using environmental modifications in the nursery in support of infant development and 80% used Neuro-Developmental Treatment (NDT). As noted previously, however, Rapport did not find that APTA best-practice recommendations for inservice education applied. For example, most special care nurseries did not have education requirements for staff, with the exception that therapists were often required to have NDT certification.

The Section on Pediatrics competencies stress that therapists provide physical therapy that is developmentally and physiologically appropriate for the infant as well as sensitive to the environmental and social needs of the family.[4] Physical therapy in the NICU must also be sensitive to the demands and characteristics of the NICU environment itself, including the competencies of other staff members, such as nurses and occupational therapists,[11] and the unique culture of the unit.[12–14] Given such sensitivity, the therapist can act as a team member and change agent, lending expertise in developmentally appropriate care to a service that has as its first commitment the provision of medically necessary care to promote the growth and survival of fragile infants.

Given the high-technology characteristics of the NICU and the fragility of its patients, the first competency addressed in the APTA guidelines is the prevention of harm.[4] Competency in this area of practice ensures the safety of the infants by emphasizing the importance of understanding physiologic monitoring systems and reading infant cues that signal stress, approach, or avoidance. The guidelines also promote injury prevention and optimally nurturing parenting through education and anticipatory guidance for families. Other areas of competency related to patient care addressed in the APTA statement include infant assessment; the design and implementation of plans of care; and consultation (education and information sharing, coordination, and collaboration with other services and community agencies). Rapport reported that examination of infants was performed by 100 percent of the therapists she surveyed, whereas 75 percent implemented parent education, gave inservice training to nurses, and provided consultation to a follow-up clinic.[10] Direct services provided by more than 80 percent of therapists included positioning of infants, range of motion (ROM) exercises, and therapeutic intervention.

Research evidence in support of practice related to the topics that have been introduced is discussed in this chapter in conjunction with a series of patient cases. The advent of new models for understanding the needs of fragile infants, new diagnostic and evaluative tools, and recent research on efficacious and cost-effective interventions allows us to review these cases and reflect on how our contemporary knowledge base, best-practice guidelines, and the Hypothesis-Oriented Algorithm for Clinicians (HOAC)[15] might be used to improve the management of high-risk infants and to suggest an agenda for future research. First, a model of service delivery designed to construct a nurturing environment for the growth and development of fragile infants is described. This section is followed by information on the identification of infants at risk for developmental disabilities, the assessment of sensorimotor development, and the effects of positioning, movement therapy, and parent education programs. Each section contains case examples and reflection on practice in light of information in the current research literature. The chapter ends with a suggested critical pathway for developmental follow-up examination, advice for novices, and an agenda for the future.

THE NURSERY: CONSTRUCTING A NURTURING ENVIRONMENT

When therapists, nurses, and psychologists first became involved in attempting to foster the development of infants at high risk for developmental morbidity, the theoretic model suggested that infants were deprived of stimulation as a result of early birth and thus in need of special attention involving handling.[16] As pioneers in the area of developmental neonatology began to study the reactions of these infants to typical caregiving,[17] and the actual levels of stimulation from light, sound, and manipulation experienced by the babies in a typical day,[18] the theoretic framework was transformed from a model emphasizing the need for stimulation to one of protection from overstimulation. Sweeney provides an excellent review of the research on environmental overload experienced by infants in special care nurseries with specific attention to studies of physical therapy effects on physiologic stability.[19] Examples of negative effects on infants described by Sweeney include decreased oxygenation, increased blood pressure, and increased heart rate during chest therapy; increased heart rate and mean arterial pressure during hydrotherapy; increased heart rate and blood pressure with skin mottling during neurologic assessment; and increased heart rate (but no change in oxygen saturation) during developmental intervention.[20]

Avery and Glass summarize current thinking by indicating that the common goal of well-conceived developmental interventions is *physiologically* appropriate sensory input.[21] They describe the brain of the 24-week fetus as barely one-fourth the size of the term infant's brain, with a smooth surface nearly devoid of gyration, a metabolically inactive cerebral cortex, and undifferentiated sleep states. These infants have minimal ability to cope with external stimuli; responses are global rather than differentiated, and activity leads to loss of autonomic control. By term-equivalent age, the brain should quadruple in size, the cortex becomes active, behavioral states become differentiated, and the ability to shut out aversive stimuli is characteristic of the well-organized infant. Interest in the environment typifies this vastly more complex organism, and *appropriate* stimulation is quite different from that needed by the 24-week infant. Thus babies who are medically stable and older are able to respond to more complex stimuli and to engage in sustained social interaction with caregivers. As a result of the rapidly changing development of infants born prematurely, as well as the effects of various medical conditions, the task of the developmental therapist is to match interactions and stimuli to infant characteristics and responsiveness.

As a result of research on infant development and the stress of neonatal intensive care, attempts ensued to recreate boundaries and environments for fragile newborns similar to those that would have been experienced had the infant remained in utero.[22] Sweeney writes that in light of this new protective approach, physical therapists must combine their traditional movement science perspective with a less familiar reflective, observational, behavioral science approach.[19] Furthermore, rather than "do something" interventions, focus has switched to assisting nursery staff and family members to recognize and interpret infant cues related to readiness to receive and profit from interactions and to altering the environment to support infant developmental progress.[23] For example, Miller and colleagues showed that cycled lighting in an NICU produced greater weight gains for infants when compared with control subjects in noncycled lighting conditions.[24] Experimental group infants also had earlier oral feeding, fewer days on the ventilator and on phototherapy, and better motor coordination than control group babies.

Research is gradually accumulating to indicate that infants of low birth weight who are cared for in a carefully structured environment that limits stimulation and supports behavioral organization based on individualized assessment of responsiveness to intervention have a lower incidence of brain hemorrhage and chronic lung disease, grow faster, are discharged from the hospital sooner, and have better cognitive, motor, and behavioral outcomes in late infancy than those cared for under a traditional medical model.[25] Infants with chronic lung disease benefit in terms of briefer stays on a respirator, improved oxygenation, shorter time to achieve complete breast- or bottle-feeding, and better developmental outcomes after discharge.[26] Furthermore, despite the high costs of the training involved in implementing such programs (approximately $97,000 per year for 2 years in 1995 dollars), annual cost savings of from $80,000 to $129,000 *per child* are reported from the use of this approach to care.[27] Employment of this approach, called the Neonatal Individualized Developmental Care and Assessment Program (NIDCAP), should be considered standard practice in the NICU environment and incorporated into APTA best-practice guidelines. One caveat to this recommendation is that another research group failed to replicate the findings previously described.[28] In a controlled clinical trial of the NIDCAP provided for very low birth weight (VLBW) infants, no effects on sleep at 3 months or on motor and cognitive development at 4, 12, and 24 months were found. Further replications are needed.

Neonatal Individualized Developmental Care and Assessment Program

In the NIDCAP, nursery team members receive training in assessing the infant's response to typical caregiving in the NICU environment. Assessment results are used to develop a care plan to foster individual development. Reassessment over time reveals how the infant is accomplishing his or her developmental agenda and what stimulation the infant invites and can handle without undue stress. Physical therapists who have been trained in this approach can play a role in

1. Assessing the infant's reactions to caregiving or developmental examination
2. Suggesting environmental modifications for the individual infant and for the nursery environment as a whole
3. Making or recommending use of various commercially available materials, such as the Wee Thumbie pacifier and positioning equipment available from Developmental Care Products (Children's Medical Ventures, Inc., 541 Main Street, S. Weymouth, MA 02190; telephone, 800-377-3449), which have been found useful in providing a supportive environment for the fragile infant
4. Educating parents in understanding their infant's signals for welcoming or discouraging interaction and in responding in a developmentally appropriate way to promote cognitive and motor development
5. Initiating physical therapy plans of care for infants with especially high risk for CP or delayed motor development that are sensitive to developmental and physiologic readiness to participate in movement therapy

Because all members of the NICU team can be trained to assume the first four of these roles in the NIDCAP approach, those services are not unique to the role of the physical therapist. The lead role is typically played by the infant's primary nurse, but it is necessary that *everyone* involved with the infant's care be consistent in using the prescribed management approach, so the therapist must be knowledgable about this method of care in order to become a fully functioning member of the team. The fifth role listed is the unique province of the physical therapist and should be carried out based on reliable and valid physical therapy examinations and the use of interventions with scientifically documented efficacy and cost effectiveness.

The following case describes the NIDCAP report on an infant who was evaluated by a physical therapist using the NIDCAP behavioral assessment. As is typical of an NIDCAP assessment, the report describes (1) the initial environmental conditions, both of the overall area and of the infant's personal space; (2) the results of a baseline behavioral observation; (3) observations during caregiving; (4) postcaregiving observations; (5) a summary of the goals on which the baby appears to be working, based on the behavioral observations; and (6) recommendations for care to facilitate the infant's ability to achieve his or her personal developmental agenda.

CASE STUDY

NEONATAL INDIVIDUALIZED DEVELOPMENTAL CARE AND ASSESSMENT PROGRAM ASSESSMENT AND REPORT

Observation Conditions

Michael was observed from 1:20 to 2:14 PM in the transitional nursery during his usual care. He sleeps in a six-bed room that was partially lighted; one bank of lights was on directly over his unshielded isolette. The room was exposed to a fair amount of noise from frequent sounding of physiologic monitoring alarms as well as construction outside the unit involving occasional hammering and drilling. It was otherwise a calm afternoon with few people about and infrequent low-volume conversations; there were three observers in an NIDCAP teaching session. Michael lay in his isolette in the supine position with his face turned toward the room on a quilt-covered waterbed with the head elevated. In his bed space were a stuffed bear, a baseball, his hat, and a chest percussion tool. Michael wore nasal prongs for oxygen flow at 0.1 liter, had an orogastric (OG) tube in place, and was monitored with a cardiorespiratory monitor and oximeter. He wore a T-shirt and diaper.

Behavioral Baseline

Michael was observed in a nondisturbed state for 10 minutes before his caregiving session, lying supine in the unshielded isolette. At the beginning of the observation he was in a drowsy state but soon settled into light sleep, making occasional whimpering sounds. He rested with arms and one leg flexed and one leg extended and showed active hand-to-face, hand-to-head, and hand-to-mouth behavior, grasping and holding onto the nasal tubing, at one point pulling out the prongs. He smiled twice in a drowsy state. His breathing rate ranged from 32 to 72 per minute with occasional pauses; his heart rate ranged between 141 and 155 beats per minute (bpm) with oxygen saturation 96 to 98 percent. His color was pink with occasional tremors and twitching.

Behavior During Caregiving

Michael was observed for a total of 34 minutes during routine caregiving consisting of the taking of vital signs, diapering, the changing of an OG tube, and of the oximeter probe; being swaddled, removed from the isolette, and held for OG feeding; and then being returned to the isolette, first in the supine position and then turned to the prone position. His breathing rate continued at 25 to 54 per minute, heart rate 131 to 158 bpm, and oxygen saturation 94 to 99 percent. His color remained pink except (1) for a brief period of flushing 10 minutes into his feeding when he attempted visual alerting and (2) just before a self-resolved period of bradycardia when he showed facial pallor. Michael awakened very gradually into a drowsy state and sustained a brief awake period, even attempting alerting when his nurse shielded his eyes from the overhead light. He then returned to a light sleep state. In the supine position during the taking of vital signs, Michael showed active flexion and extension of limbs with some finger and toe splay and hand-on-face activity plus some foot grasping. Once swaddled and held for feeding, he awakened and was quite expressive with eyebrow raising, smiles, and frowns. He actively mouthed the OG tube during the first half of his feeding. While briefly in a supine position as he was placed back in his isolette, Michael showed dramatic leg extension and grasping of his oxygen tubing. He was left in his isolette in the prone position on his waterbed.

Behavior After Caregiving

Michael was observed for 10 minutes after caregiving while prone in his isolette with his face toward the center of the room. His breathing rate ranged from 32 to 34 per minute, heart rate 136 to 142 bpm, and oxygen saturation 98 percent. Throughout the observation he remained in light sleep in a flexed posture with his left hand under his face and mouth. He was inactive except for occasional mouthing and some twitching.

Summary

Michael was born at 30 to 31 weeks of gestational age (GA) and is currently 17 days old (32.5 weeks postconceptional age), having been delivered by spontaneous vaginal delivery weighing 1415 g (40th percentile). Apgar scores were 8[1] and 9[5]. He may be developing bronchopulmonary dysplasia and receives oxygen by nasal canula. He developed hyperbilirubinemia, which resolved after 2 days under Bililites. He now weighs 1388 g (10th percentile), is fed via OG tube every 3 hours, and receives some breast milk. As assessed by changes in heart rate, breathing, color, and oxygen saturation, Michael is able to maintain physiologic stability well during the clustered caregiving that is typical for him, although oxygen saturation does decrease slightly from baseline during manipulation. He uses postural activity, such as foot grasping and hand grasping of his tubing, to maintain motoric stability during manipulations.

Current Goals

From this observation and Michael's history, it appears that Michael is working toward stabilization of breathing, heart rate, and color despite his need for supplemental oxygen. His behavioral state range is from light sleep to brief availability and alertness. He seeks social interaction by trying to come alert and demonstrating attractive facial expressions when assisted by shielding from light or by being swaddled. His bradycardia and flushing during interaction, though, indicate that this attempt was costly when it occurred during his feeding. In terms of motor control, Michael is somewhat successful in working toward maintaining a flexed posture and using hand-to-mouth and grasping with feet and hands to cope with stimulation but still needs support in the supine position when he is positioned without boundaries.

Recommendations

In order to support Michael in achieving his current goals of (1) physiologic stability, (2) social interaction, (3) greater robustness and range of behavioral states, and (4) active participation in his care through motor control of posture, consider and review

1. The environment at large in order to
   a. Maintain consistently low levels of staff activity and voice levels in Michael's room
   b. Maintain consistently low overhead light levels in Michael's room or provide diurnal variation simulating day and night
   c. Provide comfortable, reclining seating for the parents and caregiver to sit with Michael for feeding
   d. Support Michael's family in continuing to personalize his bed space to show their pride in him and demonstrate his individuality

2. Bed space and bedding in order to
   a. Provide consistently low light levels in Michael's immediate caregiving space and to shield him from light because of fatigue and the need to develop more mature sleep states
   b. Support active participation in care by parents, perhaps asking them to bring in a quilt or thick towel for use as an isolette shield for sound and light reduction
   c. Optimize the time spent prone as it may be beneficial to avoid the supine position in which Michael is less able to obtain a stable posture
   d. Explore bedding and positioning options such as a nest to facilitate Michael's ability to use foot grasp and flexion postures to maintain behavioral state control

3. Specific caregiving in order to
   a. Explore positioning options during caregiving as it may be beneficial to avoid supine positioning or, when the supine position is needed, to use hands-on containment or provide something for Michael to grasp in order to facilitate his participation in his caregiving
   b. Explore periods when eye shielding from light and invitation to social interaction can be successful in supporting Michael's attempts to achieve visual contact and alerting
   c. Evaluate Michael's ability to use a pacifier and something to grasp during feeding or for self-consoling as an assist to his attempts to maintain or conserve energy during interventions
   d. Increase opportunities for Michael to regulate the balance of his postural

> control by containing the infant on the caregiver's chest, and support the parents in swaddling and close holding of the infant
> e. Explore parents' interest in feeding and holding Michael on the parents' body
> f. Facilitate the parents' understanding of Michael's competence through demonstrations of his ability to maintain color during interventions; smile and use appropriate facial expressions during brief social interactions; and use hand grasp and body flexion to maintain energy during manipulations.

REFLECTION ON PRACTICE

Here the therapist has assumed roles 1, 2, and 4 described on page 263, that is, assessing Michael's response to caregiving, recommending environmental and caregiving modifications in support of Michael's current developmental agenda, and developing goals for educating Michael's parents in recognizing his cues. During an NIDCAP assessment, the observer attempts to ascertain when functioning is smooth, how much stress and energy depletion are seen, how much handling can be tolerated, and whether the infant has energy for social interaction and invites it. The infant's approach and avoidance signals, described succinctly by Lawhon, are identified.[29] Typical recommendations include (1) a means to facilitate consistency and appropriate pacing of caregiving in a quiet, soothing environment, (2) clustered, collaborative care within a 24-hour structured day, (3) support during transitions between positions or activities, (4) appropriate positioning and individualized feeding support, (5) developmental support for infant, staff, and family, and (6) opportunities for skin-to-skin holding and other aspects of family comfort and education.[30] In summary, important aspects of the NIDCAP behavioral assessment and report include

1. Observation before, during, and after routine caregiving
2. Analysis of physiologic, motor, and behavioral state self-regulation (efforts and successes) to determine the infant's developmental agenda or goals
3. Recommendations tailored to the infant's goals and needs for support that are described as *opportunities* for the caregiver to explore in support of the infant's developmental agenda

Specific recommendations are avoided in the report in order to encourage the creativity of the caregiver and engage the caregiver in developing an appropriate plan of care that fits into the infant's medical and physical caregiving and supports. In Michael's case, the report aims to facilitate the nurse's role as the infant's primary caregiver, but the parents are gradually encouraged to take over the care of Michael as much as possible. The focus of a future report on Michael might be the mother as caregiver in order to ready the infant and family for discharge. By the time of discharge, a goal for family members is successful ability to read the infant's approach and avoidance signals. Having this ability enables family members to respond to the infant's cues with appropriate support and the just-right challenge to facilitate further development of motoric and physiologic stability, robustness of behavioral states, and social interaction capabilities.

Sweeney and Swanson suggest, however, that the conceptual framework for parents' education is not just one of teaching parents skills.[9] Rather a model of hope and empowerment is a useful conceptual framework. "In a hope-empowerment framework, parent participation in neurodevelopmental intervention allows sharing of power and responsibility and promotes continuous, mutual setting and revision of goals with reality grounding."[9] (p 186) Hope includes the ability to adapt to what is and later to find peace of mind whatever the infant's outcome. Hope gives parents the energy to cope, and if hope is destroyed, parents withdraw in order to protect themselves from further emotional pain.

In summary, an NIDCAP-trained professional views infants as active collaborators in their own care.[30] In keeping with the HOAC model,[15] an NIDCAP assessment asks the infants to first reveal their developmental goals through observation of behavior. Then the infants' behavior provides the information base from which care is designed to best support the baby's overall development in a setting involving necessary medical and nursing interventions. A therapist trained in the NIDCAP approach can support nurses in developing plans of care, consult on design of the infants' bed space and the nursery environment as a whole, and educate families in how to identify their infant's needs and provide responsive, developmentally appropriate care for their babies.

Neonatal Individualized Developmental Care and Assessment Program Training

Training in the NIDCAP approach is available at three levels, labeled I to III.[31] Level I consists of education in infant behavioral observation and developmental care based on the behavioral observation, such as those illustrated by the case of Michael. Level II education provides consultation on the nursery integration of developmental care. This training must involve all appropriate members of the team because Als found that implementation of the approach is unlikely unless physicians, nurses, and other important personnel, including people who provide custodial services, are all on board. This is true because the NIDCAP involves both modifying the environment for the individual infant (based on assessment results) and sheltering the entire nursery environment from excessive noise and other disturbing influences on infant behavioral organization. McGrath and Valenzuela provide helpful suggestions for incorporating developmentally supportive care into a nursery service, including the use of newsletters and bulletin boards and written notes "from the baby" to the baby's nurse when particularly useful supports have been provided to the infant.[14]

Finally, level III education enables an NICU team to qualify as an NIDCAP Training Center. Information on NIDCAP training is available from Heidelise Als, National NIDCAP Training Center, Children's Hospital, Boston, 320 Longwood Avenue, Boston, MA 02115; telephone, 617-355-8249; fax, 617-35-7230; e-mail, als@a1.tch.harvard.edu.

SCREENING FOR DEVELOPMENTAL RISK IN THE NEONATAL INTENSIVE CARE UNIT AND PLANNING FOLLOW-UP

Despite improved environments to support development, new ways to prevent premature birth[32, 33] and to reduce the incidence or severity of brain damage[34, 35] and of lung disease,[36] many medical conditions continue to result in high risk for developmental morbidity. A role for physical therapists in the NICU that is within the unique province of their specialized skills is screening infants for risk for disability in the sphere of sensorimotor function. The therapist plays a role in determining how infants at risk will continue to be managed during the period of uncertainty before a definitive diagnosis or a presumption of normal development. Suggestions in the literature for engaging in this role include primarily using the medical history of the infant as a guide to risk. For example, criteria such as the birth weight, the GA at birth, Apgar scores, the time on a ventilator, brain insults, seizures, and maternal factors such as drug or alcohol use are frequently used to develop a roster of infants who should be closely followed in the nursery or in an outpatient follow-up clinic for assessment of risk for developmental disability.[9, 37] Children with documented syndromes, such as Down syndrome, are also obvious candidates. Rapport reported that deformity or postural deviation, a significant length of hospital stay, and low birth weight were common criteria for services identified in her survey.[10]

How well does this list of criteria hold up to current knowledge? An example is given in a study by Piper and colleagues, who selected high-risk children for random assignment to NDT or no therapy on the basis of medical risk factors (birth weight less than 150 g at birth, or evidence of central nervous system [CNS] dysfunction, or an Apgar score less than 4 at 1 minute and requiring more than 3 minutes of assisted ventilation in the newborn period).[38] Despite being considered high risk for CP, 66 percent of these children were rated normal on a neurologic examination at 12 months and 70 percent at 24 months. Only 10 and 14 percent, respectively, were definitely abnormal. The prospect of a normal outcome, however, varied greatly by the GA at birth, from 46 percent normal at 24 months for those born at less than 28 weeks of GA, to 84 percent for those born at 28 to 31 weeks, 89 percent for those born at 32 to 36 weeks, and 67 percent for those born at greater than 36 weeks. The relatively low rate of normal outcomes in the latter group probably reflects the presence in the group of full-term children with perinatal asphyxia, seizures, or a prolonged need for resuscitation.

If one considers that depending on the medical condition and degree of prematurity, as many as 80 to 90 percent of infants treated in the NICU are likely to turn out to have motor development within normal limits (although, as we shall see, normal does not mean developmentally *equal* to low-risk infants), the cost-effectiveness of regularly assessing the development of all these infants in an NICU or a clinic using high-cost specialty services, such as physical therapy, occupational therapy, and developmental pediatrics, does not seem to be an appropriate use of resources in these times of health care reform focused on cost reduction. A review of the literature on the developmental outcome of infants with perinatal medical complications suggests the types of infants most likely to have developmental morbidity. This information can be used to narrow the criteria for referral to physical therapy services or for frequent developmental screening of motor performance.

Risk Related to Premature Birth

Infants born prematurely or with compromising medical conditions are at risk for transient or long-term poor motor performance.[39] CNS dysfunction expressed as CP is among the most physically disabling of the potential outcomes, found with a prevalence of approximately 2 per 1000 in school-aged children.[40] In a recent national sample of 280 infants born weighing less than 1501 g, 10 percent were diagnosed with CP at 36 months.[41] The proportion was 13.8 percent for those weighing less than 1001 g. Despite the relatively low overall prevalence of CP in the population, about 40 percent of those with CP were born prematurely.

In addition to the risk of CP, children born prematurely typically have lower gross and fine motor performance scores on standardized tests in infancy than full-term controls even when age is adjusted for the degree of prematurity. For example, in a population-based sample of infants from eight counties in North Carolina, standard scores on the 1969 edition of the Bayley motor scale[42] at 12 months averaged 110 for infants weighing more than 2501 g at birth, 102 for those weighing 1501 to 2500 g, and only 95 for those weighing less than 1500 g.[43] It is important to note that these data were obtained based on old norms on the Bayley scales,[42] and scores would probably average about 10 points *lower* on the new Bayley II scales.[44] Furthermore, Goldstein and colleagues demonstrated that despite lower scores on the Bayley II when compared with the 1969 Bayley scales, children are similarly classified as normal, borderline, and abnormal on both the new and the old cognitive scales, but only fair agreement between diagnostic outcomes is achieved when the two motor scales are compared.[45]

Reporting of average scores for groups, of course, obscures the fact that many high-risk infants have age-appropriate motor performance, but Piper and colleagues found that *all* infants weighing less than 750 g at birth had depressed gross motor performance at later ages.[46] Case-Smith also reported delayed fine motor performance in prematurely born infants at 2 to 6 months of adjusted age, as well as less organized postural control in those preterm infants with many medical risk factors.[47] Churcher and colleagues reported that a group of high-risk prematurely born infants that excluded those with definite neurologic problems had an average performance on the Peabody Fine Motor Scale[48] that was more than 1 standard deviation (SD) below the mean at 2 years of age, and one-third of the group scored below 77 (compared with a normative mean of 100 and an SD of 15).[49] Furthermore, Ross demonstrated that premature infants consistently perform less well on motor development tests than on those assessing cognitive function.[50]

In summary, children born with the greatest degrees of prematurity are at high risk for low motor performance although the risk of CP is small. Motor development should be followed in these babies, but this could be done with developmental assessments that do not require the skills of the physical therapist. Michael, for instance, had a low risk of developing CP and, after NIDCAP management in the NICU, could reasonably have been followed after discharge by a developmental pediatrician, nurse, psychologist, or early-childhood specialist trained in assessing infants at risk for possible poor developmental progress. A service delivery plan for such infants might then appropriately include referral of infants for physical therapy who score lower than −1 or −2 SDs below the mean on a normative motor development test such as the Bayley II.[44]

Risk Related to Hemorrhage and Hypoxic-Ischemic Events

Prime factors associated with especially poor motor function in infants, in addition to a very low GA and birth weight, include the presence of intracerebral hemorrhage or ischemic lesions leading to periventricular cysts in preterm infants, and hypoxic-ischemic encephalopathy (HIE) in newborns of all gestational ages.

Intraventricular Hemorrhage

In follow-up of 90 preterm infants and 22 full-term controls, 24 percent of the infants with grades III or IV intraventricular hemorrhage (IVH), and no other infants in the study, were neurologically abnormal at 5 years.[51] Although the cognitive outcome in the entire cohort was related to the socioeconomic status (SES) of the family, there was no relationship of the SES to the neurologic or perceptual outcome. Overall, the duration of hospitalization contributed the most in explaining the variance in the developmental outcome. Sostek and colleagues have also reported a poor outcome on the 1969 edition of the Bayley motor scale for infants with grade III and IV bleeds (an average of 80 and 72, respectively, at 1 year, and 92 and 81 at 2 years, compared with a normative mean of 100).[52]

The smallest babies are at the greatest risk of hemorrhage.[53] The rate of CP is 25 to 30 times higher in VLBW infants (<1500 g) than in full-sized infants,[54] and Papile and colleagues reported that the 16 percent of the VLBW infants who sustained the most severe grades of bleed (III and IV) represented 51 percent of those with severe developmental handicaps and 61 percent of those who were multiply handicapped.[55] In a 1984 report on infants born weighing less than 1000 g (extremely low birth weight) in which 54 percent of infants survived the neonatal period, Kraybill and coworkers, reported one postdischarge death and a 28 percent handicap rate at 12 to 34 months.[2] In a similar more recent cohort of 36 extremely low birth weight infants in which 58 percent survived, only 31 percent demonstrated normal development on the McCarthy Scales at about 4 years of age.[1] Both subgroups with and those without chronic lung disease and/or grade III or IV intracerebral bleeds showed a *decline* in the average developmental performance relative to age-appropriate norms between 19 months and 4 years of age. Possible reasons for this finding include the fact that (1) different aspects of development are assessed at different ages and reflect the development of different parts of the brain, (2) test norms for older tests are more out of date at younger than at older ages, and (3) adjusting for the GA at birth plays an increasingly smaller role in boosting standard scores relative to age norms as the infant gets older. In summary, relative to prematurity alone, the additional presence of grade III or IV IVH doubles or triples the probability of CP. Physical therapists should closely follow the development of babies with severe grades of IVH, both in the NICU and after discharge. A later section describes tests appropriate for this purpose.

Periventricular Leukomalacia

With advances in ultrasound technology, the presence of ischemic lesions resulting in periventricular leukomalacia (PVL), evidenced early in the perinatal period as dense echogenicity on ultrasonography and later as echolucencies if cystic lesions develop, provides an even more sensitive marker than the grade of IVH for those who are likely to have a poor neurodevelopmental outcome. Cystic lesions occur in 3 to 7 percent of VLBW infants, resulting across multiple studies published up until 1990 in an outcome of CP in about 80 percent.[54] In those with echodensities only (40 to 100 percent of VLBW babies based on various reports), 67 percent developed CP. In a report on 232 babies born at less than 32 weeks of GA and screened systematically for periventricular defects, Sinha and colleagues reported an overall incidence rate of 17 percent with PVL.[56] Developmental scores on the Griffiths scale at 18 to 48 months averaged less than 80, and of 6 survivors in an early-lesion group, 4 (67 percent) had major disabilities (3 with spastic diplegia). In a group with later-appearing lesions, 7 (50 percent) of 14 survivors had major disabilities (5 with spastic diplegia). In summary, the risk of CP is over 50 percent for preterm infants with ischemic brain lesions, and physical therapists should definitely follow these infants for developmental progress.

Perinatal Asphyxia

Although the incidence of intrapartum asphyxia is only about 2 percent of births and most children whose charts contain this notation show normal development,[57] asphyxia is believed to contribute to about 25 percent of cases of CP.[40] A problem in accurately documenting the degree of risk associated with this condition has been an unclear definition of asphyxia and the need to demonstrate a series of indicators, including exposure, a clinical response, and an impact on the brain and other organs.[58] Recent efforts to provide strict rules for applying this term to a distressed newborn are likely to result in clarification of the expected outcomes.

If all the following criteria are present, a poor neurologic outcome in survivors is extremely likely: (1) a pH less than 7 in umbilical cord arterial blood, (2) an Apgar score of zero to 3 for more than 5 minutes, (3) clinical neurologic sequelae (e.g., seizures, hypotonia, coma) in the immediate neonatal period, and (4) evidence of multiorgan system dysfunction (e.g., oliguria, meconium aspiration, hypoglycemia, shock).[59] This definition of perinatal asphyxia has been endorsed by the American Academy of Pediatrics and the American College of Obstetricians and Gynecologists.[60] In our work with this definition, we find that children meeting the criteria for asphyxia are often severely damaged and may not even be candidates for assessment or treatment in the NICU because of fragile health status and a high risk of death. Using somewhat less restrictive markers, such as a severe base deficit, a low 5-minute Apgar score, and fetal heart rate abnormalities, Carter and colleagues reported a positive predictive value for abnormal neurologic outcome of 88 percent and a negative predictive value of 73 percent.[59] Table 7–1 summarizes the scoring system used by these investigators; a total of six or more points on the three items in the table constitutes a risk for an abnormal outcome.

We use these as well as some of the following criteria to predict a greater than 50 percent risk of CP:

1. Intracranial Doppler sonography cerebral vessel high diastolic flow with a resistive index below 60.[61]
2. T_1 shortening more than 3 days after injury or T_2 shortening more than 6 days after injury on magnetic resonance (MR) imaging in the deep gray matter, cerebral cortex, periventricular white matter, or a mix of these, or an MR pattern of localized atrophy of cortex with cystic changes, gliosis, and tissue loss of adjacent white matter, and a band-shaped lesion in areas bordering the central sulcus in a term infant.[62, 63]
3. A ratio of lactate/*N*-acetylaspartate greater than 6.22 in the brain (thalamus) based on proton MR spectroscopy.[64]
4. The presence of *all* three of the following in a term infant:[65]

   a. An Apgar score at 5 minutes less than or equal to 5
   b. Neonatal seizures

Scoring System for Predicting Abnormal Outcome

Clinical Sign	Score			
	0	**1**	**2**	**3**
5-min Apgar	>6	5–6	3–4	0–2
Base deficit (mEq/L)	<10	10–14	15–19	>19
Fetal heart rate tracings	Normal	Variable decelerations	Severe variation or lates	Prolonged bradycardia

TABLE 7–1

    c. *Two* of the following signs:
      1) Decreased activity after the first day of life
      2) Incubator care for 3 or more days
      3) Feeding problems
      4) Poor sucking
      5) Respiratory difficulties
   5. Stage 3 HIE (severe tonus abnormality, seizures, and coma or stupor) for 72 hours[66, 67]

Assessment of developmental progress by a physical therapist is definitely appropriate for these infants.

It could be argued that physical therapy in addition to an NIDCAP plan of care should begin in the nursery immediately for those with documented brain insults and especially high risk of poor developmental outcome. The typical premature infant, with NIDCAP support, is able to develop motor skills independently as physiologic stability is achieved. Infants with a brain lesion, however, typically have poverty of movement and abnormal postural tone. These babies may benefit from the assistance of physical therapy to develop their primary repertoire of movement skills. Research investigating this hypothesis is needed.

Risk Related to Bronchopulmonary Dysplasia

Intraventricular hemorrhage is implicated in the relatively poor outcome of infants with bronchopulmonary dysplasia (BPD), a chronic lung condition occurring in infants recovering from respiratory distress syndrome (RDS) with sustained oxygen dependence.[68, 69] Mean cognitive scores for 27 patients with BPD were 85 (compared with a normative mean of 100); 22 percent had major neurodevelopmental abnormalities at 2 to 4 years of age. Skidmore and colleagues reported that 40 percent of VLBW infants in their hospital in 1985 developed chronic lung disease.[70] Bayley motor scores in their 1983–1984 cohort averaged 81 at the outcome assessment; 15 percent had CP compared with an overall CP rate of 6 percent for VLBW infants. A recent study of 122 infants with BPD revealed an 8 percent rate of CP at 3 years of age versus 2 percent for 84 VLBW infants without BPD.[71] About one-quarter of the subjects with BPD had motor performance scores more than 2 SDs below the mean. Factors typically found in those with poor developmental outcome were periventricular abnormalities[69] and seizures.[72] Others have implicated VLBW, IVH, and Apgar scores of less than 7 at 1 and 5 minutes as comorbidities in those with especially poor outcome.[73] Whether or not specific neurologic deficits are present, however, the total group of survivors of RDS tend to have significantly lower scores than control infants in areas such as gross motor and manual performance.[74] In summary, children with BPD are at high risk for delayed motor development, but an elevated risk of CP is related to IVH or PVL comorbidity. Because of their generally poor endurance for physical activity, infants with BPD should be followed by a physical therapist both for developmental progress and for the physiologic appropriateness of their response to exercise. If they are treated, a goal of developing endurance for movement, particularly in relation to oral feeding, is appropriate.

In summary, although premature birth and other perinatal complications are sufficient to increase the risk of below-average motor developmental outcome, infants at highest risk are those born younger than 32 weeks of gestation and with a birth weight less than 1500 g, especially those born earliest and smallest and with multiple medical complications and prolonged hospitalization. Those with specific CNS insults such as PVL, profound hypoxic-ischemic encephalopathy, and severe grades of intracerebral bleeding are especially likely to develop CP with risk rates as high as 70 to 90 percent, but children with birth weights less than 1000 g also have about a 15 to 25 percent risk. Finally, according to Paneth, 5 to 10 percent of children with CP experienced congenital infection, malformations, or intrauterine stroke.[40] These specific groups should be placed on a "risk register" marking a need for close follow-up in the hospital and after discharge, including routine referral for EI services if state policies allow children without a definitive developmental diagnosis to receive services on the basis of medical risk. Those with documented brain insults, such as PVL, grade III or IV IVH, or asphyxia, should receive priority for follow-up and treatment in the nursery by physical therapists, but children with chronic lung disease should also benefit. Finally, infants with congenital anomalies or genetic syndromes who can be expected to experience delayed motor development are appropriately followed by the physical therapist. Prominent among these conditions are Down syndrome and other genetic disorders, brachial plexus injury, torticollis,[75] and myelodysplasia. See other chapters in this volume and in *Physical Therapy for Children*[76] for further information on the management of these conditions.

Because research has shown that children with medical risks who are also from low SES families are in more than double jeopardy for poor cognitive and behavioral outcomes, early referral for intervention in a prevention mode might be most needed by infants with both types of at-risk history.[77–80] This is because poverty increases both health risks and the chance that the child will experience the effects of family depression, stress, poor nutrition, substance abuse,[81–83] and suboptimal parenting. Parenting education may be especially needed by families with low levels of schooling.

Risk Established by Developmental Examination

Rather than establishing a risk register for developmental follow-up based on medical or demographic characteristics, the burden of providing unnecessary assessment and surveillance services for all infants at risk may be decreased by using new screening measures with promise for predicting the risk of developmental disability based on children's actual *developmental* performance in the nursery after a compromised beginning, rather than on medical or physical characteristics alone. In this section, we examine the predictive validity of developmental assessment tools that might be used in establishing critical pathways for developmental follow-up beginning in the NICU.

Piper suggests that planning an assessment strategy requires a hard look at the theoretic assumptions underlying practice.[84] For example, she states that the assumptions underlying the idea that early diagnosis is both possible and desirable include the following: (1) children with developmental delay were delayed as infants, and (2) children who are delayed in infancy remain delayed. Piper indicates that these assumptions ignore the significant amount of research available to suggest that some delays are transient, but also that some developmental abnormalities do not appear until maturation has continued to a point at which some expected developmental milestone fails to occur. These observations might result from processes such as recovery from early insult, the transient nature of some signs of CNS insult, maturation (or failure to mature) of developmentally significant brain areas, and environmental influences on development.

Piper stresses that most screening tests of development in early infancy have reasonable sensitivity (ability to identify those who will be abnormal), presumably because children with CP or other serious neurologic abnormalities are likely to display abnormalities early and retain them, but she also indicates that many tests have poor specificity (ability to discriminate those who will be normal) and hence poor overall predictive values.[84] This is because in early infancy, many children who are normal, or are recovering from early birth, illness, or brain insult, have deviant signs, such as transient dystonia, that disappear. Piper concludes that early discrimination of *both* those children with disabilities *and* the children who will be normal may be unrealistic. Her concerns would appear to be warranted by the report of Nelson and Ellenberg on children who "outgrew" CP.[85] A careful reading of that work, however, reveals that, although many children earlier believed to have CP later did not continue to carry the diagnosis, more than half of them had some *other* type of developmental disorder, such as behavioral deviance or cognitive delay. Thus when providing feedback to families on developmental assessment results, it should be remembered that early motor deviance can be a marker for later cognitive or affective impairment without the presence of physical disability.

Based on recent research, other investigators believe that the assessment of gross motor milestones[86] or qualitative aspects of movement[87] can be used to identify infants at high risk of CP. Next, therefore, a selection of tools for assessing neonates and young infants is described along with specific information on their predictive validity for discriminating between those with developmental disabilities and those who are normal. Only tests that have been studied for their predictive validity or are under investigation for their predictive validity are included in this section in order to emphasize the equal importance of accurately identifying those with disabilities *and* those who are normally developing during the neonatal period. The reader should consult Sweeney and Swanson for more detailed information on a variety of infant examinations.[9]

Noninvasive Observational Tools

Because of the fragility of most premature infants, the availability of noninvasive developmental assessments has been considered particularly valuable in protecting infants from stress resulting from the physiologic challenges of testing itself.[88] Prechtl and colleagues have developed a qualitative assessment of general movement in the premature or term infant that involves videotaping the baby over at least an hour during the period of development up to term age.[89] From a review of spontaneous activity on the videotape, an infant's movement is assessed for variety, fluidity, elegance, and complexity. Poverty of movement is a prime indicator of brain *insult* in the early weeks after premature birth but is not a specific indicator of permanent CNS dysfunction. A specific quality of movement called *cramped synchrony* appears to be most predictive of spastic CP when it is observed in the early weeks of life and persists on repeated assessment.

When children reach the age of about 2 months past term, a new quality of movement should appear that can be captured in videotapes of spontaneous movement (with *no* handling or other external stimuli) lasting only about 15 minutes. This quality of movement is called *fidgety*.[90, 91] It consists of small, moderate-amplitude, continuous movements of all parts of the body that are seen when children are relaxed, awake, unfocused, and unstimulated. Fidgety movements incorporate individuated movements of the digits and have elegant rotational components at the wrist, forearm, and ankles. They disappear from the infant's repertoire when goal-directed movements become increasingly dominant around 3 to 4 months of age (past term).

At any age, normal general movements are characterized by gradual onset; waxing and waning of intensity; participation of the whole body with variable activity in the many body segments; fluency; and complexity, incorporating rotations with flexion and extension movements.[91] A child who instead consistently demonstrates cramped synchrony and fails to develop fidgety movements is almost certain to develop spastic CP. Specificity of 96 percent and sensitivity of 95 percent for the prediction of 2-year neurologic outcome was demonstrated based on assessments of the presence or absence (or abnormal quality) of fidgety general movements in infants at between 6 and 20 weeks past term-equivalent age (both preterm and full-term infants were included in the study).[89] A videotape titled *Spontaneous Motor Activity as a Diagnostic Tool* that illustrates the definitions of qualitative aspects of movement assessed in the examination devised by Prechtl and colleagues is available from Christa Einspieler, Department of Physiology, University of Graz, Harrachgasse 21/5, A-8010 Graz, Austria; telephone, +43 316-380-4266; fax, +43 316-380-9630; e-mail, christa.einspieler@kfunigraz.ac.at. Training is needed to use the general movement assessment.

Clinical Tests Involving Handling for Item Administration

Als and colleagues developed the Assessment of Premature Infant Behavior (APIB)[92] as an extension of the Brazelton Neonatal Behavioral Assessment Scale[93] for the specific purpose of identifying the premature infant's behavioral organization in a variety of interacting subsystems based on what Als terms a *synaction principle*. The subsystems assessed include the autonomic, motoric, state organizational, attentional-interactional, and self-regulatory systems.[22, 25] The principle of synaction "proposes that development proceeds through the continuous balancing of approach and avoidance, yielding a spiral potentiation of continuous intraorganism subsystem interaction and differentiation and organism-environment interaction aimed at bringing about the realization of a hierarchically ordered species-unique developmental agenda."[94, (p 6)] As a realization of this developmental principle, the APIB uses a systematic sequence of manipulations to reveal (1) the infant's level of balance of subsystem function, (2) the infant's threshold of disorganization demonstrated by defensive avoidance behaviors, (3) the degree of differentiation within the infant's level of integrative functioning (i.e., the limits of organized behavior), (4) the degree of modulation and regulation of behavior the infant exhibits as stimulation changes, (5) self-regulation capabilities, and (6) the type of environmental support the infant needs to reestablish smooth functioning or facilitate optimal functioning and developmental progression.

In the APIB, packages of stimulation are provided that are increasingly intrusive (stimulation during sleep through vestibular stimulation during movement), and the subsystems' functioning are graded on scales from 9 for disorganized performance to 1 for well-modulated performance. The examiner also gathers information on how much support the infant requires from the examiner or environment in order to maintain the stability of behavioral organization. Because the test requires extensive training and about 30 minutes to administer and another 45 minutes to score, it has not been extensively used in clinical practice by physical therapists and remains primarily a research tool.

Als and colleagues used the APIB and other assessment tools to demonstrate that behavioral organization differed in different GA groups, but also that apart from the GA, infants could be separated into three reliably identified groups: well-modulated babies, moderately well modulated babies, and low-threshold, highly reactive, sensitive babies.[94] Although the specificity and sensitivity of classification were not reported, cluster membership concordance based on the use of the APIB in the newborn period to predict performance on a mental test at 5 years was statistically significant with a τ of 0.69. APIB concepts have been incorporated into the development of the infant observational assessment used in the NIDCAP program, a tool that was previously described in Michael's case and is feasible for use in routine clinical practice for planning NICU care. Sweeney also recommends the use of this assessment by physical therapists during nurse caregiving in order to identify whether an infant is appropriate for additional examination involving handling by the physical therapist.[88]

The Dubowitz Neurological Assessment of the Preterm and Full-Term Newborn Infant[95] has been demonstrated to have validity for predicting normality when used at term-equivalent age in high-risk infants but has less capability for differentiating between infants who will recover and those who go on to have permanent disabilities when infants demonstrate abnormal neurologic signs on testing.[96] A positive predictive validity of 64 percent was obtained based on the use of abnormal results on the Dubowitz assessment at 40 weeks of GA to forecast the 1-year developmental outcome; the negative predictive validity of a Dubowitz normal or borderline performance was 93 percent. The sensitivity was 83 percent and the specificity 84 percent.

Other investigators have attempted to provide means for improved evaluation of results on the Dubowitz assessment. For example, in a study of 129 infants born younger than 34 weeks of GA, specific criteria were used to document neurologic risk based on the Dubowitz assessment at 40 weeks of postmenstrual age.[97] Abnormal neurologic status was defined as marked trunk hypotonia plus head lag or three abnormal signs from among the following: arm flexor tone greater than leg flexor tone; head control abnormal; increased tremors plus startles; persistently adducted thumb; abnormal Moro reflex (extension only); abnormal eye movements; poor orientation to visual stimulation in the alert state; irritability; and asymmetry consisting of more than two points in one limb or one point in all limbs. Combining Dubowitz test results with ultrasound imaging increased the predictive validity for both the normal and the abnormal outcome.

Molteno and colleagues used a different approach to evaluating Dubowitz assessment results.[96] After testing 100 low-risk infants and developing percentile rank scores for performance on each item of infants in three different age ranges (30 to 33 weeks, 34 to 36 weeks, and 37 to 40 weeks of corrected age), another group of 100 infants at high risk for developmental disability were compared with the normative group and scored for numbers of deviant (i.e., scores below the 5th percentile) items. When the risk defined as having 2+ deviant scores was compared with the developmental outcome at 1 year, the authors obtained a sensitivity of 91 percent, a specificity of 79 percent, a positive predictive validity of 76 percent, and a negative predictive validity of 92 percent. In this study, the addition of information from cranial ultrasonography did not improve the prediction of outcomes. The use of the Dubowitz assessment for documenting the recovery of children with perinatal asphyxia and predicting poor long-term outcome is demonstrated by the case of Lee.

CASE STUDY

USE OF DUBOWITZ NEUROLOGICAL ASSESSMENT

Lee was born past term at 43 weeks of GA weighing 3850 g (average for GA). Resuscitation was needed because his Apgar scores were 1^1 and 3^5. The medical diagnosis was severe perinatal asphyxiation with meconium aspiration and persistent fetal circulation. Neonatal seizures were successfully treated with phenobarbital. At 3 days of age, he was referred for physical therapy examination. He was on room air and received feedings by nasogastric tube every 3 hours. Lee was assessed with the Dubowitz assessment. His resting posture consisted of flexed wrists and elbows, clenched fists with adducted thumbs, and "frogged" legs. His arms showed no traction or recoil responses; only minimal, brief flexion of hips and knees was seen in the legs. Popliteal angles were the only nearly normal responses noted during the entire examination. Total flaccidity of the neck and trunk muscles was present, and all reflexes were absent or minimal. Attempts to elicit sucking produced only weak attempts with some jaw clenching. No behavioral states other than sleep were observed, and the only spontaneous movements were rapid eye movements. Attempts to elicit responses to auditory stimuli and to a cloth over the face resulted in mouthing, brief neck extension, right elbow flexion, and an altered respiratory rate. Physiologic monitors revealed no abnormal responses to handling. Spontaneous yawning occurred after the examination was finished, accompanied by bilateral elbow flexion and slight hip flexion. The physical therapy diagnosis was generalized flaccidity and stupor with an absence of typical postures and alert states for his age; physiologically stable enough to tolerate gentle movement without color changes or respiratory or cardiac difficulty. His Dubowitz test results met the criteria for the prediction of an abnormal neurologic outcome.

At 8 days, Lee remained on room air, was in an open crib, and continued to receive feedings by nasogastric tube. A repeat Dubowitz examination revealed a normalized resting posture and hip flexor recoil to extension of the legs. Other recoil and traction responses were only slightly below normal for his age. A weak, briefly sustained palmar grasp was obtained. Neck and trunk muscles remained flaccid. Lee achieved a drowsy state accompanied by stretching movements. Further handling elicited arm and leg cycling and mouthing with no startles or tremors. Tactile stimulation of the face elicited mouth opening, and insertion of the examiner's finger into the infant's mouth elicited five cycles of regular sucking with good tongue stripping. The only response to auditory and visual stimuli was left eye opening at the sound of the examiner's voice. The physical therapy diagnosis was improved motor status with normal extremity postures but continued poverty of movement; decreased alertness and behavioral responsivity; and oral skills appropriate for oral feeding if alertness with physiologic stability was attainable. He continued to meet the criteria for the prediction of an abnormal neurologic outcome based on poor head control and trunk hypotonicity, as well as poor visual responsivity.

At 3 weeks of age, Lee remained hypotonic but had normal trunk and extremity postures in all positions except when held in an upright sitting position. Antigravity neck flexion and extension could not be performed. In the supine position, he was able to turn his head from midline to either side but not 180 degrees; orient to visual or auditory stimulation with his head and eyes turning 60 degrees; and bring his hand to his mouth if his head was turned to one side. He was able to suck and swallow adequately for efficient oral feeding and was discharged home with a weight appropriate for his age.

REFLECTION ON PRACTICE

Despite documentation of significant recovery on the Dubowitz assessment,[95] Lee remained at risk for developmental disability because of his medical history and continued hypotonia, poverty of movement, and limited availability of alert states. According to current definitions of perinatal asphyxia, Lee had an 80 to 90 percent risk of having CP. Unfortunately, at the time Lee was tested, his Dubowitz test performance could not be quantified or compared with normative expectations for his age over time. The test is also appropriate for use only in the neonatal period, so it could not continue to be used to follow his development after hospital discharge. We return to Lee's story in the section on posthospitalization developmental follow-up of infants at high risk for disability, where we learn about his outcome. As we reflect on clinical practice today, however, it is important to ask whether the use of other tests would have been more helpful than the Dubowitz scale in quantifying Lee's degree of risk for CP in the newborn period based on his motor performance rather than on medical factors alone.

Prechtl's general movement assessment[87] would have documented his poverty of movement, but Lee did not have cramped synchrony, so even if the test had been available, a strong risk for CP would not have been documented with this assessment in the perinatal period. It is unknown whether he developed normal fidgety general movements at the appropriate age.

As for improving the assessment of change over time with the Dubowitz test, Eyler and colleagues[97] and Molteno and coworkers[98] have developed systematic means for evaluating Dubowitz assessment results. Morgan and associates have also developed a newborn test based on the Dubowitz scale that allows quantification of results.[99] Although these assessments would have allowed quantification of risk based on neurologic signs and behavioral responsivity, I believe that tests such as these, with their heavy concentration on the assessment of posture and tone during passive manipulation, may have little relationship to the postural control needed for functional movements in infancy. Although they may have diagnostic relevance, the fact that the head is fixed in a midline position when testing many items on these examinations provides less than adequate information for planning treatment. A similar problem exists with another recently published test for neonates by Korner and colleagues.[100] A look at a new test under development by my research group that has been shown to contain items with relevance to daily caregiving demands for movement is considered next as an example of the new generation of functional assessments for newborns.

A Functional Motor Performance Scale: The Test of Infant Motor Performance

The Test of Infant Motor Performance (TIMP) is under development for therapists' use in identifying children with poor motor performance and for planning and evaluating treatment.[101, 102] Version 3.3 of the TIMP consists of two scales, one for recording observations of spontaneous movements (observed scale—28 items) and one that poses functional movement problems for the infant to solve (elicited scale—31 items). Figures 7–1 through 7–3 illustrate three observed scale behaviors recorded on the TIMP: selective movements of the digits (Fig. 7–1), centering the head along the midline of the body (Fig. 7–2), and head lifting in the prone position) (Fig. 7–3). The observed scale also provides the ability to document the presence or absence of qualitative characteristics of movement based on research on general movements, including fidgety, ballistic, and oscillating movements.[91] Observed scale items are scored pass or fail.

Elicited scale items on the TIMP involve the assessment of postural control needed for functional movements in early infancy.[102] Postural control is assessed in a variety of contexts, including numerous different positions in space and by stimulation of visual and auditory senses. Scoring for each item uses 5-, 6-, or 7-point rating scales. Figure 7–4 illustrates assessment of antigravity postural control of the legs when the hips and knees are flexed, an activity infants experience frequently during diapering. The legs are positioned in flexion (Fig. 7–4A) and released (Fig. 7–4B), and observation is made of the ability to maintain or regain an antigravity posture (Fig. 7–4C).

Another TIMP item is used to assess changes in the use of functional strategies for responding to auditory stimulation over the course of maturation. With the infant placed prone with the head turned to one side, a series of three successive sounds (rattle, squeak toy, voice) is made near the back of the infant's head. The young infant responds by turning the head, often dragging the face across the surface to orient the eyes toward the sound (Fig. 7–5). An older infant extends the trunk or pushes up on the hands and forearms and raises but is not able to turn the head, an unusual strategy because it is unsuccessful and the use of a less mature strategy would succeed. The most mature level of performance on this item is illustrated when the infant pushes up on the forearms and once again is able to turn the head to visually fixate the sound source. Finally, the item shown in Figure 7–6 assesses the infant's ability to maintain an upright head when supported in the sitting position.

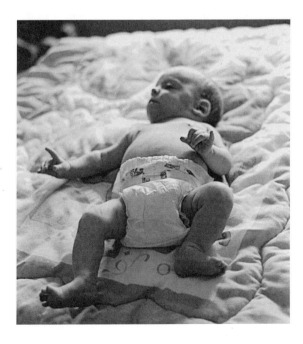

FIGURE 7–1. Spontaneous behavior scored on the Test of Infant Motor Performance (TIMP) observed scale: selective control of the index finger on the right hand and the fifth digit on the left hand. (Courtesy of Kristine Johnson, Allyson Meyer, and Dena Winkleman, Department of Biomedical Visualization, and Laura Zawacki, Department of Physical Therapy, University of Illinois at Chicago.)

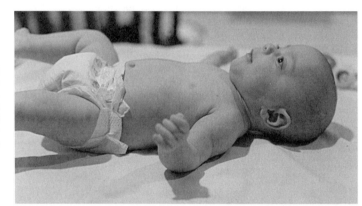

FIGURE 7–2. Spontaneous behavior scored on the TIMP observed scale: ability to center the head along the midline of the body. (Courtesy of Kristine Johnson, Allyson Meyer, and Dena Winkleman, Department of Biomedical Visualization, and Laura Zawacki, Department of Physical Therapy, University of Illinois at Chicago.)

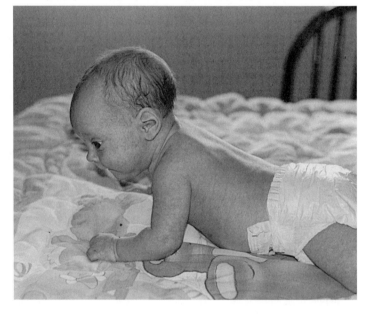

FIGURE 7–3. Spontaneous behavior scored on the TIMP observed scale: ability to lift the head more than 45 degrees in the prone position. (Courtesy of Kristine Johnson, Allyson Meyer, and Dena Winkleman, Department of Biomedical Visualization, and Laura Zawacki, Department of Physical Therapy, University of Illinois at Chicago.)

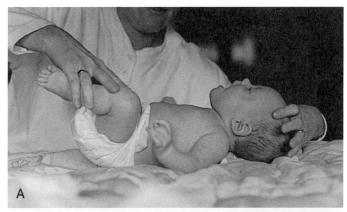

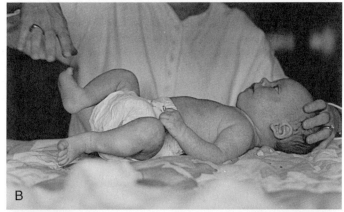

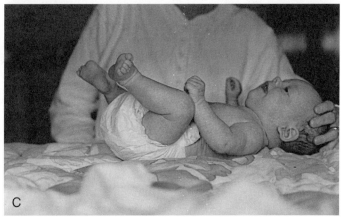

FIGURE 7–4. Assessment of antigravity postural control of the legs on the TIMP elicited scale: The examiner flexes the infant's hips and knees (*A*), releases the legs (*B*), and observes the ability to regain antigravity hip and knee flexion (*C*). This item's rating scale is as follows: 0=both thighs, knees, and feet fall immediately to the support surface; 1=both feet fall to the support surface, but the thighs and knees remain off the surface; 2=one foot falls to the support surface, but the knee remains off the support surface; the other foot and leg remain off the support surface; 3=both feet and legs remain off the support surface for at least 5 seconds making kicking movements and occasionally touching the support surface; 4=both feet return to the support surface, followed by heel pounding with the knee extended or bridging against the surface. The infant received a score of 3. (Courtesy of Kristine Johnson, Allyson Meyer, and Dena Winkleman, Department of Biomedical Visualization, and Laura Zawacki, Department of Physical Therapy, University of Illinois at Chicago.)

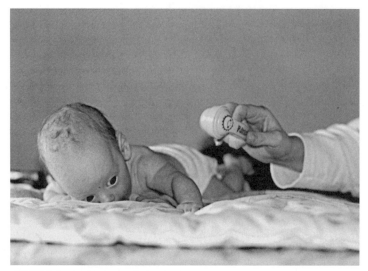

FIGURE 7–5. Assessment of visual orientation to a sound made at the back of the head on the TIMP elicited scale: The infant finds the sound source by turning the head and orienting the eyes to the sound source. This item's rating scale is as follows: 0 = no response; 1 = quiets or brightens with no movement or movements of the extremities or trunk with no attempt to lift or turn the head; 2 = initiates a head lift or turn but does not turn the head completely to midline; 3 = lifts and turns the head, but only to midline; 4 = lifts and turns the head to the opposite side; 5 = lifts the head 45 to 90 degrees and attempts to localize the sound with the eyes but cannot turn the head; 6 = lifts and turns the head, maintaining the head in an upright position to turn 45 degrees toward the source of sound. Because the infant completed his head turn, he received a score of 4. (Courtesy of Kristine Johnson, Allyson Meyer, and Dena Winkleman, Department of Biomedical Visualization, and Laura Zawacki, Department of Physical Therapy, University of Illinois at Chicago.)

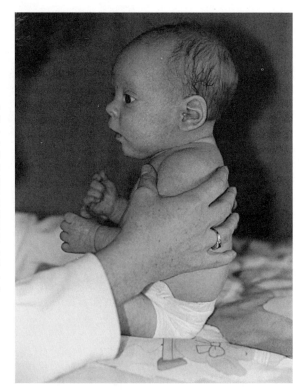

FIGURE 7–6. Assessment of upright head control in supported sitting on the TIMP elicited scale: The infant maintains an upright head position with midline alignment. This item's rating scale is as follows: 0 = no response, head hangs; 1 = attempts to lift the head twice within 15 seconds; 2 = attains an upright head position at least once but sustains it for less than 15 seconds; 3 = maintains the head in midline with the head tipped in up to but no more than 30 degrees of forward flexion for at least 15 seconds; 4 = maintains the head upright in midline for 15 to 30 seconds; 5 = maintains the head upright for greater than 30 seconds, moving the head freely with control. This infant received a score of 4. (Courtesy of Kristine Johnson, Allyson Meyer, and Dena Winkleman, Department of Biomedical Visualization, and Laura Zawacki, Department of Physical Therapy, University of Illinois at Chicago.)

**Test of Infant Motor Performance Mean and Standard
Deviation of Total Raw Scores for Infants by Age**

TABLE 7–2	Age Range	Mean Score	Standard Deviation	*n*
	Entire sample	87	32	173
	32 wk 0 days to 33 wk postconceptional age (PCA)	49	19	21
	34 wk 0 days to 35 wk PCA	64	15	31
	36 wk 0 days to 37 wk PCA	75	16	27
	38 wk 0 days to 41 wk PCA	83	16	29
	42 wk 0 days PCA to 5 wk past term	94	23	18
	6 wk 0 days to 9 wk past term	114	16	22
	10 wk 0 days to 13 wk past term	133	23	25

The TIMP has been documented to be sensitive to differences in the development of infants from 32 weeks of postconceptional age to 3.5 months past term, and children with high degrees of risk of disability based on medical complications typically score less well than same-age peers.[102] Typical performance for infants from 32 weeks of postconceptional age through 13 weeks past term age is presented in Table 7–2.

Because the construct underlying the TIMP is the postural control and alignment needed for functional movements in early infancy, a study by Murney and Campbell was conducted to show that items on the TIMP reflect challenges to postural control imposed on infants by caregivers in typical interactions, such as dressing, bathing, and playing.[103] The model infant in this study experienced demands similar to about 37 percent of the TIMP elicited scale items during a typical caregiving interaction. Demands related to TIMP items occurred, on average, 1.5 times per minute.

Norms for the TIMP are not yet available, but a study of its predictive validity to the 1-year motor outcome is under way. Preliminary analysis of the relationship between TIMP test scores at 0.5 to 1 month of adjusted age in 46 infants showed a correlation of 0.38 (P < .01) with Alberta Infant Motor Scale (AIMS)[104] percentile rank scores at 3 to 7 months. In an assessment of predictive validity (Table 7–3) using a TIMP cutoff score of 70 (1 SD below the mean for infants in a previous study) and Alberta scores below the 5th percentile at 3 to 7 months, the sensitivity was 43 percent, the specificity 97 percent, the positive predictive validity 75 percent, and the negative predictive validity 90 percent. At this point, therefore, the TIMP, like the Dubowitz assessment, appears most capable of identifying children at 1 month who will be normal (high specificity and negative predictive validity), but 75 percent of children with low TIMP scores in the first month continued to have poor motor performance at 3 to 7 months of age. Study of a larger sample for a longer period of time and at different ages is needed to strengthen the validity of these results.

Figures 7–7 and 7–8 illustrate the developmental course of two infants followed longitudinally with the TIMP whose outcomes in later infancy were different. Infant 1 (see Fig. 7–7), born at 37 weeks of gestation weighing 3139 g with perinatal asphyxia and Erb's palsy, shows a continuously improving steep course of weekly change on the

**Fourfold Table for Assessment of Screening Validity
of Test of Infant Motor Performance (*n* = 46)**

TABLE 7–3	Test Performance	Alberta < 5th Percentile	Alberta > 4th Percentile
	TIMP <70	3	1
	TIMP >69	4	38

TIMP, Test of Infant Motor Performance.

Case 047 — Perinatal asphyxia

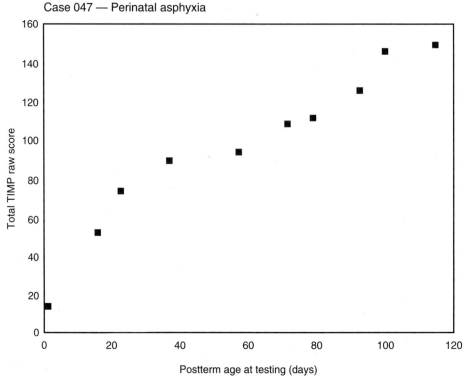

FIGURE 7–7. Longitudinal development on the TIMP of an infant with an excellent developmental outcome. (Support for longitudinal data collection was provided by a grant to the author from the National Institutes of Health, Project R01 HD32567, A Motor Test for Pediatric Rehabilitation.)

Case 071 — Grade III Intraventricular hemorrhage

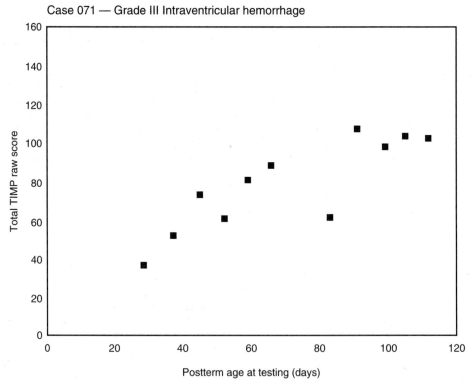

FIGURE 7–8. Longitudinal development on the TIMP of an infant with poor developmental outcome. (Support for longitudinal data collection was provided by a grant to the author from the National Institutes of Health, Project R01 HD32567, A Motor Test for Pediatric Rehabilitation.)

Suggested Score Ranges on the Test of Infant Motor Performance for Typical and Atypical Performance

TABLE 7–4	Age (wk)	Average Range*	Below Average†	Far Below Average‡
	32–33 PCA	30–68	11–29	<11
	34–35 PCA	49–79	34–48	<34
	36–37 PCA	58–91	42–57	<42
	38–41 PCA	67–98	51–66	<51
	2–5 past term	70–117	47–69	<47
	6–9 past term	97–130	81–96	<81
	10–13 past term	111–156	88–110	<88

PCA, postconceptional age.
*Score within ± 1 SD of the mean for the age group.
†Score between −1 and −2 SD below the mean for the age group.
‡Score more than −2 SD below the mean for the age group. Note that 47 as the cutoff for far below average seems unusual for the 2 to 5 weeks past term age group because it is a lower cutoff score than that for the previous age group. This group had a large variance compared with other groups, perhaps because it was a mix of normal full-term infants and infants who were prematurely born and had reached the equivalent adjusted age. These two types of infants may be developmentally different. This anomaly reveals the weakness of the TIMP for definitive developmental diagnosis at its current stage of development. Because means and standard deviations presented in Table 7–2 are based on only 18 to 31 infants per age group, the data in this table should be used as a guide to identifying children who might profit from intervention rather than for definitive developmental diagnosis.

TIMP over a 4-month period after a very low score shortly after birth; her TIMP score at 1 month was above 70. This infant's development at 12 months on a validated gross motor assessment, the AIMS,[104] was at the 90th percentile for age or in the normal range. Infant 2 (see Fig. 7–8), born at 26 weeks of gestation weighing 578 g, is also an infant with a CNS lesion—grade III IVH. She shows lower levels of performance across time and a flattening trajectory of later development (slowed rate) on the TIMP when compared with infant 1. Her TIMP score at 1 month was below 70, and her motor outcome at 6 months of age on the AIMS was at the 1st percentile, indicating that development was delayed and predicted to be abnormal at 18 months. Her especially low score at 80 days is unexplained.

Based on the performance of the infants in Table 7–2, TIMP scores documenting below-average performance as illustrated in Table 7–4 are recommended for use until formal norms are available to identify those infants, such as the infant in Figure 7–8, who might benefit from intervention in the NICU or from close follow-up.

Because norms and firm evidence of predictive validity are currently lacking, the TIMP cannot be used for definitive developmental diagnosis at this time. Data on typical TIMP performance of infants at various ages (see Table 7–2) along with the presence of strong medical evidence of brain damage, however, supports the use of the TIMP to follow the development of such infants by providing a quantitative indicator that has been shown to reflect different levels of motor development during early infancy and to reflect demands for movement infants typically experience. A further advantage of the TIMP is that it can be used in the NICU for infants as young as 32 weeks postconceptional age as well as for the 3- to 4-month-old infant in an EI program or follow-up clinic. Current work is aimed at shortening the test to facilitate examining the most fragile infants and to increase the overall efficiency of its use. A CD-ROM self-instructional program is under development for training therapists in scoring the TIMP.

The use of the TIMP to document performance far below the typical range in a full-term infant is illustrated in the case of Madonna.

CASE STUDY

USE OF THE TEST OF INFANT MOTOR PERFORMANCE

Madonna was the firstborn daughter of a 22-year-old Latino woman with mental retardation who had completed high school in a special education program. The baby was delivered at term weighing 3222 g (appropriate for the GA) after an uncomplicated pregnancy; labor and delivery, however, were complicated by fetal tachycardia, a need for a vacuum extraction, and late passage of meconium. The baby's Apgar scores were 4^1, 7^5, and 8^{10}, she required bagging, and she was hypothermic with a pH of 7.21 in cord blood. Although her pH level and Apgar scores were short of the current criteria given earlier for a diagnosis of perinatal asphyxia, she had postnatal seizures (frontal and temporal ictal events on the right side) and oliguria giving evidence of multiorgan system dysfunction. Evidence of serious brain injury, however, was provided by MR imaging and cranial ultrasound assessments, which revealed total liquefaction of the cerebral tissue and hyperechoic periventricular white matter suggesting prenatal brain damage. She also had a right facial palsy and subarachnoid hemorrhage.

Madonna was hospitalized for approximately 1 month. Therapy consisted only of positioning and environmental protection using an NIDCAP-type approach although formal assessment of the infant's tolerance for stimulation was not made in order to determine her specific individual needs. She went home to her mother after arrangements were made for them to stay with a relative. This was necessitated by the fact that the mother was not believed to have sufficient cognitive ability to fully understand the infant's needs. Concerns were raised, for instance, by the fact that the mother did not always appear at the hospital when she said she would and once fell asleep while holding and feeding Madonna. The infant was referred to an EI program in the community.

Shortly before Madonna's discharge from the hospital, she was recruited for involvement in a study of the test-retest reliability of the TIMP. At 32 days of age, spontaneous movements observed and recorded on the TIMP observed scale included hand-to-mouth movement in the prone position and antigravity arm movements and reciprocal kicking in the supine position. During observation of spontaneous movements, Madonna was noted to have cramped synchrony. Her postural tone was hypotonic in the trunk; her neck, head, and eyes were maintained toward the right consistently; and her thumbs were adducted. Her passive ROM was within normal limits throughout the body. On the TIMP elicited scale, Madonna showed minimal visual tracking (only toward the right) for a score of 3 on a scale of zero to 4, no upright head control for a score of zero, the presence of neonatal neck righting toward the left (1/5), an inability to hold her head in midline alignment (zero), trunk hyperextension and asymmetry of performance when rolling was facilitated from the arms (2/5 to the right and 3/5 to the left), but no neck and trunk extension when held in prone suspension (zero), and no head lifting or ability to flex the arms from an extended position in prone lying (zero). The infant was alert and content throughout the test but showed no smiling or other social interaction capabilities. Madonna obtained a total TIMP raw score of 40. In research on development of the TIMP, an average score for a 1-month-old infant with many medical complications was 83, so Madonna's performance was much lower than expected. Based on Table 7–4, her score of 40 at 1 month of age places her in the far-below-average range.

Although Madonna was scheduled for imminent discharge and had been referred to an EI program in the community, the mother was interviewed, and information was shared with her regarding the baby's test results. In keeping with the HOAC[15] decision-making model, she was also asked before intervention was planned (but not before TIMP testing) what she would like her baby to be able to do. Madonna's mother indicated that she was bothered by the fact that the baby kept her eyes turned toward the right and did not look at her. She also expressed her hopes that Madonna would be able to learn to walk and talk. It was evident that she did not completely understand the seriousness of the infant's brain damage, but she was very interested in attending the EI program and asked to have a report on the infant's test results sent to the center as well as a copy of the letter to her.

Given the brief opportunity to work with this mother, a goal of finding ways for Madonna's mother to engage the infant's visual attention was established. Together the therapist and mother discovered that if the baby's head was gently turned completely toward the left in the supine position and held until she relaxed, Madonna's eyes stabilized and she was able to visually fixate on her mother's face. Madonna's mother was excited about this and was later observed working independently to elicit this behavior as she cared for the baby. She was also taught how to support the baby in the sitting position while cupping the baby's chin in her hand, then release the head briefly so that Madonna could practice upright head control with a level of challenge appropriate to her current abilities. Finally, Madonna's mother was shown how to position the baby in the prone position (with warnings about doing this at home only when the baby was awake and supervised) and to use her voice to encourage head lifting. Madonna briefly accomplished this task during the session. These activities were described in simple language in a letter to the mother that was also sent to the EI program along with information on Madonna's TIMP test results. It was not deemed appropriate at the time to engage in further discussion about Madonna's ultimate prognosis, given the mother's limited understanding and the fact that she would soon enter the long-term care provided by the EI program where further support and education would be available.

REFLECTION ON PRACTICE

A general NIDCAP approach to environmental protection in the NICU for Madonna was deemed to be helpful in facilitating as much recovery from her brain trauma as possible because it was likely to reduce unnecessary movement, an important factor in lowering the oxygen cost and brain activity that could have contributed to increasing her brain damage after birth.[105] Given her low level of responsiveness to stimulation, however, use of the actual NIDCAP assessment protocol would have been helpful to document the appropriateness of specific interventions in keeping with Madonna's physiologic stability and needs as a full-term baby who would normally be significantly engaged in social interaction periodically throughout the day. This partial application of an NIDCAP approach is common in an NICU when only some staff have been trained or commitment is low and often reflects the provision of protection from stimulation based on early assessment of the baby's ability to tolerate and respond to handling but limited understanding of the need to progress the program with age or developmental change. That is, infants need repeated behavioral assessment in the NIDCAP to identify changes in their readiness for stimulation. Handling should be progressed to provide the just-right challenge to ensure both physiologic stability and proper nurturance of brain and musculoskeletal development.

An NIDCAP assessment could also have been used during an NICU trial of physical therapy in order to establish whether the infant would be able to tolerate handling to improve her postural control for functional movement while in the nursery. If so, the NDT strategy using tactics described by Girolami and Campbell would have been appropriate for this baby in the nursery.[106] The study on the use of the NDT approach with preterm infants showed that infants benefited most in achieving head-in-midline postural control, an evident need for Madonna. (This and other effective intervention approaches are described more thoroughly in the next section.) Positioning as used in the nursery was not apparently helpful in assisting the baby to develop a more symmetric posture in the supine position, in keeping with information in the literature showing little support for the efficacy of positioning in facilitating development.[107, 108]

Use of the TIMP earlier in the course of Madonna's hospitalization would have been helpful in demonstrating her severe motor delay and asymmetries, which were conducive to the development of contractures. Although the TIMP has not yet been normed, raw scores far below the mean for children tested in a previously published study, as found in this case, are the best available quantitative data to support a referral for early treatment based on testing functional skills. The test could also be used to document progress later in the EI program, especially for promoting symmetry and ability in visual tracking and fixation, goals of importance to the baby's mother.

Earlier interaction with the mother to help her establish appropriate goals for her baby would have been desirable and in keeping with the HOAC model of clinical decision making.[15] Given the special needs of this mother, administering a Brazelton scale[93] to demonstrate the baby's social interaction capabilities would have been useful as soon as the baby became physiologically stable.[109, 110] The Brazelton scale or an NIDCAP assessment could have been used to teach her how to monitor the infant's approach and avoidance responses in order to promote appropriate handling.

Madonna's mother would also benefit from having a series of snapshots illustrating handling of the baby for the facilitation of head control and other movement skills. Having a set of photographs to share with EI program providers would have facilitated communication for a mother with limited cognitive skills in order to promote continuity of care from the physical therapy provided in the hospital to the community-based intervention program. The mother would have been further empowered to act as an advocate for her baby as she entered the EI program with knowledge of her baby's plan of care that she could share with personnel in the community-based program. Finally, given the nursing concerns about the mother's feeding of Madonna, she could have been evaluated while feeding the infant using the Nursing Child Assessment (NCAST) Feeding Scale (a manual, test forms, and teaching videotapes are available from NCAST, University of Washington, CDMRC, Box 357920, Seattle, WA 98195-7920; telephone, 206-543-8528; fax, 206-685-3284) so that interaction skills could be assessed for both the baby and the mother.[111] Results could be used to develop a feeding program to be conveyed in simple terms and used to promote the mother's understanding of, and response to, Madonna's signals.

Madonna's referral to an EI program was appropriate given the certain outcome of severe neurologic dysfunction documented on MR imaging and the mother's cognitive limitations and social situation, but more intensive involvement with this mother during the infant's hospitalization might have provided a more comfortable transition to home and community for Madonna and her mother. The APTA competencies document suggests that the physical therapist can play a useful role in interagency coordination and collaboration.[4] The greatest usefulness in this role comes in helping the parents and baby make the transition from nursery care, where medical concerns are paramount, to community-based EI settings, where developmental concerns are addressed for children with disabilities. Although many roles described for therapists in the NICU are not unique to their skills and disciplinary knowledge, the role of transition to physical therapy in the community can be greatly facilitated by a therapist who has established a relationship with a family in the hospital. In Madonna's case, the transition was assisted at the mother's request, enabling a sensitive response to the parent's goals and concerns, even before Madonna's mother understood the full extent of her child's brain damage.

Parents in a study by Dodds-Azzopardi and Chapman reported experiencing stress associated with transitions from the NICU to a community-based hospital.[112] Factors contributing to stress included a lack of knowledge of procedures for transfer and a lack of continuity of care practices between environments, especially in feeding procedures. Families with low SES were more content with the transition than those with higher economic status, perhaps because their expectations were lower.

Similarly, a chief complaint of community-based EI program staff is the paucity of information shared with them by hospital personnel (typically only of a medical nature) at discharge from the nursery. The physical therapist can make a difference by clarifying, for both the family and community service providers, the previous plan of developmental care, sharing information on test results and parent education already provided, and indicating when follow-up developmental assessment, if any, is scheduled. Use of the TIMP by therapists in the nursery *and* in the community could provide continuity in understanding the infant's developmental progress. Earlier involvement of a physical therapist would have increased the ability of Madonna's mother to identify her infant's capabilities and areas of need to make her a stronger partner in determining the EI program to come. The family physician should also receive copies of information provided to the EI program, and written copies should be shared with the family. Parents can be encouraged to keep a baby book with medical and therapy information on the infant, along with the names and telephone numbers of individuals and agencies providing assessment and care. Mothers with limited cognitive skills, such as Madonna's, would find this especially helpful to aid participation in case management for their infants.

INTERVENTION STRATEGIES AND OUTCOMES IN THE SPECIAL CARE NURSERY

The case of Madonna and her mother demonstrates that even short-term intervention in the NICU has the possibility of being responsive to family goals and facilitating mother-infant interaction despite an especially ominous prognosis. Is there evidence, however, for sustained benefits from nursery treatment provided by physical therapists? In this section, we explore the evidence in support of interventions by therapists and other professionals.

Despite several decades of involvement of therapists in special care nurseries, little research exists to document the effectiveness of their services. The early literature on intervention with high-risk infants by other types of professionals suggested beneficial effects on cognitive and social development and on weight gain, but reports of effects on motor outcomes were equivocal.[16] Before the late 1980s, most intervention studies in which the motor outcome was assessed included as subjects those now considered to be at relatively low risk of poor motor developmental outcome. Of those studies, five evaluated the gross motor developmental outcome on the 1969 Bayley Scales of Infant Development[42] and only two reported significant results in favor of the experimental group.[113, 114] Two studies reported significant differences on the Brazelton scale or the Graham-Rosenblith test dimensions related to neonatal motor functioning,[115, 116] whereas two others had negative results.[113, 117] In none of these studies were specific interventions delivered by specialists in motor development, such as occupational therapists or physical therapists.[16] Furthermore, most of the studies were undertaken before it was recognized that infants benefit from protection from overstimulation and that parental training in being responsive to infant signals is likely to be a more effective support for developmental progress than packaged, nonindividualized stimulation or direct treatment by a professional. Successful strategies for improving motor developmental outcomes in infants born prematurely, that is, those strategies documented with research evidence, include parental education, the NIDCAP approach, tactile-kinesthetic programs such as infant massage,[118] and NDT. These strategies are described next.

Typical of recent interventions by professionals other than therapists are studies of multimodal packages by Resnick and colleagues,[119] parental education on contingent responding for parents of low SES by Kang and colleagues[120] and Parker and colleagues,[121] and the previously described behavioral support methods used by Als and colleagues[22, 25] to protect infants from overstimulation and to educate caregivers in reading infant cues.

Parent Education

Parker and colleagues provided weekly sessions with each experimental group infant's mother and an infant developmental specialist in the NICU.[121] Together they observed the infant's behaviors and related them to the baby's developmental needs, using the NIDCAP scale for fragile infants or the APIB for those who could tolerate the handling of assessment. The mother learned to interpret her baby's behaviors and then to modify her caregiving appropriately, including protecting the infant from overstimulation. She was encouraged to advocate for her infant's needs with the NICU staff. Infants in both the control and the experimental groups received individualized care by nurses, physical therapists, and occupational therapists based on NIDCAP assessment, so the major difference for the experimental group was parental training. No intervention was given to either group after discharge from the NICU. Infants in the parental education group scored better than control group infants at 4 and 8 months on the 1969 Bayley mental scale and at 4, but not 8, months on the Bayley motor scale (average motor scores were 111 at 4 months and 104 at 8 months versus 95 and 96, respectively, for control subjects, compared with a normative mean of 100). Mental scores were lower than motor scores, but only the control group's mental scores averaged more than 1 SD below the 1969 normative mean. Parents of experimental group infants reported them to be less difficult in temperament than control group infants.

A study by Kang and colleagues was based on Barnard's Child Health Assessment Interaction Model as a conceptual framework for parental education.[120] According to this model, the developmental outcome is a product of an interaction among the characteristics of the infants, the adaptive styles of the mothers, and the quality of the family environment, including income, supportive family relationships, and the amount of stimulation available in the home. The interactive goal for mother and infant from birth to 3 months of age is primary modulation of the behavioral state. The intervention, therefore, consisted of teaching mothers to read their infants' behavioral cues and to modulate the infants' states of consciousness during feeding in the hospital. All infants in the study were discharged from the hospital at less than 36 weeks postconceptional age, and at 1.5 months of corrected age, infants whose mothers received training in cue reading gave clearer cues during assessment with the NCAST feeding scale.[111] Mothers receiving the training program were more sensitive and responsive to their infants.

In summary, each study found significant effects of intervention when experimental subjects were compared later with control babies. The specific characteristics these interventions have in common with each other and the previously discussed NIDCAP approach is parental education on infant development, recognizing infant cues, and tailoring suggestions for intervention to the infant's readiness to actively participate.

Multimodal Stimulation Packages

Much evidence exists documenting the effectiveness of tactile-kinesthetic and auditory stimulation programs in promoting the growth and development, particularly physiologic and cognitive development, of preterm infants.[122–125] In a meta-analysis of 37 studies published since 1979 that used physiologic parameters, such as growth, as outcome measures, the use of rocking beds or waterbeds, tape recordings, or hammocks increased physiologic development by 38 to 62 percent in infants whose birth weight averaged 1524 g; interventions such as breathing bears and nonnutritive sucking improved physiologic development from 20 to 80 percent in infants whose birth weight averaged 1260 g. A further conclusion of the authors was that the data seemed to support the idea that younger infants are overwhelmed by too much stimulation and respond differently to intervention than older infants.

The results of a particularly intensive NICU intervention program for infants born weighing less than 1800 g may support this conclusion. Resnick and colleagues provided at least two per day of the following types of interventions for infants during their NICU stay: tapes of heartbeats, parents' voices, or classical music; total body massage; passive ROM exercises; a flotation waterbed; rocking exercises; face-to-face social stimulation; or oral massage before feeding.[119, 126] Parental involvement was included. At 6 months of age, treated infants were no better than controls on the Bayley mental and motor scales. This intervention project continued after hospital discharge with home visits; at 12 months, treated infants were better than controls on the mental, but not the motor scale. Better cognitive outcomes occurred for infants who had better parent-child interaction measures, again testifying to the importance of parental involvement in the production of the best infant outcomes.

The interventions provided in the studies reviewed were not specifically aimed at improving motoric functioning, and motor development was often less affected than cognitive development. Whether an approach structured to address the development of postural control enhances motor development more than other approaches, particularly when applied to children at especially high risk for CP during the neonatal period, is not established. Many studies explicitly exclude children with documented brain damage. Successful intervention, however, would logically be predicated on the motor abnormalities most likely to be observed in the infants of interest. The general problem of developmental delay in motor skills demonstrated by infants born prematurely has already been described, and effective interventions by non–motor specialists suggest that the special skills of a physical therapist are not necessary for preventing developmental delay in most infants. A therapist's assessment could be used to justify referral for EI by early educators, but to justify direct treatment by a physical therapist, problems of postural control, congenital contractures,[9] a tendency to the development of musculoskeletal abnormalities, or other specific problems within the province of treatment by physical therapists should be identified. In the next section, therefore, information is provided on the characteristics of poor motor performance in infancy demonstrated by infants at risk for developmental deviance with a view toward developing a prevention model to guide treatment during the period of nursery care. A movement therapy with scientific evidence of efficacy for preterm infants at moderate risk for disability is also described.

Characteristics of Poor Motor Performance in Infancy

In addition to the general motor developmental delay described previously as characteristic of many infants born prematurely, those infants at especially high risk for CNS dysfunction typically demonstrate poverty of movement in the neonatal period.[87] Those infants who go on to develop spastic CP have movement characterized by cramped synchrony—stiff, stereotypic movement in which body parts tend to move simultaneously rather than in alternating patterns with high degrees of complexity and variability. General movements may also demonstrate monotony, always beginning with the same body segment. Children with BPD tend to use the accessory muscles of respiration extensively and have a high energy expenditure. Infants such as those Als describes as low-threshold, highly reactive, sensitive babies show highly disorganized movements characterized by repetitive, uncontrolled activity that is inefficient and exhausting as they struggle to defend against the overwhelming effects of stimulation and to obtain positions of comfort, usually with limbs tucked in or braced against environmental supports.[94] These types of impairments may lead to (1) weakness of trunk and extremity muscles from a lack of activity; (2) hypoextensible musculature, especially tight two-joint hip and knee muscles and ankle extensor muscles; and (3) atypical postures, such as shoulder elevation and retraction,[127] neck hyperextension, and pronounced asymmetric head postures. Although these children may continue to show transient dystonia during the early months of life, those who go on to typical development gradually have normalized postural tone and movement. Children with spastic CP, on the other hand, do not lose the characteristics of immature movement, such as coactivation of muscle antagonists, and they fail to develop normal anticipatory postural reactions and selective control of movement while retaining cramped synchrony in abnormal synergic patterns.[128] Less is documented about the early development of children with dyskinetic types of CP, but clinical experience suggests that they often have low postural tone in early infancy.

Environmental Support for Development

Improvement of disorganized movement can be achieved with an NIDCAP approach,[22, 25] and all therapists working in NICUs should have at least enough understanding of this approach to engage with nurses in supporting its use. Therapists who are trained to assess infants' abilities to tolerate and profit from stimulation are best prepared to engage in neonatal developmental care and to teach these skills to parents. The therapy role in the past has included ROM exercises and positioning primarily designed to prevent musculoskeletal deviance,[9, 10] but only one study of positioning by therapists in the NICU for infants born at 24 to 28 weeks of GA demonstrated better hip adduction and neutral rotation for positioned infants versus control subjects.[129] Sweeney and Swanson anecdotally report that a program of intermittent taping is effective for reducing mild congenital foot deformities during the early postnatal period when hyperelasticity of structures exists, but research evidence of efficacy is lacking.[9] Furthermore, evidence in the literature does not support the value of positioning using waterbeds in improving postural performance as measured with the Dubowitz neurologic assessment.[107] Without further evidence of the usefulness of positioning in the prevention of musculoskeletal impairments, it should perhaps be more appropriately seen as effective in creating boundaries of comfort for children as well as promoting state modulation and efficient oxygenation.[106, 130, 131] Deiriggi, for example, found that when infants were used as their own controls, sleeping on a nonoscillating waterbed produced longer durations of quiet sleep, less active awake and fussy states, and fewer state changes and awakenings than sleeping on a regular mattress.[130] Heart rates were higher after infants were taken off the waterbed, suggesting that the beds reduced energy expenditure. The use of waterbeds to provide vestibular-proprioceptive stimulation for preterm infants promoted improved attention, more motor activity, and more normal postural tone.[132] Other reported effects of the use of waterbeds include a decreased incidence of apnea and bradycardia and a more normal head shape.[133–135] Long and Soderstrom believe that these effects of indirect positioning, that is, through the use of equipment, result from the vestibular stimulation provided by an environment that the infant can also act upon.[108] That is, the infant's movement creates a reaction in the waterbed to which the infant in turn can respond.

Movement Therapy

When children have achieved sufficient medical stability to be off a ventilator and tolerate handling without respiratory compromise or oxygen desaturation, many physical therapists believe that movement therapy can increase strength and endurance, prevent musculoskeletal impairments, promote the development of age-appropriate antigravity postural control, and improve functional uses of movement for exploring the environment and interacting with caregivers. Despite the fact that Rapport reported that 82 percent of respondents to her survey provided direct therapy and 71 percent used handling techniques in nursery-based care,[10] the current trend seems to be more hands-off in keeping with the protective model shown to be effective by Als and colleagues.[22, 25] Although the NDT approach is the most commonly used model for the provision of interventions to children in NICUs (80 percent used NDT, according to Rapport's study[10]), only one controlled clinical trial has examined the effect of this intervention on infants while *in the nursery setting.*[106] As a result, nurses and physicians may need to be persuaded that movement therapy is appropriate in the nursery. The clinical trial by Girolami and Campbell suggests that NDT can be an effective intervention,[106] but research is needed that investigates the combined effects of an NIDCAP approach with an NDT approach added to care at a point when the infant's assessment results indicate that (1) the child can tolerate and invites such intervention, and (2) brain imaging, the general movement examination results of Prechtl and associates,[89] or other evidence of high risk for permanent musculoskeletal or nervous system dysfunction exists to justify the need for involvement of a physical therapist.

To be cost-effective, therapists need to concentrate on managing infants who truly need their special expertise. The literature on research done by members of other professions clearly shows that interventions they have designed can promote motor development in typical nursery patients (although less well than cognitive development and effective parenting), so it would be difficult to justify the use of physical therapy for this purpose unless less costly alternatives to direct treatment are unavailable, or unless the physical therapist is the designated developmental specialist for the special care nursery, that is, the person responsible for meeting the developmental needs of all nursery patients. Physical therapists should otherwise concentrate on roles as consultants and educators of parents in relation to the needs of the typical nursery patient and reserve their direct services for those at greatest risk for CP or with other serious forms of motor dysfunction, such as children with Down syndrome or myelodysplasia (see Chapter 5) and those with congenital anomalies that would benefit from splinting, other assistive technology, or motor training, such as brachial plexus injury (see Chapter 6) or torticollis.[75]

In the pilot study of the effects of NDT administered in the NICU setting for 1 to 2 weeks to 34- to 35-week-old infants with neurologically abnormal responses on the reflex section of the Brazelton Neonatal Behavioral Assessment,[93] a positive response to therapy was found when the TIMP was used to assess functional motor outcomes.[106] Version 1.0 of the TIMP (then called the Supplemental Motor Test) was used by raters blind to randomized group assignment to assess the outcome of NDT provided to 9 infants versus a control intervention involving social interaction with 10 infants. At 37 weeks of postconceptional age, the treated infants performed significantly better than their preterm control group on TIMP items involving responses to handling of the infant. They were also significantly better on observed spontaneous behaviors than preterm controls as well as outperforming a second untreated control group of 8 full-term infants. The exercised preterm group demonstrated greater average weight gain than the control preterm group, but that difference was not significant in this pilot study with limited numbers of subjects. Nonetheless, the trend provides important information suggesting that growth was not impaired by mild exercise.

Unfortunately, the long-term outcome of the infants in this investigation of nursery-based physical therapy was not studied so it is unknown whether early NDT provides lasting effects on motor performance or prevents or reduces developmental deviance. The sample size was also small, and results need to be replicated with a larger clinical trial. Previous research has not suggested that NDT provided *after* nursery discharge has a role in the prevention of CP or motor delay; however, the sample size in these studies was insufficient to quantify such an effect because so few children had abnormal neurologic outcomes.[38, 136] At present, therefore, therapists should not make claims for improvements in motor control over the long term or for the possibility of limiting the effects of disability in those with permanent brain damage but can use the evidence in the literature in support of a case for assisting preterm infants to achieve current motor development that is more similar to that of the full-term newborn than to that of untreated peers, especially for those with a moderate risk of a poor developmental outcome.

An illustration of a plan of care using NDT for improving postural control in support of functional motor performance immediately after hospital discharge in a neonate with motor delay is provided in the following case history. The protocol for NDT for high-risk infants was published in Girolami and Campbell[106] and is illustrated in photographs of Girolami and the infant in the figures accompanying the case.

CASE STUDY

NEURO-DEVELOPMENTAL TREATMENT STRATEGY

Annalee was born with mandibulofacial dysostosis (Treacher Collins syndrome),[137] an autosomal dominant gene defect on chromosome 5 associated with bilateral conductive hearing loss (extent as yet unknown), full cleft of the palate, and a microscopic cleft of the lip. She also has a ventriculoseptal defect. Annalee was a full-term baby born via vaginal delivery and weighing 2993 g after a pregnancy with no problems noted. She spent 23 days in the NICU because of breathing problems and went home with an apnea monitor and pulse oximeter. Problems with anemia required transfusion after hospital discharge. Since birth she has been fed primarily through nasogastric tube, taking only about 2 mL orally per day. Vomiting occurs frequently after both oral and nasogastric feedings, and she sometimes gags and vomits upon nipple insertion.

Annalee began physical therapy once a week and speech therapy two to three times weekly at 5 weeks of age. Her parents were concerned about her feeding problems and about the fact that, because of asymmetric nares, she preferred to keep her head turned toward the left for ease of breathing and became anxious and agitated with rapid and loud breathing when her head moved voluntarily or passively out of this position. The physical therapist found Annalee to have low postural tone, little antigravity movement, and the aforementioned asymmetry of head position, which she altered only briefly in the prone position before going back to her preferred posture. She demonstrated poor attempts at orientation to visual or auditory stimuli. In the prone position she could lift her head only briefly. In keeping with the parents' concerns, the physical therapist's overall objective was to improve Annalee's muscle strength and motor skills in order to improve head and trunk control and reduce asymmetry as a postural base for motor development. Specific functional goals to be achieved by 3 months of age were established:

1. In the supine position, Annalee will hold her head in the midline to look at an object placed at chest level.
2. In the supine position, Annalee will bring both hands to the midline and reach out toward objects suspended above her at chest level.
3. In the prone position, Annalee will lift her head 45 degrees and track toys placed in her visual field while supporting on her forearms.
4. In lap sitting, Annalee will hold her head upright and in the midline while visually tracking her mother's face.
5. In lap sitting, Annalee will reach both arms forward to touch a toy held approximately 6 to 10 inches in front of her at chest level.

The strategy for intervention selected by the therapist was NDT using the treatment tactics described in Girolami and Campbell.[106] When observed in a therapy session at 3 months of age, Annalee was able to center her head consistently and maintain visual contact with toys but was not yet reaching for them consistently. She actively rolled out of a sidelying position and could maintain a stable, upright head in the prone position. She did not have enough head control to rotate her neck while maintaining upright stability of the head when sitting and lacked sufficient strength to raise her arms to shoulder height to reach for toys, so not all 3-month goals had been achieved.

Annalee was highly social and kept track of where her mother was throughout the treatment. The therapist used toys and social interaction to encourage Annalee to move independently throughout the therapy session. Support for postural control was provided as needed, based on an NDT approach, and manual guidance and proprioceptive stimulation were used to facilitate active movement and Annalee's ability to solve the postural control problems posed by small perturbations to her stability in various positions. For example, while Annalee was engaged in looking at a toy with her head up in the prone position, the therapist created slight weight shifts at the pelvis, which the infant accommodated by reorganizing the posture of other body parts so as to maintain her visual contact with the toy. When Annalee tired of looking at the toy, she responded to the therapist's manual guidance by allowing her body to *follow* the weight shift with a roll to the supine position. A second means of stimulating active postural control in the prone position was use of the environment: moving the toy to elicit visual tracking caused Annalee to organize the posture of her body so as to maintain stability of the trunk while moving her head (goal 3).

The speech therapists' initial goals included assisting the family to determine an optimal feeding position and nipple for Annalee, to improve the strength and coordination of sucking, swallowing, and breathing, and to increase the quantity of feedings taken orally. The speech therapist noted resistance to the insertion of a nipple, strong tongue retraction upon nipple insertion after lip stimulation to achieve mouth opening, and poor sucking ability. Repeated cycles of sucking could not be obtained without a period of intraoral stimulation. Control of liquid flow was poor.

In a speech therapy session, the therapist began with oral desensitization with Annalee's upper body elevated in the prone position. The therapist offered her finger for Annalee to suck and then inserted the infant's own finger into her mouth. These activities resulted in a gag and brief hiccoughing. With the infant's shoulders brought forward and supported in a reclining sidelying position, Annalee could get her own hands into her mouth or hold them up to look at them. Her mother reported that she frequently used sucking on her hand for self-consoling during the day or to get to sleep at night. When a bottle was introduced, Annalee took small amounts of liquid in between being allowed to simply play with the nipple in her mouth. She showed brief periods of organized suck-swallow-breathing activity but ingested little milk.

REFLECTION ON PRACTICE

Annalee left the hospital at 4 weeks of age with limited ability to suck and ingest food and developed anxiety reactions to certain positions and movements. It might have been advantageous to have begun regular oral motor and gross motor therapy during her 23-day hospital stay with the goal of improving her oral intake before discharge and to facilitate the postural support of ingestion that an ability to engage in the "suck posture" of adducted shoulders with flexed elbows would have afforded her. A variety of approaches to treating the feeder with disorganized suck-swallow-breathing patterns are described in the literature.[138–140]

Assessment with the TIMP would undoubtedly have resulted in a score that would have justified her involvement in physical therapy while still in the hospital and could have been used to quantify her functional motor performance at the time outpatient therapy began. Quantitative measurement of Annalee's oral motor status would also have been desirable. One possible scale for this purpose is the Neonatal Oral Motor Assessment Scale.[141]

The approach of Horn and colleagues to establishing goals and measuring outcomes would suggest that each of Annalee's therapy goals should be accompanied by a list of activities that would demonstrate that generalization of learning has occurred.[142] For example, goal 2 could be expanded to indicate that the infant would do this activity spontaneously at home in her crib or while with her grandmother during a visit to the family's home. This type of goal setting and outcome assessment ensures that the infant's therapy goals are truly functional for the needs of daily life.

The speech therapist's approach to treatment, using oral support to increase sucking efficiency, has been shown to produce an immediate increase in the amount of milk ingested,[143] but a modern task-oriented approach to intervention suggests that the infant should always be actively involved in a task because the environment plays a role in posture and movement organization. Movements, posture, attention to the task, and an emotional response to the activity are programmed together by the brain, so better results are expected when the infant becomes active, both in terms of motor activity and in terms of attention to the task. A sense of control facilitates a positive emotional response. During her speech therapy at 3 months of age, Annalee was observed to look at and actively use her hands for sucking, so the observer suggested that the speech therapist try allowing Annalee to hold her own bottle (with assistance to manage the weight) in order to see if more active participation would help to organize Annalee's suck-swallow-breathing activity. When she was assisted to hold the bottle, her oral motor patterns briefly became more organized and her face softened as she retained control of the situation. Her mother was encouraged to try this at home.

During the course of observing Annalee's therapy sessions and through reading the infant's records, it became obvious that the family was involved with more than a dozen service providers: a speech therapist, an audiologist, a physical therapist, a hematologist, an ophthalmologist, a plastic surgeon, a cardiologist, a geneticist, a nurse who visited the home, a homeopath, and the family pediatrician, as well as the numerous staff members of the developmental follow-up clinic. One can easily imagine how overwhelmed even this well-organized and financially stable family might become in the face of dealing with all these specialists. At the time of observation, the mother was involved in interviewing pediatricians because she believed that her family doctor was not sufficiently knowledgeable about Annalee's condition and with a busy practice lacked the time to become more informed. The family subsequently changed doctors when a physician was identified who demonstrated more knowledge.

Therapists need to remain alert to the demands on families that complicated medical problems produce in order to prioritize services and goals in conjunction with family needs and paramount concerns. The therapists in this case planned strategies and tactics to meet the parents' own goals in keeping with a family-centered approach[7, 144] and the HOAC.[15] Parents can also be provided with useful guides for consumers that help families to be sure services are as cost-effective and family-friendly as possible. An example is the *Consumer's Guide: Therapeutic Services for Children with Disabilities.*[145] The guide provides a list of questions that parents can ask themselves to be sure that services their children receive are beneficial. Questions include whether the services make sense and how outcomes are being measured. The guide is available from the Human Services Research Institute, 2336 Massachusetts Avenue, Cambridge, MA 02140; telephone, 617-876-0426; fax, 617-492-7401; e-mail, JWalkrHSRI@aol.com.

CASE STUDY

NEURO-DEVELOPMENTAL TREATMENT PROTOCOL WITH TEST OF INFANT MOTOR PERFORMANCE AND ALBERTA INFANT MOTOR SCALE ASSESSMENT OF OUTCOME

Breathing difficulty and airway congestion were obvious throughout Annalee's therapy sessions at 3 months of age. Her respiratory difficulties continued to increase, resulting in a 3-week hospitalization and a tracheostomy. Outpatient therapy was temporarily suspended, but weekly speech therapy and periodic physical therapy were provided in the home in order to limit her exposure to other people.

On her return to outpatient treatment at 5 months of age, Annalee was observed to have achieved the following 3-month motor goals: holding her head in midline to look at an object and reach out toward objects suspended above her chest (goals 1 and 2) (Fig. 7–9), tracking (and reaching for) toys when prone on her forearms (goal 3) (Fig. 7–10), and tracking her mother's face when sitting (goal 4). Although she was able to reach toward a toy in the supine and sitting position, strength in her arms still precluded obtaining objects suspended high above her chest or at shoulder height, so goal 5 was only partially obtained.

New goals that Annalee's parents articulated for her were rolling over, pushing up on extended arms in the prone position, independent sitting, and improved reaching and grasping. Based on these family goals, the therapist developed the following new short-term therapy objectives:

1. Annalee will independently prop on her forearms and reach for a toy held by her mother.
2. Annalee will roll from the prone to the supine position to observe or interact with a family member calling her name.

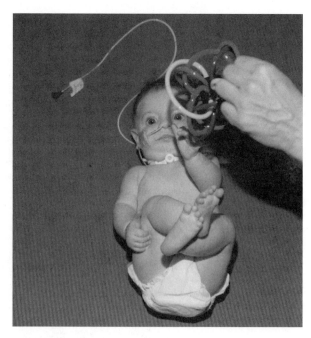

FIGURE 7–9. Annalee demonstrates achievement of 3-month goals 1 and 2: In the supine position, Annalee will hold her head in the midline to look at an object placed at chest level and reach out toward objects suspended above her at chest level. (Courtesy of Gay Girolami and Marv Chait, Pathways Center for Children, Glenview, Ill.)

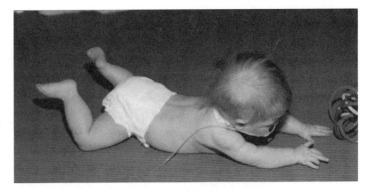

FIGURE 7-10. Annalee demonstrates achievement of 3-month goal 3: In the prone position, Annalee will lift her head 45 degrees and track toys placed in her visual field while supporting on her forearms. She also reaches for the toy. (Courtesy of Gay Girolami and Marv Chait, Pathways Center for Children, Glenview, Ill.)

3. In a supported sitting position on a parent's or caregiver's lap, Annalee will reach for an object suspended at chest height while maintaining her head upright and in midline.
4. In the supine position in her crib, Annalee will reach out to play with her feet.

At 5 months of age, Annalee was still delayed relative to age peers, who would typically be able to support themselves on extended arms when prone, sit alone, and perhaps roll over in both directions. Figures 7-9 and 7-11 show that Annalee *has* achieved the typical 5-month-old's ability to grasp her legs in the supine position. Figures 7-11 through 7-15 show Annalee's performance on several TIMP elicited scale items: Figure 7-11 shows her centering her head in the supine position while looking at a toy; Figure 7-12 shows a lack of head righting during a lateral tilt to the right; Figure 7-13 shows active head control but a lack of chin tuck during a pull-to-sit maneuver; Figure 7-14 shows neck extension just beyond the horizontal plane in prone suspension; and Figure 7-15 shows support on extended legs in the standing position for less than 5 seconds. Overall her motor performance was most like that of a typical 3- to 4-month-old but with diminished strength and endurance.

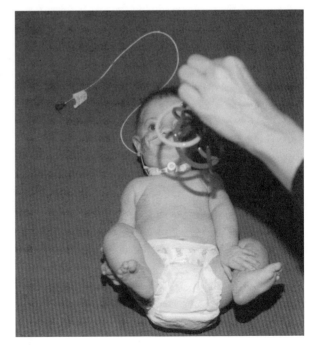

FIGURE 7-11. Assessment of the ability to center the head to look at an object on the TIMP elicited scale: Annalee received a score of 4 on a scale from zero to 4. (Courtesy of Gay Girolami and Marv Chait, Pathways Center for Children, Glenview, Ill.)

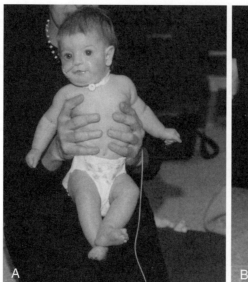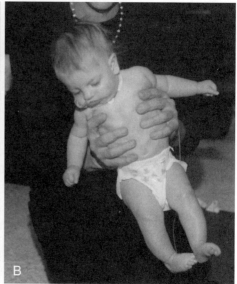

FIGURE 7–12. Assessment of head righting after a lateral tilt (movement from position in *A* to that in *B*) on the TIMP elicited scale: Annalee received a score of 1 on a scale from zero to 4. The tension in her hands and feet (*B*) shows her discomfort with the position. (Courtesy of Gay Girolami and Marv Chait, Pathways Center for Children, Glenview, Ill.)

Figures 7–16 through 7–21 illustrate some of the tactics used in Annalee's physical therapy to achieve her movement goals based on the use of an NDT strategy for intervention. Figure 7–16, the therapist facilitates rolling from the supine to the prone position over the left side using manual guidance for pelvic rotation (Fig. 7–16*A*). Annalee participates actively by using trunk flexors, righting, and controlling her head (Fig. 7–16*B*), using her right hand (Fig. 7–16*C*) to control her progress toward the prone position as the therapist applies traction on her right leg, and she ends on her forearms with her neck extended (Fig. 7–16*D*). Rolling over the right side is not as advanced because she has continued asymmetry of functioning related to the original head-turning preference. It is much more difficult for Annalee to activate her trunk and neck muscles for rolling to the prone position toward the right. During this sequence of treatment, Annalee produced her first independent roll from the prone to the supine position (Fig. 7–17).

In Figure 7–18*A* through *D*, the therapist provides postural fixation at the pelvis and assists with extending the left arm forward as she provides proprioceptive input into the shoulder to prepare Annalee for support on extended arms (Fig. 7–18*A*), provides proprioceptive stimulation at the trunk to activate trunk muscles and produces small weight shifts for the baby to accommodate (Fig. 7–18*B* and *C*) as she prepares Annalee for moving into sidelying (Fig. 7–18*D*) as a prelude to coming into a sitting position. Annalee actively participates by looking at toys, grasping a toy, using her abdominal muscles, and controlling her head and arm postures. In Figure 7–18*E* through *H*, movement into sitting occurs. The therapist provides support and manual guidance at the left shoulder and uses her right hand to activate the trunk muscles with propriceptive input (Fig. 7–18*E*). Annalee actively participates by controlling her arms, and the environment incorporates an interesting stimulus, the toy penguin. In Figure 7–18*F*, the therapist assists at the pelvis to begin the rotation into sitting. Annalee loses the toy as well as her trunk muscle activation (Fig. 7–18*G*), completing the movement into sitting with much assistance from the therapist, and then switches to using her left hand to grasp the toy (Fig. 7–18*H*). Because the movement into sitting is too challenging for Annalee's current abilities, the therapist will concentrate on working on the positions shown in Figure 7–18*E* and *F* to activate and strengthen the trunk muscles.

Annalee now discovers her toes (Fig. 7–19), and the therapist follows her lead, allowing her to play with her feet while providing proprioceptive stimulation to the trunk

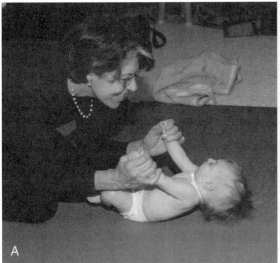

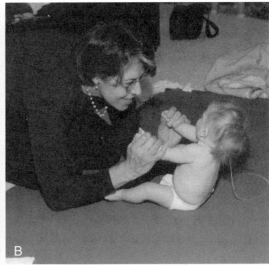

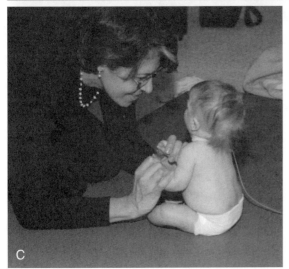

FIGURE 7–13. Assessment of head control during a pull-to-sit maneuver on the TIMP elicited scale: Traction on the arms (*A*) is used to elicit the infant's attempt to pull up to a sitting position. Annalee controls her head during the movement from the position in *A* to that in *C* but lacks capital flexion to achieve a "chin tuck." Annalee received a score of 2 on a scale from zero to 5. (Courtesy of Gay Girolami and Marv Chait, Pathways Center for Children, Glenview, Ill.)

FIGURE 7–14. Assessment of neck and trunk extension in prone suspension on the TIMP elicited scale: Annalee lifts her head slightly above the plane of the trunk and received a score of 3 on a scale from zero to 4. (Courtesy of Gay Girolami and Marv Chait, Pathways Center for Children, Glenview, Ill.)

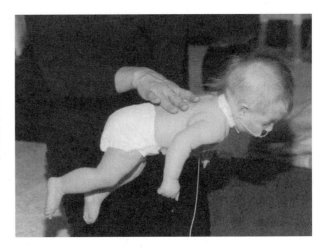

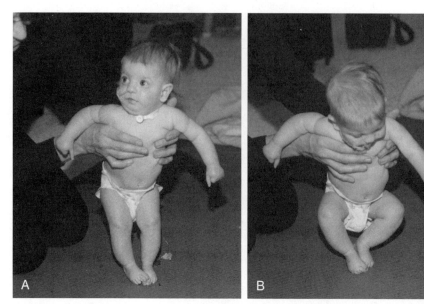

FIGURE 7–15. Assessment of supported standing on the TIMP elicited scale: Annalee supports her weight (*A*) for less than 5 seconds before collapsing into flexion (*B*) and received a score of 1 on a scale from zero to 5. (Courtesy of Gay Girolami and Marv Chait, Pathways Center for Children, Glenview, Ill.)

muscles to promote an erect posture. In Figure 7–19*B,* slight rotations of the trunk, lateral weight shifting, and stimulation of abdominal muscle activation are used to increase the strength and endurance of the trunk muscles, along with backward displacement (Fig. 7–19*C*) to activate equilibrium reactions and develop the necessary muscle activity to improve stabilization of the trunk for independent sitting. Annalee actively participates by continuing to play with her feet and by accommodating her posture to the internal and external perturbations created by her own movements and those of the therapist.

In the supine position (Fig. 7–20), the therapist works toward hands-to-feet movement by providing proprioceptive stimulation to the infant's trunk and elevating the pelvis to facilitate hip flexion and pelvic rotation (Fig. 7–20*A*). The goal of this work is to develop trunk extensors and abdominal muscles for trunk stabilization, and trunk and pelvic rotation for rolling and pushing up to a sitting from a prone or supine position. The technique proceeds with a shift of the key points of control to the hands and feet (Fig. 7–20*B*), and Annalee's mother facilitates active trunk rotation and weight shifting by attracting the infant's attention (Fig. 7–20*C*). In Figure 7–20*D,* the therapist provides slight traction to the left arm, and Annalee lifts her head and moves toward her mother to sit up. In Figure 7–20*E,* the therapist again shifts her key point of control to the infant's hands, allowing Annalee to play with pelvic rotation and the weight shifting created by turning to look at her mother (Fig. 7–20*F*). In Figure 7–20*G,* the therapist brings Annalee's pelvis back to a midline orientation and reactivates her abdominal muscles with proprioceptive inputs. Annalee is able to continue to maintain her attention on her mother while also grasping her foot. This activity develops selective control of the upper and lower body segments needed for rolling, crawling, and reaching for objects in the sitting position.

In lap sitting (Fig. 7–21), the therapist positions Annalee in a semireclining position with her knees above her hips (Fig. 7–21*A*). She provides proprioceptive stimulation to activate the trunk flexors, and Annalee actively participates with neck flexion and hand clasping. The therapist needs only two fingers at the infant's back to assist trunk stabilization. Various tactics are used throughout this activity to promote postural adjustment to movement, including trunk rotation (Fig. 7–21*B*) and lateral weight shifting (Fig. 7–21*C*). The latter is too challenging for Annalee, although she maintains her neck in flexion.

Text continued on page 303

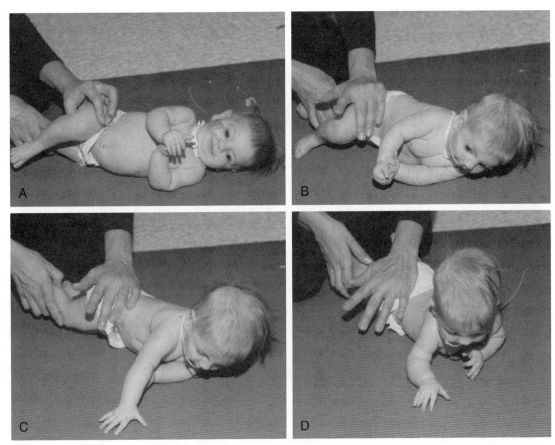

FIGURE 7–16. Facilitation of rolling to prone. The therapist provides guidance and proprioceptive facilitation at the hip (*A*). Annalee rights her head and contracts the abdominal muscles (*B*) and rolls with control (*C*) to the prone-on-elbows position (*D*). (Courtesy of Gay Girolami and Marv Chait, Pathways Center for Children, Glenview, Ill.)

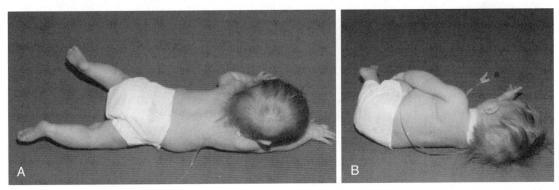

FIGURE 7–17. Annalee's first independent rolling from prone (*A*) to her back (*B*). (Courtesy of Gay Girolami and Marv Chait, Pathways Center for Children, Glenview, Ill.)

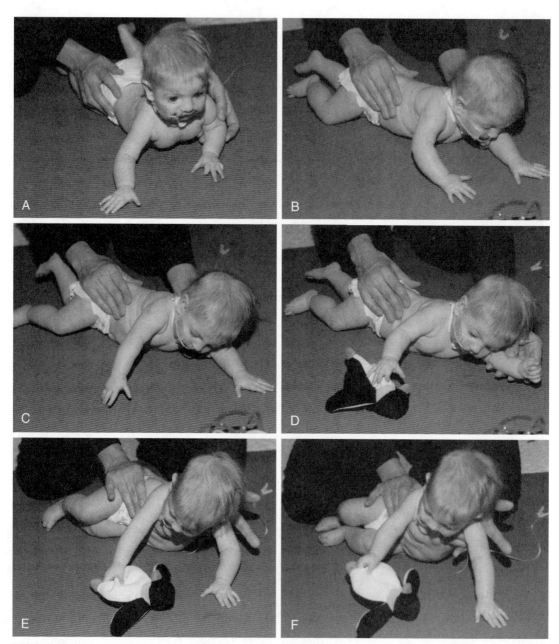

FIGURE 7–18. Preparation for the prone position on extended arms (*A*) followed by proprioceptive input to activate trunk muscles (*B*) and slight weight shifts (*C*) in preparation for moving into the side-lying position (*D*) and pushing up to the sitting position with excellent trunk muscle activation (*E* and *F*).

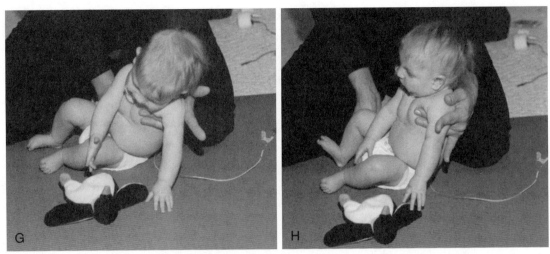

FIGURE 7–18 *Continued.* The movement into the sitting position (*G* and *H*), however, is too difficult for Annalee; she loses her trunk muscle activation as well as the toy and becomes a passive participant. (Courtesy of Gay Girolami and Marv Chait, Pathways Center for Children, Glenview, Ill.)

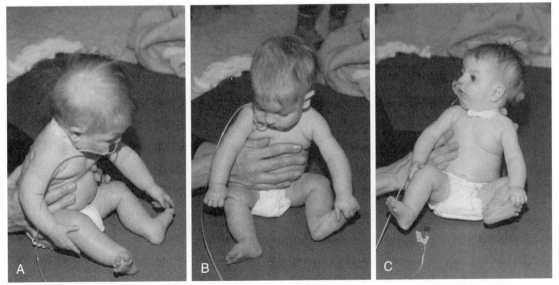

FIGURE 7–19. Annalee plays with her toes in the sitting position (*A*) as the therapist uses proprioceptive stimulation to the trunk (*B*) with weight shifting and lateral trunk rotation (*C*) to activate equilibrium reactions and develop trunk muscle strength. (Courtesy of Gay Girolami and Marv Chait, Pathways Center for Children, Glenview, Ill.)

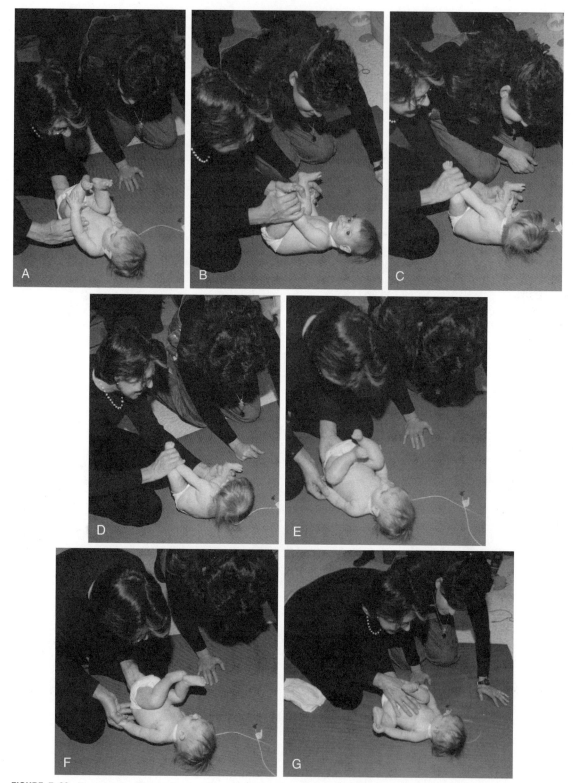

FIGURE 7–20. For play in the supine position, the therapist uses proprioceptive input to the trunk (*A*) to activate Annalee's abdominal muscles, then challenges them to work in a movement toward sitting up (*B*) as Annalee looks at her mother (*C*) and lifts her head to move toward her (*D*). Next, the therapist controls Annalee's arms (*E*) and uses small weight shifts of the body (*F*) to encourage her to play with pelvic rotation. *G*, Annalee is able to maintain a grasp on her left toes while continuing to look at her mother. (Courtesy of Gay Girolami and Marv Chait, Pathways Center for Children, Glenview, Ill.)

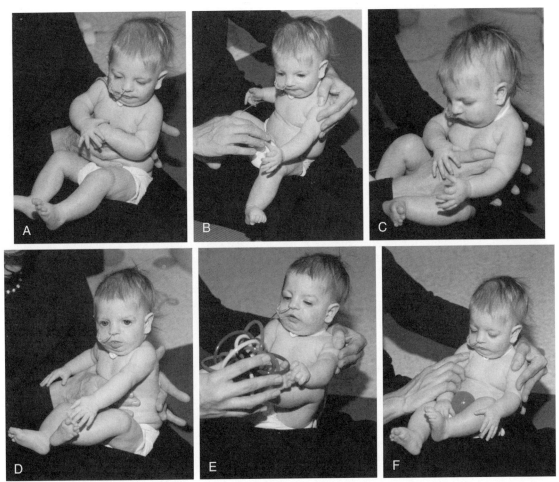

FIGURE 7–21. In lap sitting, the therapist provides proprioceptive stimulation to activate the trunk muscles (*A*) and uses trunk rotation with proprioceptive input to the shoulder (*B*) and lateral weight shifting (*C*) to improve Annalee's trunk stability. The position in *C* is too difficult, and Annalee shows her discomfort by grasping onto the therapist's hands. When moved back into a more stable position, Annalee grasps her toes (*D*), reaches for a toy (*E*), and looks at a ball (*F*). Each activity requires a different combination of trunk and neck muscle activity as well as a variety of hand and arm positions to provide Annalee with multiple options for play in the sitting position. (Courtesy of Gay Girolami and Marv Chait, Pathways Center for Children, Glenview, Ill.)

Annalee shows her discomfort by grasping onto the therapist's hands as she loses her trunk control, and the therapist must use her entire hand to stabilize the infant's trunk. When brought back toward a midline orientation, Annalee stays task oriented to playing with her feet (Fig. 7–21*D*), looking at a toy near her feet while holding her toes but with some loss of chin tuck as the therapist tilts her slightly backward, indicating poor neck flexor muscle strength (Fig. 7–21*E*), or looking at a toy between her knees (Fig. 7–21*F*), a task requiring more neck flexion than the previous activities. Throughout this sequence of activity, Annalee returns to her preferred leftward orientation of the head, perhaps because of the demanding nature of this final sequence of treatment activities. Each of the tasks used in Annalee's treatment requires a different combination of muscle activity and attention, thus providing novelty to maintain the infant's interest and the opportunity to practice a variety of movement patterns within the basic task of sitting and playing. The demands of active participation also build her cardiopulmonary and muscle endurance.

At 6.5 months of age, Annalee was assessed on the TIMP because she had still not reached the ceiling on all TIMP items. She achieved a total score of 146, which would be in the high-average range for a 13-week-old infant (Table 7–4). In order to more

accurately compare Annalee's skills with those of age peers, the AIMS[104] was administered. She obtained a score at the 5th percentile for her chronologic age (about average
for a 5-month-old infant). Because she had achieved all her physical therapy goals and
was showing signs of readiness for sitting and rolling from the supine to the prone
position, regular therapy was discontinued. Annalee will be checked once a month so
that her family can receive anticipatory guidance for continuing to promote her development. As we shall see in the next section, the AIMS, with its illustrations of developmental
milestones, is an excellent test for this purpose. Furthermore, if development falls below
the 5th percentile on the AIMS, justification for returning to a higher frequency of therapy
would be available.

In summary, a variety of intervention strategies have been documented to improve
developmental outcomes for high-risk infants. These include education on responsive
handling for parents, the NIDCAP approach, tactile-kinesthetic stimulation programs,
and NDT during the NICU stay. Unfortunately, none of these approaches have yet been
documented as successful in improving outcomes for infants with CP. Chapter 2 presents
the research results on intervention for older children, but research in the area of early
intervention for infants with brain insults is clearly needed.

Best-Practice Recommendations

Based on the research available, I would suggest that direct services in the NICU (or
during the early weeks following discharge) in which physical therapy is aimed at
improving postural control appears appropriate only for children with documented
medical syndromes or definite clinical evidence of a high neurologic risk of a poor
outcome (e.g., greater than 50 percent probability). Evidence in support of direct
treatment by a physical therapist includes (1) poverty of movement, severe asymmetry,
or cramped synchrony documented with Prechtl's videotaped general movement assessment, (2) repeated examinations with evidence of abnormal reflexes and postural tone
that do not show significant recovery during a nursery course on tests such as the
Dubowitz assessment, or (3) the documented presence of perinatal asphyxia, PVL, or
other imaging evidence of brain damage with more than a 50 percent risk of CP.

Infants with IVH in addition to BPD can also be justified as appropriate subjects
of direct treatment because of the combination of (1) poor endurance for movement
caused by severe lung disease, (2) evidence that motor development is typically delayed
in babies with BPD, and (3) a moderate risk of CP as a result of IVH. Because
infants with BPD frequently have difficulty with oral feedings because of problems in
coordinating sucking with swallowing and breathing, oral motor treatment is appropriately provided by a trained specialist, such as a physical therapist, occupational therapist,
or speech and language pathologist, in conjunction with supplemental oxygen during
feeding.[146] Similarly, infants such as Annalee with poverty of movement, asymmetry,
and feeding problems related to respiratory difficulties and craniofacial anomalies can
be justified as appropriate for treatment when motor delay and poor endurance for
feeding and other movements are documented.

Children with grade III or IV IVH might not be automatically referred to physical
therapy for direct treatment because their risk of CP is moderate as a group, but the risk
plus clinical signs based on assessment of the child's functional movement could be
used in decision making. For example, a TIMP assessment of any infant with results
more than 2 SD below the mean for age peers (see Table 7–4) could be used to support
referral for intervention, although without further research TIMP results alone cannot be
used to support a definitive diagnosis of developmental delay or to predict the risk of
CP. The TIMP has been documented as containing items that reflect typical demands
for movement experienced by infants in daily life, so an improved score with intervention
should be reflective of better functional performance, although research evidence to that

effect is currently lacking. Although the TIMP is sensitive to the effects of NDT provided for infants during their NICU stay, evidence for sensitivity to change with intervention for infants after term-equivalent age or for those with documented brain damage is not available. Research on its validity for these purposes is needed. Finally, it must be admitted that the recommendations made here stem from the evidence on the degree of certainty of a poor developmental outcome, not from evidence that early physical therapy can significantly alter that outcome. Furthermore, although the typical therapist's role in the NICU includes positioning and ROM exercises,[10] evidence is lacking for their effectiveness in promoting development or preventing contractures in those with CNS dysfunction.

MONITORING THE POSTDISCHARGE DEVELOPMENT OF HIGH-RISK INFANTS

After discharge, the typical special care nursery provides for developmental follow-up of infants, usually selected from among those with the lowest birth weight and others with documented risk of developmental disability, such as infants with BPD, PVL, or imaging evidence of other brain insult. Therapists in these outpatient settings are likely to use standard developmental assessments such as the Bayley II[44] or Peabody Developmental Motor Scales[48] at ages established for a return to the clinic primarily on the basis of a need for immunizations and other health care or screening. In this section, we review other screening and motor assessment tools that show promise for early definitive diagnosis of those with developmental motor delay or CNS dysfunction. The reader is referred to Sweeney and Swanson for more information on these and other tests.[9] In addition, we address the question of whether one test, used repeatedly at multiple follow-up points during the first year, represents best practice, or whether an assessment algorithm reflecting knowledge of child development that uses different assessments at different points in time would be more useful. An educational model of assessment as intervention[9] would also suggest that tests for potential use in monitoring infant development should be evaluated for their value in providing anticipatory guidance for families regarding their child's developmental progress and prognosis.

Bayley Infant Neurodevelopmental Screener

The Bayley Infant Neurodevelopmental Screener (BINS) is a 10-minute screening test for developmental delay or neurologic impairment in children from 3 to 24 months.[147] The purpose of the test is the identification of infants who need further diagnostic testing. The test was standardized on 600 infants and includes items in several domains, including basic neurologic integrity (muscle tone, asymmetries, head control), sensory receptive functions (visual and auditory sensation and perception), expressive functions (fine, gross, and oral motor skills), and cognitive processes (memory, attention, problem solving). Emphasis is placed on the processes of development, that is, *how* the child performs, rather than simply whether a competency is demonstrated. Items are arranged in sets of 11 to 13 items for use at key ages: 3, 6, 9, 12, 18, and 24 months. Cut scores are given for each age to delineate infants at low risk, moderate risk, and high risk for developmental delay or neurologic impairment. Those at high risk should receive further diagnostic testing with the Bayley II,[44] those at moderate risk should be reassessed with the BINS in 3 months. Sensitivity for identifying infants who will score more than 1 SD below the mean on a concurrent administration of the Bayley II motor scale is highest at 24 months (60 percent with 87 percent specificity) using the cut score for high-risk performance, while specificity peaks at 18 months at 98 percent (with sensitivity for predicting abnormal developmental performance on the Bayley motor scale at 43 percent). The concurrent validity for predicting cognitive performance on the Bayley II is better than that for motor performance: at all ages, the sensitivity for identifying children who score more than 1 SD below the mean is 50 percent or better, and the specificity is 88 percent or better. The predictive validity to a later outcome using the BINS cut scores has not been reported. It is recommended that examiners using the BINS possess a master's degree, with education in standardized assessment and infant development.

Harris Infant Neuromotor Test

The Harris Infant Neuromotor Test (HINT)[148] is a 20- to 30-minute screening test developed by a physical therapist for infants from 3 to 12 months of age. The HINT is under investigation for reliability and predictive validity. It is notable for having questions directed to parents regarding their beliefs about their child's development, which are taken into account in the scoring. Although primarily a motor test, the HINT contains items for assessing infant behavior as well.

Alberta Infant Motor Scale

The AIMS,[104] like the general movement assessment of Prechtl and colleagues, is a gross motor scale that is scored based on observation of the spontaneous motor activity of infants. The test was normed on more than 2000 Canadian infants selected to represent the characteristics of the population of the province of Alberta. Rater reliability in the high 0.90s is easily obtained with only minimal training, and the test can be done in 20 to 30 minutes. The AIMS has a pictorial display that is useful in explaining results and providing anticipatory family guidance on gross motor development. Performance relative to age norms is plotted on a graph that is similar to those used for growth measures, so the reporting device is familiar both to parents and to other professionals. A recent article on the test's predictive validity reported that use of the 10th percentile as a cutoff criterion for the identification of a high risk of abnormal development at 4 months of age produced a sensitivity of 77 percent and a specificity of 82 percent for prediction of the neurologic outcome at 18 months.[149] Use of the 5th percentile as a cutoff at 8 months produced values of 86 and 93 percent, respectively.

Movement Assessment of Infants

The Movement Assessment of Infants (MAI) is a test with four dimensions: muscle tone, reflexes, volitional movements, and postural reactions.[150] The item reliability is variable, and research has concentrated only on prediction of motor outcome from the numbers of abnormal items (risk score) at 4 and 8 months.[9] Norms are not available for the MAI, so it cannot be used to document a delay in relation to age peers.

Piper and colleagues explored the sensitivity, specificity, and predictive values of the MAI for predicting abnormal or suspect neurologic outcomes at 18 months of adjusted age from 4-month assessments of prematurely born infants.[151] Testing both at 4 months of age when adjusted for prematurity and at 4 months chronologic age was done in 75 babies. They concluded that failing to adjust for premature birth on a 4-month MAI assessment produced low specificities and recommended that testing at 4 months of *chronologic* age *not* be used for identifying children at risk for CNS dysfunction. To predict 18-month abnormal outcome, the following prediction values were obtained for the use of a cutoff score of more than 4 risk points on the MAI at 4 months of adjusted age: sensitivity, 100 percent; specificity, 80 percent; positive predictive value, 63 percent; and negative predictive value, 100 percent. If predictions were made for *either* a suspect or an abnormal outcome at 18 months, the best combination of validities for high risk was obtained using a cutoff score of more than 9 high-risk points on the MAI: 67 percent sensitivity, 94 percent specificity, 67 percent positive predictive value, and 94 percent negative predictive value. Note that the positive predictive value indicates that if one used the MAI to identify children who needed more detailed assessment or referral for intervention, approximately two of three babies would be correctly identified as having poor neurologic performance at 18 months, but 1 of 3 would be normal. Thus sensitivity and specificity document the accuracy of a screening test, but the positive predictive validity indicates to the clinician how many children will receive unnecessary further assessment or services as a result of using the identification protocol. Both financial and personal costs for families in time and the stress of unnecessary treatment are involved and must be taken into account when developing a decision-making model or critical pathway for service delivery.

Here we return to the case of Lee, who was identified as at high risk for CP based on his medical history and on the basis of abnormal performance on the Dubowitz neurologic assessment[95] despite some recovery on repeated testing. In this case, we see the value of longitudinal tracking of both motor and cognitive development and also consider whether tests available today would be more useful.

CASE STUDY

LONGITUDINAL ASSESSMENT OF DEVELOPMENT

Lee's motor development was followed using the 1969 edition of the Bayley Scales of Infant Development motor scale[42] and the MAI.[150] At both 2.5 and 4 months, his Bayley standard score, the Psychomotor Developmental Index, was 80 or slightly lower than 1 SD below the mean or below the 16th percentile for his chronologic age. At 7 and 12 months, Lee's Psychomotor Developmental Index was 1.5 SD below the mean; by 18 months it was 2 SD below the mean or below the 2nd percentile and clearly outside the normal range. At 12 months of age, Lee was able to bunny hop as a means of locomotion, could get to the sitting from the supine position, pulled to stand at furniture and cruised sideways, and took steps with hands held. He was able to lower himself to the floor from standing without falling. At 18 months, few new gross motor skills had been obtained, but in terms of self-help skills he had learned to brush his own hair and wash and feed himself. He achieved independent walking at 20 months of age.

A diagnosis of CP had been suspected at Lee's first clinic visit and was confirmed by a developmental pediatrician at 4 months when he received 23 risk points on the MAI. He was hypotonic and used compensatory postural fixations during play, had an obligatory asymmetric tonic neck reflex to both sides, and had frequent startle responses to loud sounds or sudden movements. He was unable to maintain his head erect for more than a few seconds in supported sitting but could hold it up fairly well in the prone position. CP was not, however, mentioned to Lee's parents until 7 months of age because the diagnosis of CP was considered by the conservative physician to remain uncertain in the sense that data on children who outgrew CP were fresh in his mind[35] and the risk points on the MAI were discounted because the test was not normed. Throughout this period, monthly home visits from a community-based physical therapist were Lee's only direct treatment; the therapist provided a home program for the parents to follow between visits.

REFLECTION ON PRACTICE

This case was frustrating to the clinic therapist because the diagnosis appeared clear but the physician remained uncertain that Lee would not recover. During the 1980s, when Lee was born, it was only beginning to be clear that the Bayley scales' norms were seriously out of date. Once the Bayley scale was renormed, it was clear that on the older scale, scores were being given that were at least 10 points higher than was appropriate.[44] Had a more recently normed test, such as the Peabody scales,[48] been used, Lee would probably have looked much more delayed. If Lee had obtained a standard score of 70 at 4 months, almost any physician would have considered him severely delayed on a test with a normative mean of 100 and an SD of 15. Today, use of the new Bayley II scale[44] would be appropriate to document Lee's early delay, but a better choice for an assessment tool might be the AIMS.[104] Research suggests that a score below the 10th percentile at 4 months is predictive of delay at 18 months.[149] Because the AIMS requires specific aspects of motor control and postural alignment to be present for an infant to pass each motor milestone, it is quite likely that his score on the AIMS would be lower than that on a Bayley II scale completed at the same time. Furthermore, the illustrations of motor milestones on the AIMS would be useful in providing anticipatory guidance to Lee's parents regarding expectations for continued development. Once a diagnosis of abnormal motor performance was made, however, the AIMS would no longer be appropriate because a child with CP can never attain normal performance according to the postural control standards expected of typically developing infants on the AIMS. His parents also do not need to be repeatedly reminded that his performance continues to fall further and further behind age peers. One instance in which an AIMS might be recommended for use with a child with CP, however, is when a specific normative score is needed on a one-time basis for diagnosis to justify intervention or placement in categorical programs. Otherwise, switching to a functional motor scale, such as the Gross Motor Function Measure,[152] is more appropriate. The Gross Motor Function Measure has been documented as sensitive to change with physical therapy in children with CP and will be useful for several years to document Lee's progress and areas of strength and weakness.

Lee's case, however, points out the importance of assessing cognitive development as well as motor development. Despite the weaknesses of the Bayley norms at the time, it was clear from comparison of the Psychomotor Developmental Index and the Mental Developmental Index that Lee's cognitive development was not delayed. Although the Psychomotor Developmental Index was below average, Lee's Mental Developmental Index was above average throughout his first 2 years (e.g., 119 at both 7 and 12 months). This information is useful in planning therapy that will be mentally stimulating for Lee despite his motor delay. Giving his parents the good news about his mental capabilities is also rewarding. Armed with this knowledge, Lee's parents gave him the opportunity to learn self-care skills that might not have even been attempted if they had believed his cognitive development to be as delayed as his motor skill.

Because Lee was believed to be bright, he was given the chance to wear glasses much earlier (before 12 months of age) than might have been attempted otherwise. The unexpectedly great improvement in his eye-hand coordination when wearing glasses was important for Lee and made it possible for him to attempt self-care skills that might not otherwise have been feasible. Recently, Mercuri and colleagues have reported the high frequency of visual dysfunction in infants with HIE.[153] When a battery of visual function tests was administered to 31 full-term infants with HIE, 72 percent had abnormal results on one or more tests. Visual function was always abnormal when MR imaging demonstrated damage to the basal ganglia. As a result, the authors recommend that an extensive battery of visual tests, well described in their article, be used at 5 to 7 months of age in infants with HIE.

Unlike Lee, a full-term baby at birth, the average infant born with low birth weight is likely to have low-average cognitive outcomes. Intervention can frequently improve but not completely ameliorate the situation. For example, a recent study of intervention by early-childhood education specialists, The Infant Health and Development Program, begun after hospital discharge for infants born weighing less than 1501 g, documented a significant difference in IQ at 36 months (7.2 points) relative to an untreated control group.[41] Despite the successful outcomes reported for the group of low birth weight children as a whole,[154] CP could not be prevented, and removing children with CP from the analysis increased the difference between groups with and without intervention. The authors do not believe that intervention based on their curriculum can produce a major impact on mental development in children with documented brain damage, but they also express the opinion that physical therapy services alone have limited benefits for children with CP or at risk for CP. As a result, it is not clear that Lee's development was hindered by his lack of early direct therapy. Given other research by Palmer and colleagues suggesting that an educationally based curriculum is more effective than NDT for children with late-treated spastic diplegia,[155] research is needed on whether the combined effects of physical therapy and educational approaches have a significant impact in improving the outcome of children with documented brain damage.

The Infant Health and Development Program involved weekly home visits in the first year (every other week after 1 year), and 5 days per week of educational center–based care beginning at 1 year, accompanied by parental support groups.[154] The intervention provided is called Partners.[158] The theoretical framework for this approach is based on research documenting that effective programs involve assisting parents to understand their child's development and to learn ways to foster progress through activities appropriate to the child's readiness level. Play materials were provided. A second aspect of the program facilitated the parents' skills in coping with child care.

A similar approach that was documented to be successful with families with both high and low educational levels is the Nursing Systems for Effective Parenting–Preterm, a postdischarge program for families based on Barnard's Child Health Assessment Interaction Model, discussed previously.[120] The program consists of a highly cost-effective program of nine home visits by a public health nurse beginning at 36 weeks of postconceptional age and continuing through 5 months of corrected age. The cost of this program combined with the previously described in-hospital program was $550 per infant (1995 dollars). The goal for parents during the period from 4 to 6 months is social-affective modulation. Infants whose mothers received training were more responsive on the Teaching Scale of the Barnard assessment program[111] at 5 months, and mothers were more sensitive and responsive as well. A program such as this might have been useful for Lee's family to ensure maximal development of his excellent cognitive potential despite severe motoric limitations.

In addition to incorporating these evidence-based strategies (emphasis on parent knowledge, child readiness, and appropriate activities involving parent-child interaction) into planning of physical therapy programs, the theoretical framework for treating children with CP should include (1) gradually providing parents with increased knowledge about the child's neurologic problems and functional skills and limitations and, in coordination with the child's physician, the risk of various developmental outcomes with sensitive handling of diagnostic information, (2) coaching for managing the physical impairments and functional limitations evidenced at any point in time, including the provision of information on assistive technology options, and (3) the opportunity for families to participate in goal establishment for their child's care based on family social and cultural values,[157] resources, and lifestyle. The theoretical framework with respect to the child's plan of care includes (1) developing a range of activities presenting the just-right challenge to advance functional skills, (2) empowering the child's search for interaction with the environment for self-directed learning and activity, (3) positioning and assistive technology solutions to prevent musculoskeletal problems and facilitate functional performance, and (4) preventing disability in daily life roles involving play and exploration, while eliciting appropriate caregiving and interaction with family members and also treating functional limitations and impairments that might hinder future functioning.

The case of Claire illustrates the importance of responding to parents' needs and readiness for intervention. Unlike Lee's family, from whom information was withheld for several months, Claire's mother was given information she was not ready to handle. Documenting cognitive skills was also important in this case in order to provide early intervention for communication development and to challenge the child with motor activities that reflect recognition of the child's differing abilities in the two domains.

CASE STUDY

RESPONDING TO PARENTS' NEEDS AND FACILITATING COGNITIVE DEVELOPMENT

Claire was born weighing 4250 g after a full-term pregnancy with a lack of regular prenatal care. Delivery was unattended, at home, in breech presentation. Her mother was alone when she went into labor, and a neighbor came to help only after she had partially delivered the baby. The child's head was "stuck in the birth canal for 20 minutes." She was initially cyanotic and apneic with a heart rate of 120. The neighbor reportedly gave Claire mouth-to-mouth resuscitation for 3 hours until she was finally brought to the area teaching hospital by paramedics. She was noted to be floppy but became rigid and opisthotonic when stimulated. Initially she had no reflexes except for a weak suck and weak withdrawal from painful stimuli. On the first day of life she began to have grand mal seizures, which were controlled with phenobarbital. Diagnosis was HIE with secondary multifocal seizures associated with occasional apnea. Her electroencephalogram was markedly abnormal with predominantly right and posterior dysrhythmic slowing with occasional sharp waves. By 3 days of age she was more active and able to feed independently. She was discharged at 12 days on phenobarbital and had no seizures after 10 days of age.

Claire was seen in the developmental follow-up clinic at 2 months of age. She was assessed with the Bayley Scales of Infant Development.[42] At this time she was hypotonic and could not sustain a head-up posture in the prone position for more than a second. The therapist and the developmental pediatrician told Claire's mother that they strongly suspected that Claire had CP because of her inability to sustain an antigravity position and her exceedingly low postural tone. Her mother became angry because she felt that Claire was doing fine based on her alertness and social responsivity. Concerned because Claire's mother threatened to stop coming to the clinic, the therapist pulled back and just gave suggestions for working with Claire to improve prone head control, such as placing her on a blanket roll. The baby returned to a follow-up clinic at 4 months of age, when her severely delayed motor development was verified with a diagnosis of CP.

REFLECTION ON PRACTICE

Given the likelihood that Claire's mother experienced severe guilt and perhaps depression about her lack of prenatal care and the unattended home delivery, 2 months of age was much too early for Claire's mother to hear the bad news about Claire's diagnosis. One could also question whether the professionals might have been wrong, that is, that Claire might have recovered and turned out to be normal. The therapist had little doubt about the diagnosis; the questionable behavior on her part was trying to force a mother to accept a diagnosis for which she was not ready instead of acknowledging the mother's correct assessment of Claire's excellent social responsivity while gradually leading the mother toward recognizing the motor delay herself as she became ready to do so. Claire's mother would have benefited from being linked with a parent group, such as Parents of Premature and High Risk Infants International Inc. (33 W. 22nd Street, Suite 1227, New York, NY 10036), for peer support.

In terms of developmental testing, today a better option for assessment of Claire than the Bayley scales would be the AIMS.[104] Although the AIMS is not to be used for children with CP because they can never achieve the normal postural alignment and selective control of movement required to pass AIMS items, its attractive pictorial score sheet could be used to demonstrate Claire's observed skills across time without attempting to derive a quantitative score. This unorthodox use of the AIMS would have allowed the therapist to provide anticipatory guidance to Claire's mother regarding which motor skills are next in sequence and therefore potential goals for home programming. Claire's mother would have had the chance to observe for herself the lack of progress over time, because Claire never gained skills beyond unstable sitting. Presented with sensitivity, this information would have allowed Claire's mother to draw her own conclusions, because she had a basis of knowledge of normal development as a result of having raised several children, who were teenagers or in middle school and not living with her at the time Claire was born. When the mother appeared ready to hear a diagnosis, the AIMS graph showing her performance relative to that of age peers could have been shown to Claire's mother as formal documentation of her developmental diagnosis. Once a diagnosis of delay had been made, her mother no longer would need to be shown the percentile rank, which would have fallen farther and farther below the 1st percentile with each passing month. Once development seemed to be slowing such that continued progress on the AIMS seemed unlikely (Claire never achieved an age-equivalent score on the Bayley motor scale greater than 5 months), its use would be discontinued in favor of a criterion-referenced test appropriate for Claire's skills, perhaps the Gross Motor Function Measure.[152]

Claire's mother would also have benefited from use of the Family Interest Form of the Assessment, Evaluation, and Programming System for Infants and Children.[158] This form allows parents to indicate their priorities, enabling health care practitioners to respond sensitively to the family's readiness for information at any point in time. For example, a family member who checks interest in "knowing how my child grows and learns" is in a different place than one who checks "learning about services and programs for my child." Checking a need for "counseling for my family" indicates a concern for how the family as a whole is facing the presence of a disability in their child. On the other hand, a family member who indicates interest in "volunteering with other families" has met the challenge of disability well enough to feel capable of offering to assist others.

Pathways to Diagnosis

Although therapists often hear stories from parents about the agonizing delay in receiving a diagnosis of CP when they were sure that something was wrong, the stories of Claire, Madonna, Annalee, and Lee indicate that there are many routes to diagnosis and just as many responses to the dawning recognition of a disability on the part of both families and health professionals. The qualitative research of Knafl and colleagues identified five pathways to diagnosis[159] in children with chronic diseases that are likely to be similar to those for families of children with movement dysfunction. These pathways were distinguished by the time between the onset of symptoms and the diagnosis, the problems encountered in obtaining a diagnosis, the extent to which parents took an active role in seeking a diagnosis, and the quality of the parent–health care provider relationship during the period of searching for a diagnosis.

The first pathway is *direct*—symptoms were recognized and responded to immediately by a health care provider.[159] A *delay* pathway was similar in that symptoms were recognized but they may have been explained away for a short time before a diagnosis was achieved, usually when symptoms became more severe. In each of the first two pathways, relationships between parents and professionals were generally positive. The *detour* pathway occurred when there was a setback in obtaining a diagnosis because of a problem or error in the health care system. Nevertheless, a diagnosis was achieved quite promptly, and the family recognized that errors can be made by well-meaning individuals. The pathway to diagnosis labeled the *quest* was one in which the journey was tortuous as parents actively sought answers. This route frequently occurred because the family believed that health care providers were not being helpful, and they set off to find information on their own. A search that proved particularly frustrating, long, and unproductive was identified in families whose pathway to diagnosis was labeled an *ordeal*. Here there were multiple unproductive encounters with professionals, followed by a turning point that often brought the parents to the realization of just how unhelpful their previous encounters had been. These parents sensed that good luck rather than their own active efforts, or those of health care providers, was the source of the diagnosis. In this type of story, a hero professional who uncovered the diagnosis was often heralded, but relationships with many other providers were negative. Of note is the fact that one-quarter of the families in this study changed health care practitioners early in the course of the discovery process. The results of this research, coupled with the stories of Claire, whose mother initially rejected the diagnosis of health professionals, and of Annalee, whose family found their previously satisfactory pediatrician to be inadequate in caring for a child with serious health problems, make it clear that physical therapists and others must be prepared to deal with families in flexible ways and to acknowledge their own limitations. The Family Interest Form is one way that health care providers can obtain information about how the family sees their own situation in terms of information needs and support services.[158]

CASE STUDY

INTERVENTION

Claire's early goals for treatment included (1) an ability to support herself in a prone-on-elbows position for social interaction with her mother, and (2) an ability to be seated in a stable upright position for social interaction and upper extremity play. A corner chair was used for floor-level play to provide trunk support and also to maintain hamstring muscle length. As Claire grew, her therapy incorporated assisted movement from prone to sitting to kneeling to standing so that Claire would have the opportunity to experience movement through space, develop her visual perceptual skills, and possibly be prepared for wheelchair use at a later date, because it was believed that independent or assisted ambulation was unlikely to develop. Indeed, Claire never developed an ability to independently locomote through space except by rolling. Extensive therapy was also provided to facilitate feeding activities.

Because working with Claire and previous testing seemed to indicate that she had much higher cognitive than motor skills, the Bayley mental scale was administered to Claire at 17.5 months of age. Because she lacked the motor skills to accomplish many of the tasks on the Bayley scale requiring fine motor dexterity, the test was adapted to Claire's physical abilities by providing stabilization of toys, but no other adaptations were used. With adapted test administration, Claire attained a raw score of 117, resulting in an estimated Mental Developmental Index of 89, close to 1 SD below the mean but within the average range for her age. The information from the test provided the therapist with the knowledge that Claire had skills such as object permanence, imitation of words and actions, and the concept of putting things into a container. She was also able to "mend" a broken doll and to stack three blocks when the cubes were stabilized for her and recognized shapes at a level enabling her to place square and round blocks into the Bayley puzzle board. This knowledge fit with previous Bayley testing at 11 months of age that indicated a 9-month age-equivalent for mental performance and was used to ensure that therapy activities were mentally challenging for Claire, rather than using activities appropriate to her 5-month motor level. She was not able to point at or name pictures shown to her, but she showed clear interest in looking at them so the therapist was able to reinforce her mother's belief that Claire liked to listen to stories and look at pictures in books and magazines. This activity was encouraged and supported with recommendations for books that were appropriate for Claire's estimated mental age. Armed with the information from Claire's mother that she seemed to be trying to indicate her wants and could use head nodding to indicate yes and no, a simple communication board was prepared before Claire was 14 months old, one with pictures of items of food on it that Claire liked for snacks, play activities she liked, and later one for a need to use the bathroom. She quickly learned to point to desired objects or activities, and this was the start of a passage into special education programs that led to the use of a highly complicated communication board when Claire was a teenager because she never developed usable speech despite her continued high-level cognitive performance.

REFLECTION ON PRACTICE

Perhaps the most useful thing done for Claire was to recognize her high cognitive abilities, affirm her mother's beliefs regarding Claire's excellent social skills, and begin early use of a communication device. With all the many fine pieces of assistive technology now available, Claire today would benefit from earlier fitting with a proper chair and use of switch-operated toys and equipment. One wonders about the usefulness of all the therapy to promote motor skill development. Her skills probably would have advanced to the same level on their own; with low tone she was not in great danger of developing serious contractures; and her mother was motivated enough to help her develop any skills she was capable of gaining. On the other hand, her mental abilities may not have developed as well without the challenge of problem-solving movement activities in therapy, and the activation of her multiple senses through assisted movement in space may have been influential in her cognitive development. As she grew older, therapy for Claire was also made more age-appropriate by having her wear a leotard and turning her exercises into "ballet lessions." She even participated in a dance recital with other children with disabilities. Research on the importance of meaningful and guided movement for cognitive development in infants with severe physical disabilities is needed.

CARE PATHWAYS FOR COMPREHENSIVE ASSESSMENT

In the cases of Claire and Lee, the same tests were used repeatedly across the course of development for monitoring motor and cognitive outcomes. Because it is well known that not all aspects of development proceed at the same rate and that there are sensitive periods for the recognition of important indicators of developmental progress,[160] we consider in this section whether a clinical pathway for developmental assessment that involves assessing *different* aspects of development at *different* ages would be both more efficient and more productive in achieving earlier diagnosis of either abnormality or normal development and in meeting the needs of worried families than would repeated examination with the same tests. For example, the Risk Routes Model of Aylward and Kenny suggests assessment of risk in three domains: medical-biologic, environmental-psychosocial, and behavioral-developmental.[161] A problem with this clinical care path, however, is a lack of recognition of sensitive periods and varying developmental rates across time. The degree of risk is additive across areas at each time of testing and is also cumulative across time. This means that a child who is once determined to be at risk never has the opportunity to be removed from the risk register.

Another approach is suggested by Gordon and Jens.[160] Their Moving Risk Model conceptualizes risk as noncumulative across time and as synergistic across areas of development at any single point in time. Individual domains of development are weighted at particular ages in keeping with research indicating sensitive stages for individual developmental domains. This model allows a clinic to select the tests it will use because a variety of options are suggested.

Field and colleagues formulated a cumulative risk index based on a study of predictors of mental and motor development at 12 months of age in 46 preterm infants with RDS; 46 postterm, postmature infants; and 59 infants born at term.[162] Although retrospective in nature and not tested with a new group of prospectively followed infants, their work illustrates that at different ages, risk may be best predicted by different types of variables. Measures taken most closely in time to criterion outcome measures are also demonstrated to have stronger predictive validity, as would be expected. Nevertheless, even measures taken in the newborn period contributed to explaining the outcome. Bayley motor scale scores (1969 edition)[42] at 12 months were predicted by motoric process scores on the Brazelton Neonatal Behavioral Assessment Scale[93] as well as by 8-month Bayley mental and motor scores. Use of these variables to predict 12-month Bayley motor scores yielded 91 percent correct classification of infants with standard scores of less than 85 and 86 percent of those with scores greater than 84. The probability of misclassification was only 11 percent, and the strongest predictors were 8-month Bayley scores. If indicators available only at birth were used, the Brazelton motoric process score and the postnatal and obstetric complications scores of Parmalee and associates[163] were significant predictors, but misclassification probability was 22 percent. At 4 months, the best prediction was obtained with a combination of Brazelton motoric process scores, the postnatal complications score, ratings on the Denver Developmental Screening Test,[164] and the Carey[165] temperament score (misclassification probability was 20 percent). At birth and 4 months, the Brazelton motoric process score was the strongest single predictor of outcome.

Babies with RDS tended to be hyporeactive on the Brazelton scale at birth, to have poor Denver scores on both the personal-social and the motor sectors, and during interactions with caregivers, to have particular problems with inattentiveness and fussiness that correlated with "difficult" ratings on the Carey temperament scale.[165] The Brazelton scale ratings, therefore, were consistently predictive of poor 12-month motor performance; the prediction improved slightly when behavioral problems were assessed and added to the equation at 4 months but improved still more when the 8-month Bayley performance was known. The latter became the strongest predictor, as would be expected because it is a measure taken closer in time to the 12-month scores. Although the babies with RDS tended to score lower in motor performance (average, 80) than in cognitive performance (average, 90), it is interesting to note that poor Brazelton motoric process scores were also significant predictors of Bayley *mental* performance scores at 12 months when combined with a poor Carey temperament score at 4 months. Poor motor performance as a newborn, therefore, is a nonspecific indicator of developmental outcome. By 8 months these variables were no longer significant predictors of the 12-month cognitive performance.

Finally, in contradistinction to assessment models using normative scales for diagnosis are systems that stress the use of criterion-referenced scales in what is purported to be a more family-friendly and efficient approach.[166] Typical of such systems is extensive family involvement in assessment and goal setting, emphasis on measuring infant and family competencies rather than weaknesses, and the integration of assessment and intervention in a transdisciplinary approach. Although such systems are reported to be valid in identifying children with special needs and prescribing intervention,[167] little documentation of this claim exists in the peer-reviewed research literature.

Best-Practice Recommendations: A Critical Pathway for Developmental Examination of Infants at Risk for Developmental Disability

Based on the validated assessments available and what is known about sensitive periods of development in various domains, my own suggestions for assessing developmental progress across time during the first year after birth are summarized in the proposed critical pathway in Table 7–5. The philosophy underlying this proposed care pathway is that every assessment should be an intervention,[9, 168] that is, the family should learn something new about their child at each clinic visit and receive anticipatory guidance regarding how to facilitate their child's development, whether the child is normal or delayed.

The ages suggested for assessment are based on the views of Parmalee and associates that many problems of the high-risk neonate are transient, that some problems cannot be identified until a period of developmental time has passed, and that some parents provide an optimal environment that allows the infant to compensate for mild neurologic deviance in early infancy.[163] They believe that perinatal measures should be used to establish the initial risk, and then follow-up assessment should occur at two key points. The first point is a check on development at about 4 months of adjusted age, when potentially transient problems can be identified and prevented from becoming permanent, followed by a later check at around 8 to 9 months, when the environment has had sufficient time to provide assistance to the infant in recovery from nonoptimal perinatal events. A 1-year examination is included for further documentation of the attainment of major milestones such as walking and early language development. Later examinations will be needed to rule out more subtle types of developmental, perceptual, and psychosocial problems.

The recommended assessments are a minimal set at each age (adjusted for prematurity) but seem likely to identify problems in a variety of domains that could result in referral for further comprehensive assessment if needed. Each test may be done by any trained professional, but Table 7–5 recommends a logical individual. The final column in Table 7–5 illustrates some possible actions taken as the result of various examination outcomes; these listed actions demonstrate that the tests chosen can result in (1) prognostications of the developmental outcome, (2) a need for referral for further assessment or intervention, and (3) teaching plans to facilitate parenting and infant development. The critical pathway components also make it clear that both infant and family assessment are needed to facilitate the necessary partnership between the parent and the child that leads to optimal development.

At the first visit to a developmental follow-up clinic, preferably before 3 months

**Critical Pathway for Developmental Examination of
Infants at Risk for Developmental Disabilities**

TABLE 7–5

Age (mo)	Examination	Professional	Example Outcomes
2–5	NCAST Feeding Scale Carey Scale	Nurse	Training of parent in responsivity to infant cues
	AIMS	Physical therapist	Prediction of abnormal motor development at 18 mo if <10th percentile and referral for EI
6–9	AIMS	Physical therapist	Prediction of normal motor development at 18 mo if >4th percentile
	BINS Family Interest Survey	Psychologist or occupational therapist	Referral for Bayley II if high-risk score obtained
10–12	Bayley II: cognitive, motor, and behavior	Psychologist or occupational therapist	Normal mental or motor performance; referral for psychologic assessment because of low frustration tolerance
	NCAST Teaching Scale Family Interest Survey	Psychologist or nurse	Referral to maternal support program; teaching plan on infant cues

NCAST, Nursing Child Assessment; AIMS, Alberta Infant Motor Scale; BINS, Bayley Infant Neurodevelopmental Screener; EI, early intervention.

of corrected age, the NCAST Feeding Scale[111] is used to assess parent-infant partnership during the task of feeding. This scale assesses both the parent's and the infant's role in the interactive process, and results can be used to formulate a teaching plan for the infant or the parent, or both. The Carey temperament scale identifies infants with difficult-to-manage behavior.[165] The AIMS[104] is used at the same visit, or in another by 4 to 5 months of age, to assess gross motor development because scores below the 10th percentile at 4 months of corrected age have a high predictability for abnormal motor development at 18 months of age. In addition to its graph for plotting the percentile rank performance across time, the pictures on the AIMS form can be used as a teaching tool to help parents learn what to expect next and to encourage in their child's motor development. These three assessments together take about 40 to 50 minutes. A teaching session following the assessment takes another 15 to 30 minutes, depending on the test results. Along with a physician's assessment, this visit would take less than 2 hours.

A visit between 6 and 9 months of corrected age should again include assessment with the AIMS along with the BINS to assess cognitive and perceptual development (the HINT[148] might be substituted if further evidence of predictive validity becomes available). The BINS has moderate sensitivity (50 percent) and high specificity (88 percent) for predicting concurrent poor or normal performance on the Bayley II[44] cognitive scale at 6 months and suggests whether comprehensive assessment with the Bayley II scale is needed. Together the BINS and the AIMS take no more than 30 to 40 minutes. Clinical observation during the course of these tests would indicate whether a specific fine motor assessment might be needed. If so, the Peabody Fine Motor Scale[48] given by an occupational therapist would be a possible choice. Audiologic and visual screening is often done at about this age as well.

A visit between 10 and 12 months includes the full Bayley II, that is, motor, mental, and behavioral scales (45 to 60 minutes), followed by the NCAST Teaching Scale[111] (10 minutes). The latter involves selecting a task from the Bayley test that is just above the infant's current developmental level and asking the parent to teach the child how to do this task. The parent's teaching skills and the child's responsiveness, as well as how they partner together in working on the task, are assessed. The results can be used to develop a teaching plan when necessary.

If the Bayley test raises questions about the child's development of language, a specific referral for speech and language evaluation would be appropriate. Similarly, the Bayley test should reveal the possible need for a psychologic referral for sociobehavioral concerns. Finally, because the Bayley motor scale tests developmental milestones but does not assess the quality of movement, observed deficits in the quality of movement might lead to further assessment with the AIMS, which is likely to produce a lower score than the Bayley in the presence of abnormal postural tone. In a case of spastic diplegia, the Bayley motor scale, which includes both gross and fine motor items, may inadequately reflect different capabilities between upper and lower extremities. Again, either an AIMS or the Peabody Fine Motor Scale would help to document these concerns.

At the second and third of these visits, the Family Interest Survey[158] would be helpful to identify family concerns and the need for support or information. As with the tests mentioned earlier, the information provided by the survey can be used by social workers or therapists to formulate a teaching plan or to organize referrals to other services. Results of testing at each visit should be shared with other providers of health care, therapy, or early-childhood education with whom the family has contact, and parents should receive copies of all reports.

Although the critical pathway proposed in Table 7–5 is based on what is known about infant development, its effectiveness should be judged through a formal evaluation of how well it works in comparison with other possible clinical care algorithms. Further evaluation of the proposed plan should investigate how much it costs to (1) identify infants needing further assessment or intervention in any area of development and (2) provide education for parents to improve their knowledge of child development and responsive parenting. A formal database with defined expected outcomes would be useful for this purpose.

PROGRAM EVALUATION OF NEONATAL INTENSIVE CARE UNIT CARE AND DEVELOPMENTAL MONITORING OF HIGH-RISK INFANTS

Overall program evaluation is not commonly undertaken for service programs delivered by physical therapists, but the field would demonstrate important progress if such an analysis of therapy services in special care nurseries and developmental follow-up clinics were undertaken. An example of how to undertake such a program of evaluation of services is suggested by Wolery and Bailey based on the example of evaluation of EI programs.[169] These investigators proposed that a program evaluation include a search for answers to the following questions:

1. Does the method of service delivery represent the best educational practice?
2. Is the intervention being implemented accurately and consistently?
3. Is an attempt being made to objectively verify the effectiveness of intervention?
4. Does the program carefully monitor clients' progress and demonstrate a sensitivity to points at which changes in service need to be made?
5. Does a system exist for determining the adequacy of clients' progress and service delivery?
6. Is the program accomplishing its goals and objectives?

7. Does the service delivery system meet the needs and values of the community and clients it serves?

Addressing question 1 in the area of infant care would involve reviewing intervention programs in use against evidence in the literature on effective programs. These include the NIDCAP program and NDT for preterm infants, parenting education using materials like the Partners or Nursing Systems for Effective Parenting programs, and other models of effectively facilitating developmental progress. Implementation evaluation would address the question of whether (1) referrals are made appropriately and in a timely fashion; (2) sufficient staffing is available to address the appropriate components of a program of assessment; intervention planning and service delivery; and family education; and (3) the plan of care is actually being carried out as intended. Question 3 requires addressing whether the outcomes of the program fit with expectations suggested by the research literature and examples of other model nursery or follow-up programs. Evaluation of progress monitoring would include addressing whether outcome assessments are accomplished in a reliable, regular, and timely fashion, whether clinic no-show rates are unacceptably high (and if so, why), and whether coordination with community service providers and other professionals in the NICU is accomplished, documented, and satisfactory to all participants.

The transition from the medical center to community-based intervention and follow-up assessment is a critical point of much dissatisfaction on the part of parents, and it deserves specific attention. An aspect of evaluation of this component of effective care is surveying the satisfaction of families with the care provided and whether their goals have been identified and met. The use of a critical pathway would assist a program in documenting changes in services provided at important developmental junctures when expected progress has not been attained. Question 5 is being addressed in other areas of health care through collection of information from multiple service sites to form a large database on rehabilitation outcomes. The data can be used to compare outcomes across centers (or therapists) to explore both areas of excellence in performance and whether areas of deficiency exist.

A database can also be useful in addressing the question of whether a nursery program has met its overall goals and objectives. Beyond mortality and medical morbidity statistics, an NICU might set a goal that every family whose child leaves the nursery has demonstrated successful feeding and other physical care of their child as well as sensitive reading of and reactions to their child's approach and distress cues. Another goal might be that every EI program to whom a high-risk child has been referred would receive a copy of the child's developmental history, status, and developmental plan of care, including a summary of parental competencies demonstrated before infant discharge. The research literature documents the need for such standards of care: A study of mothers' perceptions of their NICU experience revealed that many families reported not having received information about developmental issues or the transfer of medical records.[170] A large variety of approaches could be used to assess the accomplishment of such goals. An article by Wyly and colleagues provides advice for establishing a seamless service system from family-centered intervention in the NICU through transition to community EI services.[171] Horbar and Lucey describe a four-step process for assessing and improving NICU practices, including (1) monitoring of practices, outcomes, and costs, (2) analysis of variation in practices, outcomes, and costs, (3) assessment of the efficacy of individual interventions, and (4) feedback and education to alter clinicians' behavior.[172]

Asking whether the NICU service delivery system, including follow-up for assessment of developmental progress and referral for needed services, meets the needs of families is essential to best practice in developing a user-friendly, responsive, and efficacious system. The use of the Family Interest Survey[158] can reveal over time, for instance, whether families express common needs that do not appear to be met by the service without special action. Rosenbaum and colleagues have also developed a system for documenting families' responses to developmental intervention services that reveals the critical components families find most helpful to them and their children.[173]

In today's health care arena, an additional question that must be included relates to the cost-effectiveness of the program and whether early intervention in nurseries or developmental monitoring in follow-up clinics has effects such as the prevention or diminution of disability or results in more effective use of medical and educational resources for children with disabilities over time (decreased use would be preferred but is unlikely given the overall high costs of developmental disability). One program for which costs and benefits have been documented is the NIDCAP approach. Shendell-Falik also describes a work redesign program that employs a case manager to oversee costs using an approach similar to a critical pathway in which a variety of outcomes are quantitatively assessed to improve the quality of care, costs, and satisfaction of clients and personnel.[174] Therapists need to be aware that today's definition of a case manager's role includes reducing costs, not just coordinating service delivery. In addition to knowledge of evidence-based effective interventions, of particular importance in justifying services is clearer delineation of the roles of occupational therapists and physical therapists than has heretofore been typical. Therapists must take an active role in identifying areas of overlap and areas of unique competencies.

In an EI program evaluation, Haley and colleagues showed that high parental education, the degree of motor delay of infants, and the therapists' availability contributed to explaining variations in service delivery characteristics for infants in EI.[175] Because none of these factors have been demonstrated by research to contribute to the *effectiveness* of intervention for infants with movement dysfunction, one must question the basis on which these services were planned and offered. Translating the questions described into forms appropriate for services to high-risk infants in nurseries and subsequent monitoring programs would be useful in identifying who gets services, to what effect, and with what cost. Again, NIDCAP investigators have begun this process with regard to supportive care for fragile newborns,[22, 25] pointing the way to effective means for assessing physical therapy programs as well.

ENTRY TO NEONATAL INTENSIVE CARE UNIT PRACTICE

Given the volumes of research literature, numerous potential assessment devices, and modest number of efficacious interventions available to aid the development of high-risk infants, what advice can be offered to the novice physical therapist hoping to enter neonatal practice to serve these fragile, tiny babies? The best place to start is the statement of the APTA Section on Pediatrics, which outlines the knowledge base needed for entry to the nursery.[4] Gaining the foundational knowledge suggested by the APTA guidelines should begin with reading book chapters and review articles such as those by Sweeney and Swanson,[9] Kahn-D'Angelo,[37] and Long and Soderstrom.[108] Although much of the knowledge base described in the APTA guidelines remains pertinent, other aspects of the statement are out of date, and it is currently undergoing revision. In addition to continuing to suggest that NICU services are an advanced level of practice, the committee working on revisions is considering including the following recommendations for a systematic entry to practice (Jane Sweeney, personal communication, March, 1997): (1) to first provide direct services for hospitalized children on physiologic monitoring equipment and supplemental oxygen or ventilators, (2) to conduct assessments and design and modify home intervention programs in NICU follow-up clinics, and (3) to complete precepted clinical training individualized to the neonatal population served and neonatal therapy procedures used in specific NICUs.

My personal recommendations for required skills to enable practice at the highest level include (1) NIDCAP level I training, (2) reliability in the use of Prechtl's general movement assessment, the AIMS, and a neonatal motor performance test, such as the Dubowitz or Morgan tests, or the more functionally oriented TIMP, (3) a continuing education course and supervised practice in the development of family-focused, interdisciplinary plans of care, and (4) an ability to succinctly describe (for both families and other professionals) the research literature on effective (and ineffective) methods of intervention in support of furthering engagement in evidence-based practice. Command of the literature and an ability to communicate its research findings to families in nontechnical terms,[176] including controversies regarding appropriate treatments, is one of the principles of family-centered neonatal care developed by consumers.[7] A literature review and analysis by Long and Soderstrom on positioning studies[108] is an excellent illustration of how therapists can succinctly summarize the strength of the evidence in favor of an intervention using a means for grading the levels of evidence provided by published research studies. Perhaps the two greatest needs of therapists preparing for nursery practice are skill in educating and empowering families to meet their infant's needs, and competencies in coordinating service delivery across multiple settings and disciplines.

AGENDA FOR THE FUTURE

The final section of this chapter addresses an agenda for future research. If implemented, this agenda will build on the current state of our knowledge and further the goal of enabling the evidence-based practice of physical therapy in the NICU environment and after hospital discharge for infants at high risk for motor delay in general, and CNS dysfunction in particular. A model for further research should assess the use of a decision model such as the HOAC, including (1) exploration of ways to engage parents effectively in developing goals for the care and assessment of their infants; (2) the use of valid assessments for the diagnosis of risk or developmental deviance; (3) planning for infants' care based on scientific evidence incorporated into a conceptual model for addressing impairments and functional limitations in infants that includes the best of what is known about brain plasticity and effective strategies for treatment; and (4) the use of valid and reliable assessments of outcome with tests or methods having sensitivity to change in infants whose progress may be expected to be slow. A suggested management model that addresses these four areas is presented next. Research is necessary to document the validity of the model.

Family-Focused Goal Setting

One approach to engaging parents in setting goals for their infants and for their own education in managing the problems of an infant at risk for disability who may also have numerous medical complications is the use of a systematic approach like the Canadian Occupational Performance Measure (available from Canadian Occupational Therapy Association, Caleton Technology & Training Center, Suite 3400, 1125 Colonel By Drive, Ottawa, Ontario, Canada K1S 5R1; telephone 613-523-2268; fax 613-523-2552) as a structured means to encourage parental involvement.[177] Although the specific interview questions developed for the measure are inappropriate for use in infancy, such an interview approach will lead the parents to express the concerns they have about their infant's functional movement development. The scoring system for the measure allows the parents to prioritize their concerns and, after intervention, demonstrates whether their satisfaction with the outcome of dealing with identified problems has improved.

Any effective program must include parental education, and the first assessment of the family's goals will include their personally identified knowledge needs. The Family Interest Survey can be useful in identifying these needs in a general way.[158] For parents who like to read as a means of gaining information, several useful books are available.[178–181] The use of parental support groups should also be a part of the model for empowering and supporting families.[182] Furthermore, parents can be helped to become better consumers of therapeutic services through being provided with consumer's guides, such as the *Consumer's Guide: Therapeutic Services for Children with Disabilities,* and the article on principles for family-centered neonatal care mentioned earlier.[7, 145]

Assessment

After the family's concerns and needs are identified, valid and reliable examination approaches should be used to explore the sources of the problems identified by the family and professional caregivers and to quantify functional performance. The general movement assessment assists in identifying poverty of movement and other abnormalities, such as the presence of cramped synchrony.[89] The latter problem should generate an immediate plan for treatment, despite the possibility that cramped synchrony may in a minority of cases resolve, because of the assessment's demonstrated sensitivity for predicting CP. The infant's capability to regulate state and behavior in the face of handling is observed with the NIDCAP assessment, and this procedure can also be used as the basis of an educational program for teaching the family about the infant's cues and how to read and respond to them.[22, 25] Finally, the TIMP provides a sensitive means of assessing postural and selective control of movement that the infant will need for functional activities, such as interacting with caregivers, changing positions, activating the motor ensemble to engage with environmental objects and events, and expressing displeasure through movement (e.g., attempting to remove a cloth placed over the eyes).[102] Scores in the far below average range (see Table 7–4) should generate a plan for intervention to promote functional motor development; timing of treatment initiation and its frequency and intensity should be based on NIDCAP assessment results indicating the infant's readiness to engage in movement therapy.

Intervention in a Task-Oriented Context

The strategy for intervention I would suggest is one incorporating the best of NDT; family-centered intervention as described by Law and colleagues[183] and based on the principles stated by consumers;[7, 184] Horn and colleague's approach to developing treatment objectives based on existing impairments, desired functional changes, and an expected generalization of learning;[142] Shumway-Cook and Woollacott's task-oriented approach to infant postural assessment[185] and intervention; and general exercise and motor learning principles incorporating the concept of overload, or the "just-right" challenge. Intervention planning for infants must incorporate current knowledge of brain development and plasticity, as well as recognition of Als' synactive model of infant systems development and integration.[94]

Analysis of Impairments and Functional Limitations in Light of Motor Development and Motor Control Theory

The typical newborn infant with a brain insult has poverty of movement, pronounced asymmetry of posture, and synchronized spontaneous movements rather than the elegant sequences characterizing normal writhing movement. A monotonous quality may be present, that is, movements tend always to begin with activation of the same body segment. Movement ranges used are often small, tending to be limited to flexion and extension without rotation, and movement is characterized by weakness, or in the extreme, by stiffness or hypotonicity. Actions in a task context are also impaired. For example, the ability to rotate the head and eyes to follow visual stimuli or search for interesting sounds is limited or impossible, and attempts to orient to environmental stimuli often result in movement reversal after a short progression in the desired direction, as if a resistance were encountered.

In the past, we believed that brain maturation drove the development of mature posture and movement patterns and that postural, that is, proximal, control preceded the capacity to engage in functional tasks. Thelen's work helped us to understand that the human infant is a self-organizing being and that multiple systems interact to create the actions of the motor ensemble, that is, the muscles, joints, neuronal components, and cognitive-emotional aspects of movement.[186] Self-organization, furthermore, occurs in a task context that also contributes to shaping the movements used to accomplish a purposeful action. Rather than brain development shaping movement, we can now consider that the primary repertoire of actions with which the infant is born is used by the baby to drive brain development. Research has clearly shown that the sensorimotor areas of the brain reorganize in response to lesions,[187] either central or peripheral, but also in response to specific practice.[188] The use of the motor ensemble is best thought of as engendering the sensory inputs that shape the organization of the sensorimotor cortex and other brain regions, thus linking action with perception through movement. Note that this differs from a therapeutic concept in which sensory inputs are used to evoke motor responses; in fact, the idea is quite the opposite.

A newborn's primary repertoire of actions includes orienting the eyes toward light; following moving objects with the eyes and projecting the arm toward them; orienting the head and eyes toward appealing sounds; seeking the hand or nipple with the mouth; sucking; tucking the body parts in for comfort; and kicking. Postural realignment of body parts occurs when muscles are stretched by the force of gravity and body weight (head and trunk righting reactions), or by segmental rotations, such as head turning. Infants also have the capacity to inhibit movement when attending to interesting visual or auditory inputs.

A serious constraint on movement is the weight of the infant's head relative to the mass of the rest of the body and the strength of muscles.[189] Anticipatory postural organization is also lacking in the newborn; hence movements occur without preparation for the internal reactive forces that will be generated by muscles acting on the bony levers. One of the few consistently used functional synergies is the "suck posture" with elbows flexed, arms tightly adducted, and legs extended.

Law and coworkers suggest that treatment goals should reflect actions for which the infant demonstrates readiness.[183] Shumway-Cook and Woollacott would then suggest a search for constraints on action.[185] A place to begin, therefore, is an analysis of how well an infant's primary repertoire matches that of a developmentally well-organized infant of a similar age. This analysis includes (1) an assessment of what actions the infant appears to be attempting, both with and without success (visual following, sucking, mouth-to-hand movement, and so forth), (2) a search for the constraints that hinder the successful accomplishment of actions (e.g., a failure to stop sucking to breathe and swallow; an inability to maintain the head centered with respect to the trunk midline to look at an interesting object; contact of the mouth with the hand but an inability to sustain the position), and (3) the development of hypotheses regarding sources of constraints and how to remove them (provide partial assistance to movement that lacks strength; impose a pause in sucking to allow a breathing break by removing the nipple periodically; change the position or the environment to make the task easier; aid positioning of body parts removed from the primary area of active movement to provide a point of stability; and so forth). Whatever the choice of intervention strategy, for example, NDT or parental education in responsiveness to the infant's cues, the aim must always be to aid the infant's spontaneously generated actions, that is, to avoid as much as possible imposed or passive movements. Brain development (and motor control and learning) will be aided by activities that occur in interaction with a developmentally appropriate environmental event (e.g., the mother's voice near the infant's ear) or self-generated action from the infant's primary repertoire (e.g., visually scanning an object in the crib, looking at the hand while assuming a fencing posture). We next consider a theory of brain plasticity and development that is a useful conceptual framework for considering intervention to promote motor and brain development.

Conceptual Framework Based on Brain Plasticity and Development*

Historically, proposed theoretic mechanisms for the development of motor control in humans involved the search for an explanation for the production of efficiently generated movement.[190] It is well known that the human motor system shows adaptability and flexibility in the presence of continually changing environmental tasks and throughout an individual's life span in response to changing biomechanical parameters, such as growth. The predominant question appears to be how the CNS works in conjunction

*I thank the graduate students in PT 462 at the University of Illinois at Chicago who assisted in developing the summary of the theory of neuronal group selection: Michael Hirsh, Kathy Kriemelmeyer, Pai-jun Mao, Phyllis Rowland, and Sharon Thompson.

with the peripheral musculoskeletal system to constrain the excessive degrees of freedom inherent in the developing and evolving organism. Several theories that were originally proposed to explain motor control have poor explanatory power as a result of their reliance on control mechanisms and feedback loops that do not allow for "instantaneous adaptability of the motor ensemble and its associated circuitry in response to biomechanical and environmental changes."[190, (p 978)] Edelman's theory of neuronal group selection is based on scientific knowledge of anatomy and function of the brain and attempts to overcome the weaknesses of other theories.[191]

Theory of Neuronal Group Selection

The theory of neuronal group selection is a comprehensive conceptualization of brain development and function that emphasizes the plasticity of the nervous system throughout life. As such, it provides a conceptual framework for considering the ability of physical therapists to improve movement function through the application of its principles. Neuronal group selection theory has three basic tenets.[191] These tenets describe how (1) the anatomy of the brain is produced during development, (2) experience selects for strengthening certain patterns of responses from the available anatomic structures, and (3) the resulting maps of the brain give rise to uniquely individual behavioral functions through a process called *reentry* that leads to formation of global maps. Global maps encompass many regions of the nervous system in organizing the response of the motor ensemble to environmental demands.

Tenet 1

The first tenet of Edelman's theory is concerned with developmental selection by which the characteristic neuroanatomy of a species is formed. The genetic code and the local operation of specific molecules establish the borders of different neuronal areas in the brain whose connections are not preprogrammed. The neural cells compete to make connections. Because of the competition and the interaction of neural elements, diversity comes about as a result of the dynamic way in which the brain is formed. Consequently, each individual has a unique brain that nevertheless is generally characteristic of its species. This neural development, along with the somatic development of muscles and joints, provides the infant with a primary repertoire of species-specific behavior. In humans, as mentioned previously, these behaviors include kicking, visual orientation to interesting sounds, and the projection of the hand toward moving objects. The ability of the newborn to engage in these types of behaviors makes it clear that regions of the brain devoted to vision and audition are, even from birth, connected with areas related to movement organization through reciprocal projections from area to area.

The behaviors of the primary movement repertoire are produced through activation of the neuronal groups that were formed by the developmental processes of cell production, migration, and death. The process by which the primary repertoire is formed does not appear to rely on experience from the environment (for example, movement in the fetus is possible before sensory afferents make synapses in the spinal cord) and is generally complete by birth. Each neuronal group receives overlapping inputs from a wide variety of afferent sources that are initially somewhat undifferentiated although limited in functional potential. The neuronal group, each consisting of hundreds to thousands of strongly interconnected neurons, is considered to be the basic functional unit of the nervous system; neuronal groups are arranged in neural maps in segregated areas of the brain. There are long-range reciprocal connections between groups that integrate activities of multiple sensory and motor areas of the brain in a process known as reentry.

Tenet 2

The second tenet of Edelman's theory proposes that through the experience of moving and thereby activating sensory receptors, a secondary repertoire of functional circuits is carved out from the many pathways of neural connections, that is, neuronal groups, available to the organism. As experience moving in the environment occurs, the preexisting neuronal groups that receive input become more strongly interconnected through the enhancement of synaptic efficacy. The developing infant's movement experiences in the context of given tasks, environments, and biomechanical factors function to competitively "select" neuronal groups that meet motor requirements efficiently. Circuit selection is dependent on enhancing adaptive or goal-directed movements. Afferent somatosensory neurons exhibit degeneracy, meaning that single neuronal groups react to many receptive fields and vice versa, through the spreading of their respective axonal and dendritic trees. Neuronal groups are selected by various inputs through temporally correlated stimulation. Because infants demonstrate very poor organization of postural responses in early infancy, part of the formation of a secondary repertoire must include the strengthening of synaptic connections that organize posture for anticipating the internal forces created by the activation of muscles, as well as anticipating the need for particular force, velocity, and patterns of muscle activation needed to accomplish intended tasks within an environmental context. Thus posture comes to be inextricably linked with movement and sensations in order to create efficient and effective actions while maintaining stability of the body in space. The selection process creates favored functional synergies, or strategies for performing the movements associated with desired actions, from among the many combinations that could be effective. The development of synergies is believed to be the means by which the nervous system solves the problem of redundant degrees of freedom in the motor ensemble; thus synergies are the fundamental units of movement.

Less frequently selected circuits continue to exist with the probability that they may be used if changes in the task, environment, or peripheral musculoskeletal system enhance their effectiveness in meeting the infant's adaptive needs. The neural connections are available in the brain; whether they are easily accessed (or selected) depends on whether their synapses are strengthened during a sensitive period of development. Nevertheless, the fine tuning of secondary repertoires continues throughout an individual's life, maintaining plasticity within the nervous system in response to changing internal and external requirements of adaptive responses. As a result, many circuits are available for selection even in the event of a brain lesion or musculoskeletal injury.

Tenet 3

Edelman's third tenet describes how the first two selectional processes interact to form neural maps. These maps connect vast areas of the nervous system such that perception, cognition, emotion, and movement control are interconnected in the organization of spontaneously emitted movements, or movements in response to the environment. The maps are formed by massively parallel and reciprocal connections because the brain is a distributed system, that is, the various characteristics of an object or a movement are represented in different parts of the nervous system. For example, moving edges have a characteristic representation in visual regions, as does color. Directional control may take place in different neuronal groups or parts of the nervous system than force production through the selective recruitment of motor units. In order to create a functional movement, that is, one that will achieve the task goal while maintaining the stability of the body as a whole, selection occurs over neuronal groups from various maps throughout particular regions of the brain and the nervous system as a whole.

The combination of neuronal groups from selected multiple maps of an area's function allows the production of a movement that is precisely tuned to the environmental demands for functional performance yet unique to the individual's capacity for receiving sensory inputs and for combining selections of neuronal groups from his or her individual regional maps. For example, a reach-and-grasp action might include selections from the hand motor area of primary cerebral motor-sensory cortex combined with selections from maps that are concerned with the receipt of visual and tactile information and ones concerned with the postural function of the neck and shoulder. As a result of the selectional process from many possible movement synergies, individuals demonstrate unique yet similar strategies for accomplishing common tasks. Because of constraints on function created by our unique structure, the movements performed by different individuals to accomplish a particular task have a characteristic appearance we can identify as human. Nevertheless, we can recognize someone's walking pattern as unique to that individual even though the basic characteristics of human gait are universal.

Edelman's theory of neuronal group selection differs from other theories in that (1) no motor programs are proposed to exist (selection from distributed maps occurs anew with each movement but more efficiently with experience), (2) the stimulus-response approach to understanding movement is turned on its head because movement is considered to be the stimulus for the activation of feature detectors (sensory receptors) leading to the creation of sensorimotor maps based on correlated activation of multiple parallel pathways, and (3) comparison of the brain to a computer is inappropriate because the nervous system is not hard-wired; neither must complex calculations be postulated for solving the redundant degrees-of-freedom problem.

Applications of Neuronal Group Selection Theory to Physical Therapy

Edelman's theory suggests the following for physical therapy: (1) repeated experience is necessary to create functional mappings that can be easily accessed for motor performance; (2) movement is the means of generating the activation of sensory receptors; (3) correlated activation of feature detectors is critical for creating movement patterns that are responsive to internal reactive forces, the requirements of stability of the body, and environmental demands; (4) active, self-generated movement is essential to improving motor coordination, accuracy, and the ability to generalize function to a variety of task and environmental demands; and (5) a variety of functional movement synergies could be used by an infant to accomplish a task demand, that is, no one right way to move exists.

Because infants with brain damage have a limited primary repertoire, finding a treatment strategy that increases movement generally and broadens the repertoire of available functional actions is essential. These infants otherwise develop a limited set of movement synergies that are applied to virtually all tasks. Their repeated use strengthens these synergies that may have been functional in supine or prone positions but can hinder progress in upright positions and lead to contractures. An NIDCAP assessment allows the therapist to assess the infant's physiologic and behavioral readiness for movement therapy. The TIMP provides a means of identifying the infant's (1) primary repertoire, (2) available postural control strategies, and (3) readiness for various functional movements. Analysis of constraints to function should lead to hypotheses regarding why task performance is compromised.

Both infants with CP and infants with Down syndrome have atypical movement. For example, Ulrich and Ulrich showed that infants with Down syndrome kick less than infants with normal development and the frequency of kicking was related to the age of walking.[192] A strategy for increasing activity in children with poverty of movement might be hydrotherapy in which the buoyancy of the water helps to relieve constraints caused by weakness as well as calming the irritable infant.[193] However active movement is achieved, extensive repetition is necessary for strengthening the appropriate connections among neural maps. Finally, another correlate of successful motor learning is attention to the task. Being active involves not just moving actively but also actively processing the elements of the activity.[194]

Employing an NDT strategy with infants means working to obtain postural stability in midline alignment with flexion of limbs and trunk in the supine position, followed by active movement away from this centered position with small, at first, then increasingly larger weight shifts of the trunk the infant must accommodate. The therapist's handling provides for correlated input from tactile, joint, and muscle receptors during guided movement. The use of toys, sounds, or a moving face provides further correlated inputs that should be helpful in forming global maps of useful movement synergies in a task context. Whenever possible, however, the therapist should follow the infant's self-generated movements rather than passively impose activity, and a variety of movement options should be practiced.

Outcome Assessment

Assessing outcomes effectively could use the approach of Horn and colleagues to evaluating the generalization of skills,[142] a need she identified after reviewing weaknesses in pediatric rehabilitation approaches for children with CP.[195] When goals for movement have been identified, specific tasks to which generalization should occur are targeted for observation. This approach ensures that goals are meaningful for daily life performance. A test such as the TIMP can also be used to document changes in functional motor performance. Outcomes related to the prevention of contractures and deformity and of the need for surgery or assistive technology must be assessed.

Ultimately, however, a means must be found to document the effects of physical therapy on parents, because family education has been shown to be so effective in promoting infant development, at least in the cognitive dimension. NCAST assessments document parental responsivity to infant cues and the use of cognitive growth-promoting strategies by parents.[111] Such an assessment approach could perhaps be modified to monitor parents' encouragement of movement activities for their infants. Some means for evaluating parents' comfort with handling their infant's needs, promoting optimal development, and advocating for their children is also needed. Such achievements are most likely to result in reduced costs of care over the long-term course of chronic disability and, as such, they are important outcomes to measure.

In summary, a research agenda for the future entails (1) documenting how best to establish goals for therapy in infancy; (2) developing new therapeutic strategies and tactics based on current knowledge of motor control and infant development, impairments and functional limitations of infants with brain damage, and brain development and plasticity; and (3) developing sensitive methods for documenting effects and costs of intervention for infants and parents. The ultimate goal is to find an answer to the question of whether early intervention can reduce the effects of prenatal or perinatal brain damage enough to justify the costs to both families and the health care system.

REFERENCES

1. Collin MF, Halsey CL, Anderson CL: Emerging developmental sequelae in the "normal" extremely low birth weight infant. Pediatrics 88:115, 1991.
2. Kraybill EN, Kennedy CA, Teplin SW, Campbell SK: Survival, growth, and development of infants with birthweight less than 1001 grams. Am J Dis Child 138:837, 1984.
3. Saigal S, Szatmari P, Rosenbaum P, et al: Cognitive abilities and school performance of extremely low birthweight children and matched control children at age 8 years. A regional study. J Pediatr 118:751, 1991.
4. Scull S, Deitz J: Competencies for the physical therapist in the neonatal intensive care unit (NICU). Pediatr Phys Ther 1:11, 1989.
5. APTA Task Force on Early Intervention, Section on Pediatrics: Competencies for physical therapists in early intervention. Pediatr Phys Ther 33:77, 1991.
6. Phillips WE, Spotts ML: Medicolegal issues in the United States. *In* Campbell SK, Vander Linden DW, Palisano RJ (eds): Physical Therapy for Children. WB Saunders, Philadelphia, 1994, p 895.
7. Harrison H: The principles for family-centered neonatal care. Pediatrics 92:643, 1993.
8. Ignatavicius DD, Hausman KA: Use of clinical pathways in a variety of health care settings. *In* Clinical Pathways for Collaborative Practice. WB Saunders, Philadelphia, 1995, p 34.
9. Sweeney JK, Swanson MW: At-risk neonates and infants. NICU management and follow-up. *In* Umphred DA (ed): Neurological Rehabilitation. CV Mosby, St Louis, 1990, p 183.
10. Rapport MJK: A descriptive analysis of the role of physical and occupational therapists in the neonatal intensive care unit. Pediatr Phys Ther 4:172, 1992.
11. The Neonatal Intensive Care Unit Task Force: Knowledge and skills for occupational therapy practice in the neonatal intensive care unit. Am J Occup Ther 47:1100, 1993.

12. Gilkerson L: Understanding institutional functioning style: A resource for hospital and early intervention collaboration. Inf Young Child 2(3):22, 1990.
13. Campbell SK: Organizational and educational considerations in creating an environment to promote optimal development of high-risk neonates. *In* Sweeney JK (ed): The High-Risk Neonate: Developmental Therapy Perspectives. Haworth, New York, 1986, p 191.
14. McGrath JM, Valenzuela G: Integrating developmentally supportive caregiving into practice through education. J Perinat Neonat Nurs 8:46, 1994.
15. Rothstein JM, Echternach JL: Hypothesis-Oriented Algorithm for Clinicians: A method for evaluation and treatment planning. Phys Ther 66:1388, 1986.
16. Campbell SK: Effects of developmental intervention in the special care nursery. *In* Wolraich M, Routh DK (eds): Advances in Developmental and Behavioral Pediatrics, vol. 4. JAI, Greenwich, Conn, 1983, p 165.
17. Long JG, Philip AGS, Lucey JF: Excessive handling as a cause of hypoxemia. Pediatrics 65:203, 1980.
18. Gottfried AW, Gaiter JL (eds): Infant Stress Under Intensive Care. University Park, Baltimore, 1985.
19. Sweeney JK: Assessment of the special care nursery environment: Effects on the high-risk infant. *In* Wilhelm IJ (ed): Physical Therapy Assessment in Early Infancy. Churchill Livingstone, New York, 1994, p 13.
20. Kelly MK, Palisano RJ, Wolfson MR: Effects of a developmental physical therapy program on oxygen saturation and heart rate in preterm infants. Phys Ther 69:467, 1989.
21. Avery GB, Glass P: The gentle nursery: Developmental intervention in the NICU. J Perinatol 9:204, 1989.
22. Als H: A synactive model of neonatal behavioral organization: Framework for the assessment of neurobehavioral development in the premature infant and for support of infants and parents in the neonatal intensive care environment. *In* Sweeney JK (ed): The High-Risk Neonate: Developmental Therapy Perspectives. Haworth, New York, 1986, p 3.
23. Bennett FC, Guralnick MJ: Effectiveness of developmental intervention in the first five years of life. Pediatr Clin North Am 38:1513, 1991.
24. Miller CL, White R, Whitman TL, et al: The effects of cycled versus noncycled lighting on growth and development in preterm infants. Inf Behav Dev 18:87, 1995.
25. Als H, Lawhon G, Duffy FH, et al: Individualized developmental care for the very low-birth-weight preterm infants. JAMA 272:853, 1994.
26. Als H, Lawhon G, Brown E, et al: Individualized behavioral and environmental care for the very low birth weight preterm infant at high risk for bronchopulmonary dysplasia: Neonatal intensive care unit and developmental outcome. Pediatrics 78:1123, 1986.
27. Als H: Developmental Care Implementation in a Newborn Intensive Care Unit (NICU): Overview of Training Process, Budget Projections, and Cost-Benefit Analysis. National NIDCAP Training Center, Children's Hospital, Boston, 1995.
28. Ariago RL, Thoman EB, Boeddicker MA, et al: Developmental care does not alter sleep and development of premature infants. Pediatrics 100(6):e9, 1997; also available at http://www.pediatrics.org/cgi/content/full/100/6/e9.
29. Lawhon g: Management of stress in premature infants. *In* Angelini PJ, Whales Knopp CE, Gibes RM (eds): Perinatal Neonatal Nursing: A Clinical Handbook. Blackwell Scientific, Boston, 1984, p 319.
30. Als H, Gilkerson L: Developmentally supportive care in the neonatal intensive care unit. Zero to Three 15(6):1, 1995.
31. Als H: Program Guide: Newborn Individualized Developmental Care and Asessment Program (NIDCAP)—An Education and Training Program for Health Care Professionals. National NIDCAP Training Center, Children's Hospital, Boston, 1995.
32. Phelan JP (ed): Prevention of Prematurity. Clin Perinatol 19:(2), 1992.
33. Dammann O, Leviton A: Does prepregnancy bacterial vaginosis increase a mother's risk of having a preterm infant with cerebral palsy? Dev Med Child Neurol 39:836, 1997.
34. Abdel-Rahman AM, Rosenberg AA: Prevention of intraventricular hemorrhage in the premature infant. Clin Perinatol 21:(3)505, 1994.
35. Plamer C, Vannucci RC: Potential new therapies for perinatal cerebral hypoxia-ischemia. Clin Perinatol 20:(2)411, 1993.
36. Long W (ed): Surfactant Replacement Therapy. Clinics in Perinatology, vol 20, no 4. WB Saunders, Philadelphia, 1993.
37. Kahn-D'Angelo L: The special care nursery. *In* Campbell SK, Vander Linden DW, Palisano RJ (eds): Physical Therapy for Children. WB Saunders, Philadelphia, 1994, p 787.
38. Piper MC, Mazer B, Silver KM, Ramsay M: Resolution of neurological symptoms in high-risk infants during the first two years of life. Dev Med Child Neurol 30:26, 1988.

39. Kitchen WH, Doyle LW, Ford GW, et al: Cerebral palsy in very low birthweight infants surviving to 2 years with modern perinatal intensive care. Am J Perinatol 4:29, 1987.

40. Paneth N: The causes of cerebral palsy. Recent evidence. Clin Invest Med 16:9, 1993.

41. McCormick MC, McCarton C, Tonascia J, Brooks-Gunn J: Early educational intervention for very low birth weight infants: Results from the Infant Health and Development Program. J Pediatr 123:527, 1993.

42. Bayley N: The Bayley Scales of Infant Development. Psychological Corporation, New York, 1969.

43. Campbell SK, Siegel E, Parr CA, Ramey CT: Evidence for the need to renorm the Bayley Scales of Infant Development based on the performance of a population-based sample of twelve-month-old infants. Top Early Child Spec Ed 6:83, 1986.

44. Bayley N: Bayley II. Psychological Corporation, San Antonio, 1993.

45. Goldstein DJ, Fogle EE, Wieber JL, Oshea TM: Comparison of the Bayley Scales of Infant Development, Second Edition and the Bayley Scales of Infant Development with premature infants. J Psychoed Assess 13:391, 1995.

46. Piper MC, Kunos VI, Willis DM, et al: Early physical therapy effects on the high risk infant: A controlled trial. Pediatrics 78:216, 1986.

47. Case-Smith J: Postural and fine motor control in preterm infants in the first six months. Phys Occup Ther Pediatr 13(1):1, 1993.

48. Folio M, Fewell R: Peabody Developmental Motor Scales and Activity Cards. DLM Teaching Resources, Allen, Tex, 1983.

49. Churcher E, Egan M, Walop W, et al: Fine motor development of high-risk infants at 3, 6, 12 and 24 months. Phys Occup Ther Pediatr 13(1):19, 1993.

50. Ross G: Use of the Bayley Scales to characterize abilities of premature infants. Child Dev 56:835, 1985.

51. Vohr BR, Coll CG, Lobato D, et al: Neurodevelopmental and medical status of low-birthweight survivors of bronchopulmonary dysplasia at 10 to 12 years of age. Dev Med Child Neurol 33:690, 1991.

52. Sostek AM, Smith YF, Katz KS, Grant EG: Developmental outcome of preterm infants with intraventricular hemorrhage at one and two years of age. Child Dev 58:779, 1987.

53. Robertson CMT, Hrynchyshyn GJ, Etches PC, Pain KS: Population-based study of the incidence, complexity, and severity of neurologic disability among survivors weighing 500 through 1250 grams at birth: A comparison of 2 birth cohorts. Pediatrics 90:750, 1992.

54. Leviton A, Paneth N: White matter damage in preterm newborns—an epidemiologic perspective. Early Hum Dev 24:1, 1990.

55. Papile L, Munsick-Bruno G, Schaefer A: Relationship of cerebral intraventricular hemorrhage and early childhood neurologic handicaps. J Pediatr 103:273, 1983.

56. Sinha SK, D'Souza SW, Rivlin E, et al: Ischaemic brain lesions diagnosed at birth in preterm infants: Clinical events and developmental outcome. Arch Dis Child 65:1017, 1990.

57. Low JA: Relationship of fetal asphyxia to neuropathology and deficits in children. Clin Invest Med 16:133, 1993.

58. Nelson KB, Emery ES III: Birth asphyxia and the neonatal brain: What do we know and when do we know it? Clin Perinatol 20:(2)327, 1993.

59. Carter BS, Haverkamp AD, Merenstein GB: The definition of acute perinatal asphyxia. Clin Perinatol 20:(2)287, 1993.

60. American Academy of Pediatrics, American College of Obstetricians and Gynecologists: Relationship between perinatal factors and neurologic outcome. *In* Poland RL, Freeman RK (eds): Guidelines for Perinatal Care, 3rd ed. American Academy of Pediatrics, Elk Grove Village, Ill, 1992, p 221.

61. Stark JE, Seibert JJ: Cerebral artery Doppler ultrasonography for prediction of outcome after perinatal asphyxia. J Ultrasound Med 13:595, 1994.

62. Barkovich AJ, Westmark K, Partridge C, et al: Perinatal asphyxia: MR findings in the first 10 days. Am J Neuroradiol 16:427, 1995.

63. Rademakers RP, van der Knaap MS, Verbeeten B Jr, et al: Central cortico-subcortical involvement: A distinct pattern of brain damage caused by perinatal and postnatal asphyxia in term infants. J Comput Assist Tomogr 19:256, 1995.

64. Penrice J, Cady EB, Lorek A, et al: Proton magnetic resonance spectroscopy of the brain in normal preterm and term infants, and early changes after perinatal hypoxia-ischemia. Pediatr Res 40:6, 1996.

65. Ellenberg JH, Nelson KB: Cluster of perinatal events identifying infants at high risk for death or disability. J Pediatr 113:546, 1988.

66. Amiel-Tison C, Ellison P: Birth asphyxia in the fullterm newborn: Early assessment and outcome. Dev Med Child Neurol 28:671, 1986.

67. Martin-Ancel A, Garcia-Alix A, Gaya F, et al: Multiple organ involvement in perinatal asphyxia. J Pediatr 127:786, 1995.
68. Luchi JM, Bennett FC, Jackson JC: Predictors of neurodevelopmental outcome following bronchopulmonary dysplasia. Am J Dis Child 145:813, 1991.
69. Winterbourn CC: Free radicals, oxidants and antioxidants. *In* Gluckman PD, Heymann MA: Pediatrics and Perinatology. The Scientific Basis, 2nd ed. Oxford University Press, New York, 1996, p 168.
70. Skidmore MD, Rivers A, Hack M: Increased risk of cerebral palsy among very low-birthweight infants with chronic lung disease. Dev Med Child Neurol 32:325, 1990.
71. Singer L, Yamashita T, Lilien L, et al: A longitudinal study of developmental outcome of infants with bronchopulmonary dysplasia and very low birth weight. Pediatrics 100:987, 1997.
72. Teberg AJ, Pena I, Finello K, et al: Prediction of neurodevelopmental outcome in infants with and without bronchopulmonary dysplasia. Am J Med Sci 301:369, 1991.
73. Piekkala P, Kero P, Sillanpaa M, Erkkola R: Growth and development of infants surviving respiratory distress syndrome: A 2-year follow-up. Pediatrics 79:529, 1987.
74. Robertson CMT, Etches PC, Goldson E, et al: Eight-year school performance, neurodevelopmental, and growth outcome of neonates with bronchopulmonary dysplasia: A comparative study. Pediatrics 89:365, 1992.
75. Karmel-Ross K (ed): Torticollis: Differential Diagnosis, Assessment and Treatment, Surgical Management and Bracing. Haworth, New York, 1997.
76. Campbell SK, Vander Linden DW, Palisano RJ (eds): Physical Therapy for Children. WB Saunders, Philadelphia, 1994.
77. Parker S, Greer S, Zuckerman B: Double jeopardy: The impact of poverty on early child development. Pediatr Clin North Am 35:1227, 1988.
78. Aylward GP: Perinatal asphyxia: Effects of biologic and environmental risks. Clin Perinatol 20:(2)433, 1993.
79. Brooks-Gunn J, Liaw F-r, Klebanov PK: Effects of early intervention on cognitive function of low birth weight preterm infants. J Pediatr 120:350, 1992.
80. Fetters L, Tronick EZ: Neuromotor development of cocaine-exposed and control infants from birth through 15 months: Poor and poorer performance. Pediatrics 98:938, 1996.
81. Arendt RE, Minnes S, Singer LT: Fetal cocaine exposure: Neurologic effects and sensory-motor delays. Phys Occup Ther Pediatr 16(1/2):129, 1996.
82. Forrest DC: The cocaine-exposed infant. Part II: intervention and teaching. J Pediatr Health Care 8:7, 1994.
83. Swanson MW: Neuromotor outcome of infants exposed prenatally to cocaine: Issues of assessment and interpretation. Phys Occup Ther Pediatr 16(1/2):35, 1996.
84. Piper MC: Theoretical foundations for physical therapy assessment in early infancy. *In* Wilhelm IJ (ed): Physical Therapy Assessment in Early Infancy. Churchill Livingstone, New York, 1993, p 1.
85. Nelson K, Ellenberg JH: Children who "outgrew" cerebral palsy. Pediatrics 69:529, 1982.
86. Allen MC, Alexander GR: Using gross motor milestones to identify very preterm infants at risk for cerebral palsy. Dev Med Child Neurol 34:226, 1992.
87. Ferrari F, Cioni G, Prechtl HFR: Qualitative changes of general movements in preterm infants with brain lesions. Early Hum Dev 23:193, 1990.
88. Sweeney JK: Physiologic adaptation of neonates to neurological assessment. Phys Occup Ther Pediatr 6(3/4):155, 1986.
89. Prechtl HFR, Einspieler C, Cioni G, et al: An early marker for neurological deficits after perinatal brain lesions. Lancet 349:1361, 1997.
90. Hadders-Algra M: The assessment of General Movements is a valuable technique for the detection of brain dysfunction in young infants. A review. Acta Paediatr Suppl 416:39, 1996.
91. Cioni G, Prechtl HFR: Preterm and early postterm motor behaviour in low-risk premature infants. Early Hum Dev 23:159, 1990.
92. Als H, Lester BM, Tronick E, et al: Toward a research instrument for the Assessment of Preterm Infant's Behavior (APIB). *In* Fitzgerald HE, Lester BM, Yogman MW (eds.): Theory and Research in Behavioral Pediatrics, vol 1. Plenum, New York, 1982, p 35.
93. Brazelton TB: Neonatal Behavioral Assessment Scale, 2nd ed. Clinics in Developmental Medicine No. 88. JB Lippincott, Philadelphia, 1984.
94. Als H, Duffy FH, McAnulty GB, Badian N: Continuity of neurobehavioral functioning in preterm and full-term newborns. *In* Bornstein MH, Krasnegor NA (eds): Stability and Continuity in Mental Development. Lawrence Erlbaum, Hillsdale, NJ, 1989, p 3.
95. Dubowitz L, Dubowitz V: The Neurological Assessment of the Preterm and Full-Term

Newborn Infant. Clinics in Developmental Medicine No. 12. JB Lippincott, Philadelphia, 1981.

96. Dubowitz LMS, Dubowitz V, Palmer PG, et al: Correlation of neurologic assessment in the preterm newborn infant with outcome at 1 year. J Pediatr 105:452, 1984.

97. Eyler FD, Delgado-Hachey M, Woods NS: Quantification of the Dubowitz neurological assessment of preterm neonates—developmental outcome. Inf Behav Dev 14:451, 1991.

98. Molteno C, Grosz P, Wallace P, Jones M: Neurological examination of the preterm and full-term infant at risk for developmental disabilities using the Dubowitz Neurological Assessment. Early Hum Dev 41:167, 1995.

99. Morgan AM, Koch V, Lee V, Aldag J: Neonatal Neurobehavioral Examination: A new instrument for quantitative analysis of neonatal neurological status. Phys Ther 68:1352, 1988.

100. Korner AF, Constantinou J, Dimiceli S, et al: Establishing the reliability and developmental validity of a neurobehavioral assessment for preterm infants: A methodological process. Child Dev 62:1200, 1991.

101. Campbell SK, Osten E, Kolobe THA, Fisher A: Development of the Test of Infant Motor Performance. Phys Med Rehabil Clin North Am 4:541, 1993.

102. Campbell SK, Kolobe THA, Osten ET, et al: Construct validity of the Test of Infant Motor Performance. Phys Ther 75:585, 1995.

103. Murney ME, Campbell SK: The ecological relevance of the Test of Infant Motor Performance Elicited Scale items. Phys Ther 78:479, 1998.

104. Piper MC, Darrah J: Motor Assessment of the Developing Infant. WB Saunders, Philadelphia, 1994.

105. Gunn A, Edwards AD: Central nervous system response to injury. *In* Gluckman PD, Heymann MA (eds): Pediatrics and Perinatology: The Scientific Basis, 2nd ed. Oxford University Press, New York, 1996, p 443.

106. Girolami GL, Campbell SK: The efficacy of a neuro-developmental treatment program for improving motor control in preterm infants. Pediatr Phys Ther 6:175, 1994.

107. Darrah J, Piper M, Byrne P, Watt MJ: The use of waterbeds for very low-birthweight infants: Effects on neuromotor development. Dev Med Child Neurol 36:989, 1994.

108. Long T, Soderstrom E: A critical appraisal of positioning infants in the neonatal intensive care unit. Phys Occup Ther Pediatr 15(3):17, 1995.

109. Nugent K: Using the Neonatal Behavioral Assessment Scale With Infants and Their Families. March of Dimes Birth Defects Foundation, White Plains, NY, 1985.

110. Brazelton TB: A window on the newborn's world: More than two decades of experience with the Neonatal Behavioral Assessment Scale. *In* Meisels SJ, Fenichel E (eds): New Visions for the Developmental Assessment of Infants and Young Children. ZERO TO THREE: National Center for Infants, Toddlers, and Families, Washington, DC, 1996, p 127.

111. Barnard K: Nursing Child Assessment Scales. University of Washington, Seattle n.d.

112. Dodds-Azzopardi SE, Chapman JS: Parents' perceptions of stress associated with premature infant transfer among hospital environments. J Perinat Neonat Nurs 8:39, 1995.

113. Leib SA, Benfield DG, Guidubaldi J: Effects of early intervention and stimulation on the preterm infant. Pediatrics 6:83, 1980.

114. Powell LF: The effect of extra stimulation and maternal involvement on the development of low-birth-weight infants and on maternal behavior. Child Dev 45:106, 1974.

115. Neal MV: Organizational behavior of the premature infant. Birth Defects 15:43, 1979.

116. Scarr-Salapatek S, Williams ML: The effects of early stimulation of low-birth-weight infants. Child Dev 44:94, 1973.

117. Brown JV, LaRossa MM, Aylward GP, et al: Nursery based intervention with prematurely born babies and their mothers: Are there effects? J Pediatr 97:487, 1980.

118. Portela ALM: Massage as a stimulation technique for premature infants: An annotated bibliography. Pediatr Phys Ther 2:80, 1990.

119. Resnick MB, Eyler FD, Nelson RM, et al: Developmental intervention for low birth weight infants: Improved early developmental outcome. Pediatrics 80:68, 1987.

120. Kang R, Barnard K, Hammond M et al: Preterm Infant Follow-up Project: A multi-site field experiment of hospital and home intervention programs for mothers and preterm infants. Public Health Nurs 12:171, 1995.

121. Parker SJ, Zahr LK, Cole JG, Brecht M-L: Outcome after developmental intervention in the neonatal intensive care unit for mothers of preterm infants with low socioeconomic status. J Pediatr 120:780, 1992.

122. Palisano RJ, Wilhelm IJ: Neonate and infant responses to and developmental effects of tactile and vestibular-proprioceptive stimulation. Annotated Bibliography. Phys Occup Ther Pediatr 1(2):71, 1981.

123. Wheeden A, Scafidi FA, Field T, et al: Massage effects on cocaine-exposed preterm neonates. Dev Behav Pediatr 14:318, 1993.
124. White-Traut RC, Nelson MN: Maternally administered tactile, auditory, visual, and vestibular stimulation: Relationship to later interactions between mothers and premature infants. Res Nurs Health 11:31, 1988.
125. White-Traut RC, Nelson MN, Silvestri JM, et al: Patterns of physiologic and behavioral response of intermediate care preterm infants to intervention. Pediatr Nurs 19:625, 1993.
126. Resnick MB, Armstrong S, Carter RL: Developmental intervention program for high-risk premature infants: Effects on development and parent-infant interactions. J Dev Behav Pediatr 9:73, 1988.
127. Georgieff MK, Bernbaum JC: Abnormal shoulder girdle muscle tone in premature infants during their first 18 months of life. Pediatrics 77:664, 1986.
128. Forssberg H: Development of motor function. *In* Gluckman PD, Heymann MA (eds): Pediatrics and Perinatology: The Scientific Basis, 2nd ed. Oxford University Press, New York, 1996, p 407.
129. Downs JA, Edwards AD, McCormick DC, et al: Effect of intervention on the development of hip posture in very preterm babies. Arch Dis Child 66:197, 1991.
130. Deiriggi PM: Effects of waterbed flotation on indicators of energy expenditure in preterm infants. Nurs Res 39:140, 1990.
131. Bjornson K, Deitz J, Blackburn S, et al: The effect of body position on the oxygen saturation of ventilated preterm infants. Pediatr Phys Ther 4:109, 1992.
132. Korner AF, Schneider P: Effects of vestibular-proprioceptive stimulation on the neurobehavioral development of preterm infants: A pilot study. Neuropediatrics 14:170, 1983.
133. Korner AJ, Ruppel EM, Rho JM: Effects of waterbeds on the sleep and mobility of theophylline-treated preterm infants. Pediatrics 70:864, 1982.
134. Korner AF, Kraemer HC, Haffner E, Cosper LM: Effects of waterbed flotation on premature infants: A pilot study. Pediatrics 56:361, 1975.
135. Schwirian PM, Eesley T, Cuellar L: Use of waterpillows in reducing head shape distortion in preterm infants. Res Nurs 9:203, 1986.
136. Goodman M, Rothberg AD, Houstan-McMillian JE, et al: Effect of early neurodevelopmental therapy in normal and at-risk survivors of neonatal intensive care. Lancet 8468:1327, 1985.
137. Edwards SJ, Gladwin AJ, Dixon MJ: The mutational spectrum in Treacher Collins reveals a predominance of mutations that create a premature termination-codon. Am J Hum Genet 60:515, 1997.
138. VandenBerg KA: Nippling management of the sick neonate in the NICU: The disorganized feeder. Neonat Network 9(1):9, 1990.
139. Shaker CS: Nipple feeding premature infants: A different perspective. Neonat Network 8:9, 1990.
140. Matthews CL: Supporting suck-swallow-breath coordination during nipple feeding. Am J Occup Ther 48:561, 1994.
141. Braun M, Palmer MM: A pilot study of oral-motor dysfunction in "at risk" infants. Phys Occup Ther Pediatr 5(4):13, 1985.
142. Horn EM, Warren SF, Jones HA: An experimental analysis of neurobehavioral motor intervention. Dev Med Child Neurol 37:697, 1995.
143. Einarsson-Backes LM, Deitz J, Price R, et al: The effect of oral support on sucking efficiency in preterm infants. Am J Occup Ther 48:490, 1994.
144. Sparling JW, Kolobe THA, Ezzelle L: Family-centered intervention. *In* Campbell SK, Vander Linden DW, Palisano RJ (eds): Physical Therapy for Children. WB Saunders, Philadelphia, 1994, p 523.
145. Human Services Research Institute: Consumer's Guide: Therapeutic Services for Children with Disabilities. Human Services Research Institute, Cambridge, Mass, 1995.
146. Lau C, Schanler RJ: Oral motor function in the neonate. Clin Perinatol 23:(2)161, 1996.
147. Aylward GP: Bayley Infant Neurodevelopmental Screener Manual. Psychological Corporation, San Antonio, 1992.
148. Harris SR, Daniels L: Content validity of the Harris Infant Neuromotor Test. Phys Ther 76:727, 1996.
149. Darrah J, Piper M, Watt M-J: Assessment of gross motor skills of at-risk infants: Predictive validity of the Alberta Infant Motor Scale. Dev Med Child Neurol 40:485, 1998.
150. Chandler LS, Andrews MS, Swanson MW: Movement Assessment of Infants. Chandler, Andrews and Swanson, Rolling Bay, Wash, 1980.
151. Piper MC, Pinnell LE, Darrah J, et al: Early developmental screening: Sensitivity and specificity of chronological and adjusted scores. J Dev Behav Pediatr 13:95, 1992.

152. Russell DJ, Rosenbaum PL, Cadman D, et al: The Gross Motor Function Measure: A means to evaluate the effects of physical therapy. Dev Med Child Neurol 31:341, 1989.
153. Mercuri E, Atkinson J, Braddick O, et al: Visual function in full-term infants with hypoxic-ischaemic encephalopathy. Neuropediatrics 28:155, 1997.
154. Infant Health and Development Program: Enhancing the outcomes of low-birth-weight, premature infants. JAMA 263:3035, 1990.
155. Palmer FB, Shapiro BK, Wachtel RC, et al: The effects of physical therapy on cerebral palsy: A controlled trial in infants with spastic diplegia. N Engl J Med 318:803, 1988.
156. Sparling J, Lewis I, Ramey CT, et al: Partners, a curriculum to help premature, low birth-weight infants get off to a good start. Top Early Child Spec Ed 11:36, 1991.
157. Barrera I: Thoughts on the assessment of young children whose sociocultural background is unfamiliar to the assessor. In Meisels SJ, Fenichel E (eds): New Visions for the Developmental Assessment of Infants and Young Children. ZERO TO THREE: National Center for Infants, Toddlers, and Families, Washington, DC, 1996, p 69.
158. Bricker D: AEPS Measurement for Birth to Three Years. Paul H Brookes, Baltimore, 1993.
159. Knafl KA, Ayres L, Gallo AM, et al: Learning from stories: Parents' accounts of the pathway to diagnosis. Pediatr Nurs 21:411, 1995.
160. Gordon BN, Jens KG: A conceptual model for tracking high-risk infants and making early service decisions. J Dev Behav Pediatr 9:279, 1988.
161. Aylward GP, Kenny TJ: Developmental follow-up: Inherent problems and a conceptual model. J Pediatr Psychol 4:331, 1979.
162. Field T, Hallock N, Ting G, et al: A first-year follow-up of high-risk infants: Formulating a cumulative risk index. Child Dev 49:119, 1978.
163. Parmalee AH, Sigman M, Kopp CB, Haber A: The concept of a cumulative risk score for infants. In Ellis NR (ed): Aberrant Development in Infancy: Human and Animal Studies. Lawrence Erlbaum, Hillsdale, NJ, 1975, p 113.
164. Frankenburg WK, Dodds JB: The Denver Developmental Screening Test. J Pediatr 71:181, 1967.
165. Carey WB: A simplified method of measuring infant temperament. J Pediatr 77:188, 1970.
166. Meisels SJ, Fenichel E (eds): New Visions for the Developmental Assessment of Infants and Young Children. ZERO TO THREE: The National Center for Infants, Toddlers, and Families, Washington, DC, 1996.
167. Erikson J: The Infant-Toddler Developmental Assessment (IDA): A family-centered transdisciplinary assessment process. In Meisels SJ, Fenichel E (eds): New Visions for the Developmental Assessment of Infants and Young Children. ZERO TO THREE: The National Center for Infants, Toddlers, and Families, Washington, DC, 1996, p 147.
168. Meisels SJ: Charting the continuum of assessment and intervention. In Meisels SJ, Fenichel E (eds): New Visions for the Developmental Assessment of Infants and Young Children. ZERO TO THREE: The National Center for Infants, Toddlers, and Families, Washington, DC, 1996, p 27.
169. Wolery M, Bailey DD: Alternatives to impact evaluation: Suggestions for program evaluation in early intervention. J Div Early Child 4:27, 1984.
170. Meck NE, Fowler SA, Claflin K, Rasmussen LB: Mothers perceptions of their NICU experience 1 and 7 months after discharge. J Early Intervent 19:288, 1995.
171. Wyly MV, Allen J, Pfalzer SM, Wilson JR: Providing a seamless service system from hospital to home—The NICU Training Project. Inf Young Child 8:77, 1996.
172. Horbar JD, Lucey JF: Evaluation of neonatal intensive care technologies. Future Child 5:139, 1995.
173. Rosenbaum P, King S, Cadman D: Measuring processes of caregiving to physically disabled children and their families. I: Identifying relevant components of care. Dev Med Child Neurol 34:103, 1992.
174. Shendell-Falik N: Perinatal Pro-ACT: Work redesign and case management. J Perinat Neonat Nurs 8:1, 1995.
175. Haley SM, Stephens TE, Larsen AM: Patterns of physical and occupational therapy implementation in early motor intervention. Top Early Child Spec Ed 7(4):46, 1988.
176. Popper BK: Achieving change in assessment practices: A parent's perspective. In Meisels SJ, Fenichel E (eds): New Visions for the Developmental Assessment of Infants and Young Children. ZERO TO THREE: The National Center for Infants, Toddlers, and Families, Washington, DC, 1996, p 59.
177. Law M, Baptiste S, Carswell A, et al: Canadian Occupational Performance Measure, 2nd ed. CAOT, Toronto, Canada, 1994.
178. Harrison H, Kositsky A: The Premature Baby Book: A Parent's Guide to Coping & Caring in the First Years. St Martin's New York, 1983.

179. Manginello FP, DiGeronimo TH: Your Premature Baby. John Wiley, New York, 1991.

180. Simons R: After the Tears: Parents Talk About Raising a Child with a Disability. Harcourt Brace Jovanovich, New York, 1987.

181. Pueschel S (ed): A Parent's Guide to Down Syndrome: Toward a Brighter Future. Paul H Brookes, Baltimore, 1990.

182. Hoelting J, Sandell EJ, Letourneau S, et al: The MELD experience with parent groups. Zero to Three 16(6):9, 1996.

183. Law M, Darrah J, Pollock N, et al: Family-centred functional therapy for children with cerebral palsy: An emerging practice model. Phys Occup Ther Pediatr 18(1):83, 1998.

184. Holloway E: Parent and occupational therapist collaboration in the neonatal intensive care unit. Amer J Occup Ther 48:535, 1994.

185. Shumway-Cook A, Woollacott M: Theoretical issues in assessing postural control. *In* Wilhelm, IJ (ed.): Physical Therapy Assessment in Early Infancy. Churchill Livingstone, New York, 1993, p 151.

186. Thelen E, Kelso JAS, Fogel A: Self-organizing systems and infant motor development. Dev Rev 7:39, 1987.

187. Byl NN, Merzenich MM, Cheung S, et al: A primate model for studying focal dystonia and repetitive strain injury—effects on the primary somatosensory cortex. Phys Ther 77:269, 1997.

188. Nudo RJ, Milliken GW, Jenkins WM, et al: Use-dependent alterations of movement representations in primary motor cortex of adult squirrel monkeys. J Neurosci 16:785, 1996.

189. Amiel-Tison C, Grenier A: Neurologic Assessment During the First Year of Life. Oxford University Press, New York, 1986.

190. Sporns O, Edelman GM: Solving Bernstein's problem: A proposal for the development of coordinated movement by selection. Child Dev 64:960, 1993.

191. Edelman GM: Neural Darwinism. Basic Books, New York, 1987.

192. Ulrich BD, Ulrich DA: Spontaneous leg movements of infants with Down syndrome and nondisabled infants. Child Dev 66:1844, 1995.

193. Sweeney JK: Neonatal hydrotherapy: An adjunct to developmental intervention in an intensive care nursery setting. Phys Occup Ther Pediatr 3(1):20, 1983.

194. Larin HM: Motor learning: Theories and strategies for the practitioner. *In* Campbell SK, Vander Linden DW, Palisano RJ (eds): Physical Therapy for Children. WB Saunders, Philadelphia, 1994, p 157.

195. Horn EM: Basic motor skills instruction for children with neuromotor delays: A critical review. J Spec Ed 25:168, 1991.

Index

Note: Page numbers in *italics* indicate illustrations; those followed by t refer to tables.